A–Z of Natural Therapies

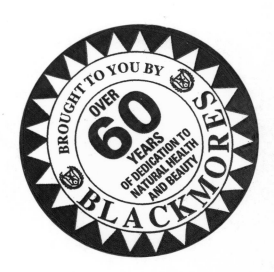

A–Z of Natural Therapies

A compendium of common ailments
and their natural treatments

Judy Jacka
N.D., Grad. Dip. H.R.E.

LOTHIAN BOOKS

A Lothian Book

Lothian Publishing Company Pty Ltd
A division of Thomas C. Lothian Pty Ltd
11 Munro Street Port Melbourne Victoria 3207

National Library of Australia
Cataloguing-in-Publication data:

Jacka, Judy, 1938.
    A–Z of natural therapies.

    Includes index.
    ISBN 0 85091 293 8.

    1. Naturopathy. I. Title.

615.5'35

Typeset from disk by Bookset Pty Ltd
Printed by Impact Printing

Preface

I have known Judy Jacka and her work for many years, and deeply appreciate the special wisdom she brings to the healing profession.

The history of medicine and healing has been characterised by controversy. Debate about the cause of disease and its correct treatment has always taken place. So too has continuing argument about who should be empowered to treat the sick. Today, these vital questions are being considered by more and more people, along with a growing awareness of the value of different, though complementary, systems of healing.

Natural therapy represents a significant contribution to the total field of medicine and healing. The relationship between the natural approach to health and that of conventional Western medicine has been highlighted in recent times. Establishment journals such as the *Lancet* and the *British Medical Journal* have carried articles on natural healing, and special interest groups, such as the British Holistic Medical Association, are involved in actively assessing the published material.

There is often a particular benefit to the client of a natural therapist in relation to the holistic approach and that is the love and attention which accompanies the treatment. At times, the spirit in which the medicine is offered may be more important than the remedies.

We should welcome the direction towards mutual appreciation and understanding between orthodox medicine and so-called alternative medicine. We sometimes deny our dark fears of illness and death with the claim that we can understand all there is to know. Too often, the term 'science' has been used to silence opposition to an accepted line of thought, or questioning of the official wisdom. In fact, it is the superior scientist who can recognise the limitations of his or her knowledge, and acknowledge contributions from an alternative approach.

This book offers information and ideas in a way which will encourage genuine healers from a variety of backgrounds to further investigate points of comparison and areas of need amenable to complementary treatment.

The book also offers esoteric interpretations for some of the disease states described. These ideas and theories challenge us to rethink aspects of health and illness from a fresh and intriguing viewpoint.

As long as there are different approaches to healing, useful debate will continue. Creativity comes from having more than one point of view, more than one description of the world in which we live. From unthinking agreement comes complacency; from discussion, even disagreement, comes true understanding.

In providing another description of disease processes, Judy Jacka gives us a chance to learn, to suspend our more conventional thinking, and to see what we might otherwise have overlooked.

James Oldham, M.D., F.R.C.P.(C)

Contents

Preface   v
Introduction   xi
Glossary of Terms   xv

Part 1
Chapter 1   What does Natural mean?   3
Chapter 2   The Subtle Causes of Disease   11
Chapter 3   The Cornerstones of Treatment   29

Part 2
Disorders Treated by Natural Therapists   42
Acne   45
Abdominal Migraine   49
Addison's Disease   51
Alcoholism   52
Allergies   53
Amenorrhoea   57
Anaemia   58
Angio-neurotic Oedema   60
Ankylosing Spondylitis   61
Anorexia Nervosa   62
Anxiety   64
Arthritis   67
Asthma   74
Atherosclerosis including Angina and Coronary
   Artery Disease   79
Auto-immune Disorders   86
Bell's Palsy   89
Blood Pressure   90
Bronchiectasis   96
Bronchitis   99

Cancer   101
Carpal Tunnel Syndrome   108
Cataracts   109
Cerebral Vascular Disease   110
Chicken-pox   111
Chilblains   112
Coeliac Disease   113
Colic   116
Common Cold   117
Constipation   119
Corneal Ulcer   122
Cramps   124
Crohn's Disease   126
Cystitis   128
Depression   131
Dermatitis   132
Diabetes   136
Diarrhoea   139
Diverticulitis   142
Down's Syndrome   144
Ear Infections   145
Eczema   146
Emphysema   149
Endometriosis   150
Epilepsy   152
Fibroids   155
Fluid Retention   157
Fractures   158
Gallstones   160
Gastritis   163
Gastro-enteritis   166
German Measles   167
Glandular Fever   168
Glaucoma   169
Glomerulonephritis   170
Goitre   174
Gonorrhoea   178
Gout   179
Growing Pains   181

Haematuria 183
Haemophilia 183
Haemorrhoids 183
Hallucinations 185
Hay Fever 186
Headache 188
Heart Disease 191
Hepatitis 192
Hernia 195
Herpes 197
Hiccoughs 200
Hodgkin's Disease 201
Hypoglycaemia 202
Immune Deficiency Disorders 205
Impetigo 206
Insomnia 207
Jaundice 210
Kidney Stones 211
Laryngitis 214
Leukaemia 216
Measles 218
Melanoma 219
Meniere's Disease 219
Meningitis 222
Menopause 223
Menstrual Cramps 225
Migraine 226
Motion Sickness 230
Mouth Ulcers 231
Multiple Sclerosis 231
Mumps 234
Nephritis 235
Neuralgia 235
Neuritis 236
Neuroses 237
Obesity 239
Osteoporosis 241
Ovarian Cysts 242
Paget's Disease 245

Pancreatitis   246
Papillomas   249
Parkinson's Disease   249
Pleurisy   250
Pneumonia   252
Pregnancy   253
Premenstrual Tension   254
Prolapse   256
Prostatitis and Enlarged Prostate   258
Psoriasis   260
Raynaud's Syndrome   263
Repetitive Strain Injury   264
Rheumatic Fever   266
Rickets   267
Scabies   269
Scarlet Fever   270
Schizophrenia   271
Scleroderma   273
Scurvy   276
Senile Dementia   276
Shingles   278
Sinusitis   280
Stomach Ulcers   282
Syphilis   285
Tachycardia   286
Thrush   288
Tonsillitis   291
Tuberculosis   292
Ulcerative Colitis   293
Vaginal Discharge   296
Varicose Veins, Varicose Eczema and Varicose
    Ulcers   298
Venereal Warts   301
Warts   303
Whooping Cough   304
Worms   306

Notes   308
Index   326

Introduction

This book is intended to be a practical compendium of natural therapies, and an aid to understanding how natural therapies are applied to individual disorders.

Over the past fifteen years the natural health profession has seen an unprecedented expansion. It has been estimated by the profession and also by a government report in Australia that at least 10 per cent of persons visit a natural therapist over a period of twelve months. In the United Kingdom similar figures for Western Europe are quoted by the Research Council for Complementary Medicine. Large sections of the public accept natural therapies as a viable part of the health care delivery system.

Attitudes within the orthodox medical profession are also changing. Reports and surveys in the United Kingdom reveal that 65 per cent of young doctors think that at least one form of natural therapies is effective and 40 per cent have referred patients to non-medical practitioners.

The continuing interest in natural therapies by the general public has stimulated another parliamentary inquiry into the area in Australia, while in the United Kingdom the British Medical Association completed a three-year investigation into the area during 1986. The British Holistic Medical Association and the British Association for Holistic Health have together pioneered regular dialogue through conferences attended by registered doctors, natural therapists and interested members of the public. There are regional groups meeting throughout the country to develop further the concepts of total health care.

A complication has followed on the heels of the extraordinary expansion of the natural health profession. Numbers of entrepreneurs have entered the field, becoming involved not only in the manufacture and sale of natural medicines, but also in training and education. Meanwhile, responsible educators have continued to develop professionally-oriented courses of study which contain the requisite basic and medical sciences to enable their graduates to become proficient as primary contact practitioners, and to make a creative and safe contribution to community health.

A–Z of Natural Therapies is designed to clarify the principles behind natural healing and their application to many health disorders.

Due to the very broad field of natural therapies, there is sometimes confusion in the minds of the general public as to where natural therapy begins and ends. As well as the key traditional internal therapies of clinical nutrition, herbal medicine and homoeopathy, an enormous array of ancillary therapies has evolved or reappeared during the last fifteen years. Examples are different kinds of massage therapy, Bach flower remedies, colour therapy, reflexology, kinesiology, aromatherapy, and bio-regulatory or bio-functional therapy.

My previous book A Philosophy of Healing (Inkata Press, Melbourne, 1979) introduced the reader to the concept of the subtle energies which form the matrix or base for the anatomy and physiology of the physical body. In general, that first book was a weaving and synthesis of ideas and, apart from explaining how the various therapies worked together, the practical application of natural medicine to particular diseases was not addressed. I have also taken up the theme of the inner causes of disease in this A–Z, as well as indicating the ways in which natural therapies can complement orthodox medicine.

A–Z of Natural Therapies has been designed primarily as a resource book for understanding natural therapies. It uses an alphabetical listing of both common and medical terms for ailments which are frequently helped by these disciplines. However, it needs to be stressed that it is not a manual for self-prescribing, and readers seeking help for health ailments should consult a well-qualified natural therapist.

Many individuals visit natural therapists for sub-clinical conditions for which there is no medical nomenclature. This field of preventive medicine is probably our main contribution to the health care delivery system. Likewise it explains why I found difficulty finding a clear-cut case history for all medical conditions listed.

There are five disease conditions which natural therapists have been advised not to treat except in association with a registered medical doctor. These five conditions are venereal diseases, cancer, diabetes, epilepsy and tuberculosis. The wise natural therapist will add heart and circulatory disorders to this list. In each of these six categories of disease pharmaceutical drugs are sometimes essential for the patient.

How to Use this Book

Part 1 of this book begins with a summary of naturopathic principles, followed by a chapter on the subtle or inner causes of disease in relation to our inner constitution. Then comes a chapter on the cornerstones of treatment, and this explains the main traditional areas of natural therapies and how they are applied to health problems. Included in this chapter is a description of the therapist/patient relationship, differing as it does from the current medical model.

The main section of the book (Part 2) contains an alphabetical listing of diseases; each problem is divided into definition, causes, treatment and case histories. There is considerable variation in the size of each section under this listing. I have gone into more detail in areas which form a large part of our practice such as arthritis or allergies, and in those health problems where it is of use to explain more fully the esoteric or subjective factors. With some conditions like anaemia or childhood fevers there is little to say, while a genetic condition like Down's syndrome is not really amenable to natural treatment.

An effort has been made to give the source of as many statements and conclusions as possible. Clinical research in the areas of vitamins, minerals, herbs and homoeopathy is very patchy. Some conditions which have been popular in the media such as atherosclerosis, premenstrual tension and asthma have been more fully researched than ailments like eczema, migraine or dyspepsia which are just as common but less fatal or dramatic. The research papers quoted are not always particularly suitable for illustration of naturopathic diagnosis or treatment, and in many areas where we are obtaining significant clinical results, I have been unable to find suitable references.

A new research model is needed for natural therapies. The usual double-blind clinical trials are not suitable for the holistic approach. It is rare that we give one substance in isolation or without suggesting changes in the life-style of the patient. A suitable research model needs to include the synthesis of pre-

scribing which we practise. On the other hand, natural therapists do not have the funds to undertake their own research.
Until there is government recognition and support it is also
unlikely that private institutions will finance our research.

In some of the case histories given it is possible that improvement would have occurred without any treatment, due to the
inherent life-force within the individual which, given a chance,
always moves us towards wholeness and health. It is for this
reason that the chapter entitled 'The Subtle Causes of Disease'
forms a large section of Part 1.

Glossary of Terms

Acupressure
Developed from the same philosophy and understanding about health and disease as that for Acupuncture but finger pressure on the points is used instead of needles.

Acupuncture
A method of treatment developed in ancient China to promote health through balancing energies by means of needles inserted into particular points on the skin which relate to the channels for energy flow known as meridians.

Alexander Technique
A technique developed by F. M. Alexander to re-educate people into more natural and healthful methods of posture with primary importance being attached to the head-neck-back relationship.

Aromatherapy
The use of essential oils and flower essences which are massaged into the skin for a healing and stimulating effect on tissues and organs.

Astral
The term is used to designate the principle of emotion/feeling in living beings and the realm or plane of the universe which expresses emotion/feeling.

Atmic/Atma
Atma is the innermost spiritual essence of man/woman which resides on the atmic plane of the universe as expressed by the Trans-Himalayan teaching about the constitution of man and the universe.

Bach Flowers
A system of therapy developed by Dr Edward Bach involving thirty-eight European flower essences which are given orally for various emotional imbalances.

Bio-Functional Diagnosis
A method of diagnosis developed during the second half of this century in Germany to evaluate the balance of energies and function of organs in the body using electronic instrumentation.

Buddhi/Buddhic plane
The principle of love/wisdom or pure reason in man/woman and the associated plane of the universe as depicted by the Trans-Himalayan teachings.

Chakras
The term which is commonly applied in esoteric teaching to the vortices of energy associated with the energy body which underlies the physical body and which transmit energies from one part of this subtle body to another.

Chi
A Chinese term for the life-force underlying the physical existence and function of organs and tissues. This life-force is regulated to promote health by means of acupuncture and related therapies.

De-armouring
A term coined by Wilhelm Reich to explain the release during therapy from tension and rigidity in muscles associated with emotional repression and suppression.

Etheric body/plane
The common term used for the subtle energy vehicle and state which underlies the physical body and the physical universe and which is understood to condition health and disease in all kingdoms in nature.

German electro-acupuncture
The use of electronic instruments to diagnose and treat illness via the acupuncture points on the body using low currents of less than one volt. The system was pioneered by Dr Rhinholt Voll and others from 1953 onwards.

Herbal medicine
The use of herbs as teas, tinctures, fluid extracts or tablets to promote and restore health in animals and mankind.

Homoeopathy
The use of animal, vegetable or mineral matter in minute doses to stimulate the immune system and the healthy function of

organs and tissues through the selection of a remedy which matches closely the disease process to be treated.

Homoeostasis
The self-regulating and balancing systems within the living organism which tend to promote a healthy equilibrium in the body.

Kinesiology
Applied kinesiology uses the application of muscle testing to diagnose physiological conditions and anatomical problems of the human body.

Kirlian photography
High frequency photography pioneered by Semyon Kirlian and which has been used to diagnose illness and to monitor energy states in the body through assessment of the variations in the coronal discharge photographed around living matter.

Manas/mental plane
The principle of mind and the thinker residing on that level of the universe which is named the mental plane or noosphere.

Mora Therapy
Therapy using a Mora electronic device is either given to the person electronically via the surface of the body or orally by means of a tincture which is patterned on the specific electrical oscillations of the patient.

Orgonomy
The name for the science and therapeutic modality based upon the discovery of orgone or life energy by Wilhelm Reich. The therapy aims at establishing orgastic potency through the release of rigid and tense muscles. See also De-armouring.

Primal screaming
A system of therapy developed by Dr Ivan Janov to release deep-seated emotional tensions which interfere with growth and development.

Prana
The Hindu term for the life-energy originally derived from the sun which according to its state in the body is responsible for health or disease. See also *Chi*.

Theratest
A form of German electro-acupuncture involving electrical

measurement at an acupuncture point as a means of translating and evaluating energy flowing in the acupuncture meridians.

Touch-for-health
A therapy for balancing energies in the body using the Chinese meridian system by means of linking the therapist with the client through touch.

Vega testing
The latest branch of German electro-acupuncture using test ampoules as part of the diagnostic measurement via an acupuncture point to evaluate health and disease states.

Vivaxis
A method pioneered by Frances Nixon to evaluate body and life energies and to rebalance and restore these energies using specific energy bands which flow through the surface of the earth.

Part 1

CHAPTER 1

What does Natural mean?

All healing is natural, and the use of the terms natural healing and natural therapist are in one sense misnomers. What then is so different about the approach of the natural therapist? Why do we prescribe vitamins, minerals and herbs instead of advocating the usual drugs and surgery which characterises modern medicine?

The answer lies in our understanding of the concept of homoeostasis in relation to health and disease. Homoeostasis is defined as the self-regulating or balancing mechanism of the body. It could also be defined as the self-recuperative processes of the body. The natural therapist is seeking to restore or enhance the equilibrium of the body through the use of vitamins, minerals, herbs, homoeopathy and other harmless means. The process of homoeostasis could be extended to psychological realms because our philosophy includes the need to treat the whole person. Balance must be restored to all levels of our being.

As a branch of generic medicine, natural therapy promotes treatment based on a holistic approach, with concern for underlying causes, rather than dealing only with the presenting symptoms. This approach is complementary to medicine and surgery and to other physical disciplines such as chiropractic, osteopathy, and physiotherapy.

The main internal therapies which are used to promote health are vitamins, minerals, herbs and homoeopathic medicines. These therapies will be described in some detail in chapter 3.

Bach flower remedies, massage, reflexology, acupressure, colour therapy, touch for health, kinesiology, the Alexander technique, and Vivaxis may be used by individual practitioners as adjuncts to the main therapies mentioned.

Practitioners often specialise in a particular area, even perhaps in one of the minor areas mentioned. In training practitioners to be professionals in the area of health science, I have found it valuable to encourage students to become proficient in the main three internal therapies of clinical nutrition, botanic medicine or herbalism, and homoeopathy. The individual then has a firm basis to meet the needs of clients with a broad range of disorders, and from that base line specialties may be added.

By staying with the basic concept of maintaining and restoring the homoeostatic mechanism of the body, any therapy can be classed as natural which tones organs and tissues, and which improves the general life-style of the patient. A number of factors which inhibit the homoeostatic mechanisms have been observed in clinical practice. These factors may be both inherited and acquired. Table I illustrates these items which include stress, negative emotions, lack of sleep, environmental pollutants and poor diet. The last factor covers the use of preservatives, flavourings, colourings, emulsifiers, bleaches and stabilisers in foods. Also chemicals are present extensively in the water, soil, and air surrounding any big city.

The various factors which contribute to imbalance and loss of homoeostasis may be grouped under two main headings — accumulation of toxins, and loss of energy or vitality. The latter in particular affects the immune system. Each of these two main factors leads to the other. For example, loss of energy through lack of sleep, fresh air, stress at work and negative emotions gives rise to accumulation of toxins throughout the tissues of the body. The mechanism for such accumulation is as follows: when our body becomes tired and exhausted and we experience loss of vitality there is a general slowing down of the normal eliminative processes through bowel, lung, kidney and skin. This results in retention of waste which may not be significant over a few days, but over months and years can lead to that condition which natural therapists have termed auto-intoxication. Our clinical findings indicate that waste products thus retained have a toxic effect on organs and tissues of the body giving rise to the many chronic diseases of modern man.

The process can also work in reverse. Refined food gives rise to

Table 1

SOME FACTORS LEADING TO DISEASE

Stress and negative emotions

Lack of rest and relaxation

Lack of exercise

Mineral and vitamin deficiencies in diet

Poor assimilation of vitamins and minerals

Pollution of food, air and water by:
insecticides
industrial effluent
food additives

Electronic pollution from:
high voltage power lines
television and video screens
xrays and ultrasound

Some pharmaceutical drugs

poor digestion, faulty elimination and consequent lack of tone or vitality in all the cells and tissues of the body. The individual may have no particular illness, but will feel generally below par and complains of tiredness and lack of vitality. This overall debility could be classed as a sub-clinical condition, yet is significant from the point of view of well-being.

These sub-clinical states are very common in the 1980s. This is the field of preventive medicine and is the area in which the natural therapist prefers to work. The medical scientist may argue that there is no proof for either the theory of accumulated toxins or of differing states of vitality. The natural therapist is satisfied that there is sufficient clinical evidence to warrant a new approach to health and disease encompassing this philosophy.

We move towards the imbalance known as disease in stages. The average baby and young child, with a good inherited constitution, has a good level of vitality. The term vitality is used by the natural therapist to mean the strength of the electromagnetic field associated with the physical body. Acceptance of this field is spreading quickly in the 1980s amongst members of the general public. A few medical scientists have been researching the electrical parameters of health and disease for several decades. The electromagnetic field associated with the physical body has been called an energy body.

In the past, the term vitality was fairly loosely used to express an energy which science had not researched in connection with health and disease. It is now more widely accepted that there is an energy body which underlies the gross physical level. Inherited and acquired factors can profoundly affect this electromagnetic field which science is beginning to research gradually. It may be that although this research is fairly isolated in a global sense, the work of Burr and more recently, the work of Australian medical scientist Dr Bevan Reid, will gradually penetrate our minds.[1]

Generally, natural therapists have accepted that inherited and acquired factors affect the shape, health and function of our organs via the energy field which underlies the physical body, and which was previously known by a vague concept of vital force. Thus we have a chain of events: inherited factors influencing the energy field which influences the homoeostatic or balance mechanisms and this state affects the biochemistry of the body and the assimilation of vitamins and minerals.

These traits of inheritance are called 'chronic miasms' by homoeopaths and can be traced back many generations by the trained practitioner. The manifestations of these inherited 'taints' vary enormously. One simple example involves tuberculosis. The parents of an asthmatic child may not be aware of any known tuberculosis in the family tree. A background of tuberculosis has been noted by natural therapists to influence the respiratory health of many generations. The natural therapist does not expect any signs of the active disease, but in many cases there are problems of assimilation with minerals such as silica and calcium. The family member who suffered tuberculosis may be four or five generations back. Perhaps there will be a legacy in the great grandchildren of bronchial weakness, night sweats and nose bleeds. The homoeopathic treatment is very important in eradicating the inherited factors which affect homoeostasis. It is the only type of natural therapy which can have a profound effect at the genetic and subtle level of the body and homoeopathic treatment can therefore influence inheritance.

Development of Chronic Disease

Imagine a typical situation where a child with healthy parents moves towards chronic disease through a misunderstanding of the factors which maintain health. Following this progression will give an understanding of the stages of disease from a naturopathic point of view. A baby of normal weight and apparent health is breast-fed for eight months. Let us assume that the woman is a fairly average mother and not particularly health conscious; beyond restricting herself from lots of sweets and rich food, she makes no particular study of the vitamins and minerals needed in her diet for healthy breast milk.

The first onslaught to the baby's immune system occurs about the age of three months with the triple antigen immunisation. The foreign antigens injected into the body require a response on the part of the baby's immune system. The expected response is the production of antibodies which will supposedly protect the baby from future development of the infectious fevers. There are arguments to suggest that this challenge to the immune system can create problems.[2] Some scientists have commented that vitamin C is essential for the immune system to function adequately, and also that it is needed in certain quantities to prevent problems from immunisation.[3] Unless a mother takes a supplement of vitamin C during lactation, it is unlikely there will be sufficient in her breast milk for the baby at this first test involving the immune system.

In the next few months, it is noticed that the baby has repeated colds and infection moves into the bronchial area. Antibiotics are now administered, and these put a further strain on the organs — in particular the liver which has to handle all drugs. The natural therapist would say that the originally healthy baby now starts to move from the acute stage of disease characterised by transient head colds, to a more insidious sub-acute stage commonly termed bronchitis. This progression towards disease occurs in spite of the original vitality and health of the baby.

The baby is then weaned, and the mother further enhances the bronchial problem by putting the baby on cow's milk. This burdens the body for the organs of many people are unable to handle dairy produce adequately. The mucus production is now increased. In attempting to eradicate the accumulating toxins caused by incomplete digestion of foods, the baby manifests high fevers each time a respiratory infection develops.

Scientists are presently studying the effects of fever on infectious illness. It has been found that immunity to infection is enhanced through fever, thus vindicating what traditional therapists have said for centuries.[4] Natural therapists would go a step further. In the movement towards balance or homoeostasis, a body wherein toxins have accumulated provides the soil for the growth of viruses or bacteria. This development triggers off the fever which in turn reduces toxins to simpler chemical forms. These are eliminated through the normal channels of skin, kidneys, mucus membranes and bowel.[5]

Natural therapists find in the type of case mentioned that the use of antibiotics reduces the response of the immune system, vitality diminishes, and toxins accumulate. Perhaps the next stage in the disease process may be asthma. This is definitely a process moving towards the stage of chronic disease, although given good inheritance and a reasonable life-style, many children have been known to outgrow the condition of asthma by about the age of eight.

Unfortunately, the incidence of chronic asthma is increasing. The usual response to this condition is to use bronchodilators to expand the breathing passages, and antihistamines to dry up the mucus. As the condition worsens, cortisone is added to the medication in various forms. This further lowers the resistance of the person. We must also consider the effect on the respiratory tree from the constant use of bronchodilators. Many asthmatics in later life develop the condition known as bronchiectasis which manifests as a loss of elastic tissue in the breathing apparatus making breathing very difficult.

This is but one example of how the body can move through the various stages of acute to chronic disease in a certain number of years. The process can be accelerated by environmental factors including diet, stress and lack of exercise. More importantly, it can be retarded or arrested by changes in life-style and by natural medication which enhances the immune system. There are also psychic factors which influence the health of the body and these causes will be explored in the next chapter and again in the alphabetical section in part 2.

Other types of disease could be traced from acute to chronic stages along similar lines. There is the chain of events involving food allergies, eczema, and arthritis, or the many nervous complaints which develop from the suppression of eczema at some stage in the family tree. This highlights the important observation that the chain of poor health is often not confined to one generation in a family, but may extend over several generations. A person with eczema which is suppressed by drugs may precipitate asthma or migraine in the next generation. The natural therapist does not see these specific disease entities in isolation as do most practitioners of the orthodox profession, but rather as a causal chain of events. The aim of natural therapies is to reverse the disease process. During the course of treatment the client moves back to the acute stage of disease. This happens as toxins are eliminated and as the vitality is improved.

The naturopathic profession does not have the type of clinical trials which would satisfy the criteria of modern scientific journals. We do have the testimony of many thousands of healthier clients who had first done the rounds of orthodox medicine without any improvement to their various conditions. These people have received lasting benefit from a combination of improved life-style, vitamins, minerals, herbs and homoeopathy, plus other useful and simple adjuncts which can be applied to enhance health and well-being.

About Diagnosis

Do natural therapists recognise any conditions which should be referred to registered orthodox doctors? Natural therapists are trained to recognise those conditions which, because of their acuteness and consequent threat to life, need immediate orthodox medical treatment. Every well-trained natural therapist knows how to diagnose such conditions and immediately refers them for appropriate medical intervention. The majority of our cases, however, do not fall into this category.

Graduates from schools accredited by responsible professional associations undertake a four-year full-time course. They study anatomy, physiology, chemistry, biochemistry, pathology and clinical diagnosis to an appropriate level for a practitioner who is in direct contact with the public. They will use the same diagnostic methods to some extent as orthodox medical graduates. These methods will include palpation or touch, auscultation or listening, blood pressure evaluation, urine analysis and, where necessary, the use of pathology tests. In addition they may use iris diagnosis, bio-functional diagnosis through measurement of acupuncture meridians, reflexology or kinesiology. It is useful to combine several methods for cross-checking. For instance, diagnosis through use of the hand can be cross-checked by the iris and again through bio-energetic diagnosis.[6] It is not wise to rely on one method alone as illness can be very complex.

The complexity of health and disease will be further explored in the next chapter where the subtle causes of disease are considered.

CHAPTER 2

The Subtle Causes
of Disease

During the last two centuries, mainstream medicine has passed through a relatively materialistic phase. The material emphasis was in keeping with nineteenth-century physics and chemistry; the reductionist approach of Newtonian physics was adopted by orthodox medicine whereby the body has been viewed as a collection of parts which tend to be studied in isolation from the whole person. In his book *The Turning Point*, physicist Fritjof Capra has skilfully traced the changes which are taking place in medicine as a result of twentieth-century physics.[1] The finding of modern science that the universe is an unbroken related whole has been further explored by physicist David Peat and science writer and poet David Briggs in their book *Looking Glass Universe*.[2]

The first branch of orthodox medicine to respond to a more holistic approach to health and disease has been modern psychology. Psychologists have investigated the interaction of life-style, thoughts and emotions with health and disease patterns. The connection between goals, motivations, emotions, thoughts and physiological processes has been observed. It has been found that emotional imbalance and disordered thought processes may have a profound influence on the endocrine and immune systems of the body. Natural therapists have always been concerned with the whole life-style and have accepted that all parts of the person must be in harmony to prevent disease.

11

The recent emphasis by an increasing number of people on having a healthy life-style, and the widespread use of vitamins and minerals, has caused us to ignore the more subtle factors of our psyche and soul which contribute to health. It is these subtle factors leading to health or disease which will be discussed in this chapter. The main thrust of the chapter will be that the majority of health problems come from conflict, suppression and blocks at the emotional or astral level, and from imbalances of energy at the etheric or subtle part of the physical level.[3] This point should be remembered as the alphabetical section is read, otherwise the mention of so many physical remedies for each condition may distract from the real causes of disease.

If modern psychology is already undertaking research into the connections between the psyche and disease, why does a naturopathic text need to bring in Eastern philosophy and terminology which some people may see as esoteric jargon? The answer lies in the fact that modern psychology has only scratched the surface of a very complex system of healing and philosophy which has been understood in the East for centuries, and which can answer many problems in medicine and psychology. The first sphere of science to vindicate the ancient Eastern traditions has been modern physics, and the first group of physicians to relate these teachings to an understanding of health and disease has been the naturopaths. Naturopaths have always recognised the existence of the life-force in the physical body as well as recognising the importance of balance at all levels of our nature.

The research of a few medical scientists who have demonstrated the existence of a life-force in all living matter has helped to explain naturopathic philosophy. We can now explore the connections between the vital force, recent medical findings, and the various levels of our psychic and spiritual constitution which have been tabulated so extensively in Eastern philosophy. Many persons now accept that health is dependent on factors reaching beyond basic anatomy and physiology. Both the general public and practising therapists are becoming increasingly interested in the possibility of subtle energy states which may influence our health. During the last ten years, workshops have introduced subjects such as meditation, psychic healing and energy centres, and groups have explored various levels of consciousness.

In Melbourne, the Australian Cancer Patients' Foundation teaches the use of meditation to its members. The Foundation now has evidence of fifty cases involving terminal cancer which have gone into remission following participation in their programme. Many of those involved with the programme combine natural therapies with orthodox treatment plus meditation techniques. Meditation is considered an essential part of the programme which also includes information on nutrition and a variety of approaches to the cancer problem.

In clinical practice, I rarely discuss these subtle factors with the patients at the first consultation. With many cases it is unnecessary to raise the subject even over a period of treatment lasting six months or more. However, the parameters of our understanding and those of our clients are broadening, and consideration of these subtle factors is becoming necessary. I find it of great value to reflect on the relationship of these subtle factors to disease and believe that appreciation of the more subtle causes will achieve increased understanding of disease processes. I have been introducing patients to the idea of attending classes in meditation and of learning to use subtle energies in various ways to improve health.

Our Inner Constitution

To summarise, it has been said that the major causes of disease are subtle factors beyond the physical, and this has been recognised for centuries in the East; psychologists and natural therapists recognise some of these factors, and a few scientists have begun to research the energies underlying the physical body. Science has no instruments to measure the most subtle parts of our nature related to emotions and mind, and this teaching is dependent on information which has come from China and India and from some of the findings of modern psychology. A few scientists have begun to research the subtle part of the physical body which is often called the etheric body. Systems of medicine developed in ancient India and China have always emphasised the role of this energy vehicle as a carrier of vital force or energy to all physical organs and tissues. The energy body mediates between our psychic or psychological functions and the physical anatomy and physiology.[4] The words for vital force or energy vary from country to country, but are interchangeable in meaning — prana in the Hindu system, chi in medical philosophy from China, and bioplasma in Russian literature on the subject.

Who are the medical scientists who have contributed research in this area? They have been mainly involved with various forms of diagnosis through exploring the life field around the physical body and have used a number of techniques. High frequency photography, measurement of the energy which flows through the acupuncture meridians of the body, and measurement of the electromagnetic field surrounding and penetrating the body, have all been the subject of experimentation. Pioneers in this area include Semyon Kirlian and Thelma Moss in the area of Kirlian photography, Wilhelm Reich and his theory of Orgonomy, Rudolf Steiner in the area of anthroposophical medicine, Harold Burr and the life fields, and Frances Nixon who pioneered the Vivaxis techniques.[5] The more recent work of Dr Bevan Reid has also been mentioned.

At present, the only subtle parts of our constitution suitable for accepted methods of scientific analysis are those which may be expressed as electromagnetic fields or radiation and which are measured accordingly. Thus a vacuum tube voltmeter was used by Burr to measure his life fields, high frequency photography has been used to measure acupuncture points, and very low voltage circuitry is used to measure body energies in bio-energetic diagnosis which is discussed below.

These unusual examples of diagnosis all demonstrate to some extent the existence of a subtle physical dimension which appears to be relevant to health and disease. Some of the most recent clinical use of this knowledge is covered by the term bio-energetic diagnosis, meaning diagnosis of life-energy. Other terms coined for this include — 'bio-functional diagnosis', 'German electro-acupuncture', and 'bio-energetic regulatory techniques'. Several diagnostic aids are available including those named Theratest, Vega, and Mora. These instruments operate on the basic principle of the Wheatstone bridge which is a method of accurately measuring electrical resistance. The method is used in this instance to measure the electrical resistance of organs via the Chinese meridian system.[6]

Quite recently, Dr Bevan Reid, a medical research scientist at the University of Sydney, has attracted world-wide attention with an experiment which demonstrated extremely low level energy fields in living matter. The field is understood to result not from variation in voltage across the cell membrane as occurs from different concentrations of salt ions, but rather as a less tangible life-force. In his experiment, the life-force from a group of bacteria was imprinted on a thin plastic film of polystyrene.

Dead bacteria made no imprint on the film.[7] The experiment may come closer to measuring the actual life-force than either Kirlian photography or the research of Burr. In collaboration with Dr Sergei Barsamion, Fellow in Physics at the Royal Prince Alfred Hospital, Sydney, a bold theory has been developed which suggests that a field pervades the entire universe, reminding us of the aether about which man has speculated for centuries. It is thought that the field is too subtle to have been detected previously. The function of the field is supported by an electromagnetic force field theory or vortex theory developed by Barsamian. The two scientists believe the field to be responsible for growth and to be the medium for transmission of patterns from one natural source to another.[8]

Dr Reid believes that alterations in this subtle electric field can be detected in pre-cancerous tissue, forming the basis for more accurate and earlier diagnosis. In this respect, his ideas about the life field concur with those of the earlier pioneers such as Burr, Moss in the area of Kirlian photography, and the exponents of bio-functional diagnosis who use Theratest, Vega and Mora instruments. Diagnosing the electrical parameters of the body has been found significant in clinical practice especially in the area of preventive medicine. The work of these scientists underscores the basic naturopathic tenet that a disturbance in the energy or life field underlying the physical organs precedes disease by months and in some cases, years. This energy field provides the pattern for development and growth of all the organs and tissues of the body and it can be changed by diet, chemical and electrical disturbances, that is, the factors leading to poor health which were discussed in the previous chapter. In the West, the term etheric body is often used for this energy field.

The Etheric Body

Having briefly covered the explorations by Western science into the electromagnetic parameters of the etheric body, we will now explore its anatomy in more detail as it has been understood in the East. In Hindu philosophy it is known as the Linga Sharira, and in Chinese medical philosophy, the acupuncture meridian known as Triple Heater expresses some of the main attributes of this subtle anatomy. It is necessary to distinguish between the actual anatomy of this energy body and the life energy called *prana* or *chi* in the East, which flows through it to all parts of the physical body. The electrical measurements taken by Burr and by those using the bio-energetic form of diagnosis may relate more to the energy flowing through the etheric body rather than to the subtle structure or mechanism itself.

The etheric body is understood to be composed of threads of energy which interlace to form a network which penetrates every organ and tissue. This extends beyond the physical skin, roughly following the shape of the body. The etheric body should not be confused with the astral aura which is described by the average astral clairvoyant, and which will be explained shortly. The etheric is part of our physical nature although this is not yet accepted by medical science. It is a body of light and is often known as the golden bowl.

The main function of the etheric body is to act as a transmitter of the energy or *prana* received from the sun to all parts of the physical body. As the mediating link between our higher levels of consciousness and the physical brain, it receives, assimilates and transmits energy via specific energy centres situated in particular areas of the etheric body. There are a number of centres and they are formed where the threads of energy interlace repeatedly.[9]

Seven major centres are formed where the lines of energy cross twenty-one times and these are the traditional *chakra*s situated at intervals along the spine. Minor centres such as those found in the palms of the hand, behind the knees and in conjunction with the various organs of the body occur as a result of energies crossing fourteen times. The tiny centres which are usually called acupuncture points occur as a result of energies interlacing seven times and they number many hundreds.

The seven main centres are the most important in terms of the basic causes of disease. Each is associated with an endocrine gland and with a particular state of consciousness. Before describing their function, it is necessary to talk briefly about another basic concept from Eastern philosophy which is gaining interest in the West — the seven states of consciousness or planes of being. It is found that each *chakra* relates to one plane.

The Seven Levels of Consciousness

The lower three worlds of expression through the mechanism of our personality cover the sum total of our usual experiences: sensations, feelings and thoughts. The three planes associated with this expression are the physical, astral or emotional, and mental levels of being. The mental level is actually divided into two parts: the concrete and the abstract. The concrete mind is part of our everyday personality and deals with facts, memory and knowledge acquired through the five senses. The abstract mind deals with concepts and creative thought. In esoteric literature and understanding it is the level on which the reincarnating soul resides.

The abstract mind is the lowest of three higher spiritual principles which form part of our inner nature. We have therefore a spiritual triad called Atma, Buddhi, and Manas, and its reflection in the personality life through the mind, emotions and etheric/physical body. The mediating influence between these two sets of principles is the soul, our inner body of sentient consciousness which is understood to reincarnate through many lives until a personality develops which perfectly reflects our inner spiritual nature. Our journey towards health is the removal of blocks within the personality life which prevent the inner creative energies flowing freely through the personality. The etheric body is said to reflect the level of soul development as it absorbs the positive qualities of each personality life.

It has been mentioned that the most common blocks in the personality which cause ill health are emotional problems and disturbances to the etheric both from the emotions and from outer environmental factors such as poor life-style. These factors then affect the homoeostasis or biochemical equilibrium of the body, gross pathology being the final expression in the majority of cases.

Many new approaches in psychology are concentrating on problems associated with the astral or feeling body. Once again, as with the etheric body, the mechanism of the astral body must be distinguished from the actual emotions which are produced, although obviously there is a close correlation between the type of astral body and the emotions experienced. Unfortunately, an increasing number of people attend psychic healers who are usually astral clairvoyants. Although astral problems may be seen as a fairly fundamental cause of physical problems, the average psychic does not have sufficient medical or psychological knowledge to diagnose and interpret meaningfully. At the same time it should be said that a few psychics who are also spiritually

Table 2

THE SEVEN LEVELS OF CONSCIOUSNESS

1 Adi — the plane of the divine

2 Monadic plane — home of our highest spiritual self
— the monad

3 Atmic — the plane of spiritual will

4 Buddhic plane — the level of pure love/wisdom or
pure reason

5 Mental plane — focus of higher mind or manas —
home of our soul
Lower or concrete mind

6 Astral plane — focus of our feelings and emotions

7 Etheric or higher part of physical plane
Physical plane of our senses — solids, liquids and gases

developed may make contributions of real benefit to the understanding of human problems.

Disordered thought processes are obviously another cause of problems in the personality but are not as common as neuroses which result from emotional problems. The mind is the integrating factor in the personality life and is of great importance to modern man. The emphasis on developing creative thought in modern education processes indicates that humanity as a whole is now more interested to achieve a meaningful life intention. The creative use of the mind links us with the higher spiritual aspects previously mentioned.

Many people now experience transcendent states of consciousness beyond that of the ordinary waking personality life. These may be fleeting or regular and can have the effect of sweeping away blockages which cause illness. The perception of beauty, the experience of love, profound thought, or the advent of a crisis, can add an extra dimension to our life, lifting us beyond ordinary consciousness. In such states we may touch the level of soul or abstract mind, the plane of buddhi or love/wisdom and the atmic plane of spiritual will. The psychologist Maslow has identified these occasions as peak experiences.[10]

There are two planes of consciousness above the atmic which complete the seven. They are the plane of our individual highest spiritual expression, the Monadic, and the plane of Divine life called the plane of Adi. As these planes of spiritual awareness are beyond even advanced states of human consciousness, they are not relevant for this book. The chart in this section shows the seven levels of consciousness.

For perfect health we need to be able to bridge the gap between our higher and lower self so that spiritual energies can be touched on a regular basis. Healing streams of energy from the higher planes can then flow through our personality and heal the physical, astral and lower mental or mind nature. Regular meditation is invaluable for achieving this aim although it needs to be understood that meditation is of many kinds and can produce differing states of consciousness.

In one sense, meditation can be understood as the best natural therapy and is to be encouraged alongside any physical supplements given. Through regular meditation, we can approach and penetrate the higher levels of consciousness in an aware and consistent manner. The mind can then be used to interpret the new experience, and the whole person will gain benefit.

The term 'meditation' is often used loosely to cover a number of states of consciousness, but there are various types of meditation and they achieve different states. A common dictionary definition is to reflect or think deeply and this is actually closer to the esoteric meaning than the popularised understanding which often equates meditation with relaxation.

Yoga schools and stress management courses mainly teach a form of meditation which promotes relaxation by systematically turning the mind to different parts of the body and training people to recognise stress and to relax consciously all areas of the body. Having achieved complete relaxation, the mind is usually allowed to drift passively or to focus on a positive thought so that the body can have a chance to recharge with healing energy.

Some schools then go a step further and encourage people to use the creative imagination to visualise achieving health and life goals in various ways. This brings in the higher level of the astral or feeling nature which is the seat of the imagination. Through a visualisation process the astral nature and the lower mind are brought together in a positive sense. Colour visualisations and music may be used to enhance the process. These techniques are promoted to lose weight, overcome smoking and drug habits, promote confidence in work situations, and to solve emotional problems.

Individuals who teach the foregoing techniques often encourage the participants to lie down and this points to the predominance of the physical relaxation and to an emphasis on the astral or feeling component of the exercise. The process is therefore not unlike that of healthy sleep. To practise true meditation, which is mainly a mental function, the person must certainly be relaxed and comfortable but the spine needs to be erect. For deep reflective thought, a brief period of relaxation and alignment with the various levels of our nature precedes deep reflection on a particular subject or seed thought. When we have explored every facet of the subject with the mind, endeavouring to penetrate the essence of the subject with the higher or conceptual mind, the thinking process is suspended. We remain, however, in a state of alertness and mental poise and it is during this stillness that spiritual impressions from higher levels can be received. These impressions can then be interpreted correctly by the mind because it is held in a state of alertness. This process relates to the intuitive impressions received by all great scientists and thinkers, and may account for their great staying power in many instances due to the healing effect of higher energies.

There is great potential for healing through this deep form of meditation. We have already discussed the seven levels of consciousness and the seven principles in man. To flood the personality with healing energies we need to bridge the gap in consciousness which exists between the personality vehicles and the three spiritual levels of the spiritual triad. Through the use of the mind in this form of creative meditation, the personality is linked with the soul, which is the mediating vehicle between the personality and the spiritual triad. The soul provides and transmits the true pattern to the etheric body and healing of even chronic illness can then take place. It is probable that no matter what technique of meditation has been used, those individuals who have experienced complete remissions from diseases like cancer have activated this healing mechanism within themselves. The works of Alice Bailey give further insights into this subject.[11]

A further benefit of meditation should be highlighted — the broader effect on our inter-personal relations and on the environment. This could be described as the positive effect of not only integrating the various levels of our own being, but developing facility through emerging wholeness and health to integrate with other people and with the environment. In this way we make our creative contribution or service to the whole planetary evolutionary process.

This brings us to the final effect on the etheric or energy body underlying the physical expression of our being. As the bridge between the higher levels of consciousness, the physical brain consciousness and physical organs, it is the etheric vehicle in the final instance which conditions our health. The energy centres or *chakras* are like doorways which transmit energies from all levels of consciousness into the physical body. They do this by alignment with the corresponding energy centres in the astral body and lower mind. This factor emphasises the need for integration in the personality life before there can be alignment with the soul and even higher levels of being.

It is in this area that the modern schools of psychology have made an impressive contribution towards the health of humanity. Assertiveness training, gestalt techniques, rational-emotive and cognitive behavioural therapies, and desensitisation procedures are instances of contributions towards producing the initial integration of the personality which must take place before meditation can be used wisely as the next step towards wholeness.

Disease may therefore have both an inner and outer cause, with the etheric as the link between the outer world and the inner. Psychological problems work downwards to the etheric body and thus condition health at the physical level. On the other hand, life-style and environmental problems such as noise, lack of rest or exercise, poor diet, and overwork, impinge from below on the etheric. A number of our therapies — for example homoeopathy, the flower essences, acupuncture and to some extent herbs and vitamins — have a profound effect on body energies. This two-way traffic provides the reason why natural therapists are often interested in esoteric subjects.

The Seven *Chakras* or Centres Influencing Health

Each level of consciousness is expressed through the seven main *chakras* as they condition and affect the physical body via the endocrine glands and surrounding tissues.

It is logical to begin this discussion with the sacral centre and work through the seven in pairs as each *chakra* has a lower or higher counterpart. Table 3 in this section shows the seven *chakras*. The basic problems which involve these energy centres in the etheric body relate to lack of balance or harmony between the centres. This in turn gives rise to over- or under-stimulation with consequent over- or under-secretion of the endocrine gland associated with the centre involved.

As with all aspects of natural healing, the main aim is to recreate balance and harmony. In terms of the *chakras* this may mean psychological help, meditation, change in life-style, plus the raw material needed by the endocrine glands to produce the appropriate secretions. For example, a severe deficiency of zinc is found to give a dwarfish stature with lack of secondary sexual development.[12] In this latter situation, there would be a reflex action back on the sacral *chakra* from the undernourished gonads or sexual organs.

The first pair of energy centres to consider are those consisting of the sacral and throat centre. The sacral centre is related to the gonads or reproductive glands — ovaries in the female and testes in the male. An imbalance of energy in this centre may result in problems with the reproductive tract in either sex, and to troubles with the last portion of the large bowel. Examples in the female include ovarian cysts, fibroids of the uterus, blocked fallopian tubes, and problems with menstruation. In the male, problems could involve cysts in the testes, enlarged prostate, and in both sexes cancer of the area, bladder infections and sexual problems may occur. A period of sterility may occur also as a result of energy transference from the sacral to the throat *chakra* during the development of mental creativity.

The overall function of this *chakra* concerns three aspects of our everyday life: sex, food and comfort. This centre is therefore associated with our appetites. At the psychological level, problems will involve the sex life, food addictions and needs for physical comfort. The reader will probably agree that the average person in our materialistic society is quite active at this level.

The higher counterpart of the sacral centre is the throat *chakra*

Table 3

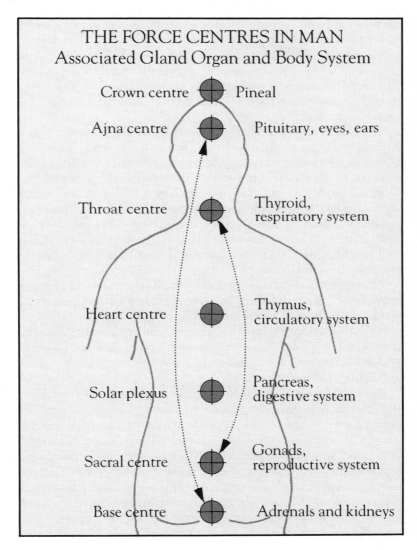

THE FORCE CENTRES IN MAN
Associated Gland Organ and Body System

Crown centre — Pineal

Ajna centre — Pituitary, eyes, ears

Throat centre — Thyroid, respiratory system

Heart centre — Thymus, circulatory system

Solar plexus — Pancreas, digestive system

Sacral centre — Gonads, reproductive system

Base centre — Adrenals and kidneys

and together these form a creative pair. The sacral expresses creativity through perpetuation of the race, and also gives the needed energy for grounding the mental creative schemes which emanate via the throat *chakra*. We should not suppress the functions of the sacral centre, but should control and direct the energies. Gold is a symbol for the sacral centre, dealing as it does with the use of physical energy, and with the use of money. From an esoteric point of view, money is crystallised *prana* or energy. We can see the possible repercussions for health if wealth is cornered for selfish purposes, and not used for the benefit of those around us. There would be a corresponding congestion in the sacral *chakra* and perhaps this is one reason for the widespread pelvic disease in a large section of humanity in this materialistic age.

The throat centre relates to the endocrine gland known as the thyroid and this is situated in the front of the neck. Problems with this centre not only include hypo- and hyper-activity of the thyroid gland, but also respiratory problems such as bronchitis, asthma, laryngitis and loss of voice. In relation to the actual thyroid, metabolic problems involving weight loss and nervousness, palpitations and hot flushes can develop. Menopausal problems of women are often related to the throat and sacral *chakra* and will be further mentioned under the heading Menopause in the alphabetical section.

At the psychological level, this *chakra* is the organ for creative thought. A generally sluggish system evidenced by depression, weight gain, boredom and lack of creative activity may relate to a sluggish or underactive throat centre. Conversely, the tremendous emphasis on hobbies, recreation, post-graduate learning and self-actualisation training indicates that this *chakra* is rapidly unfolding in humanity as a whole.

Just as the lower part of this pair expresses physical creativity, this *chakra* is intimately related to mental creativity, and its activity can be expressed through art or any mental activity involving creative planning. Such mental activity relates to the 'blueprint' whether in the field of town planning, architecture, engineering, dressmaking, landscaping, cooking, painting or writing. The individual focuses intelligence through the throat centre and it becomes the organ for distribution of creative energy. As we develop our inner potentials, energy is drawn upwards from the sacral centre as a result of the increasing activity of the throat centre. The ensuing control of the sacral centre provides extra energy for creative pursuits. Thus, our appetites related to food, sex and comfort are controlled but not suppressed, and most importantly, we learn to use money wisely and for the good of the whole. This affects the health in a positive manner.

The seven *chakras* can be grouped in three pairs plus the Ajna *chakra*. The Ajna *chakra* is the final expression of the throat/sacral axis. The Ajna centre is responsive to the impression of ideas and can mediate spiritual impressions from higher levels of consciousness which are later formulated into plans by the throat *chakra*. As one of the two head centres, the Ajna centre synthesises the whole personality life and later relates this to the spiritual energies flowing through the crown *chakra*.

The endocrine gland connected to the Ajna centre is the pituitary, situated centrally in the brain. Health problems due to an imbalance in the Ajna *chakra* may involve the eyes, ears and various kinds of headaches. As the pituitary gland provides secretions which stimulate all the glands situated below it in the body, there may also be imbalances of other glands. In terms of the effect on the inner life of the individual, the Ajna *chakra* can express either the heights of personality ambition, or become the organ for distribution of spiritual energies from both the head and heart. From another viewpoint it is the organ of creative imagination, and in this sense brings in energies from the solar plexus and from the higher levels of the astral plane.

The Ajna *chakra* is associated with the eyes and it is understood that the right eye is related to insight or spiritual vision and the left eye with the lower, material aspect of the mind. The third eye is really a synthesis of the two eyes and becomes the organ for spiritual vision. It is traditionally associated with the Ajna *chakra*, but only after a magnetic field is created between the Ajna and crown centres.

The next pair is the solar plexus and heart. The solar plexus centre is the gateway to the astral plane or world of feeling. Associated with this centre is the endocrine gland known as the pancreas. We can see how our feelings can affect the digestive processes, for the pancreas not only produces insulin but also the pancreatic juice which deals with fats, carbohydrates and proteins. All the other digestive processes involving stomach, liver, gall-bladder and the small bowel are intimately related to this centre. Examples of disorder in relation to this *chakra* would be dyspepsia, gallstones, stomach, duodenal and bowel ulcers, lack of assimilation, diabetes and many types of nervousness which stem from imbalance of the autonomic nervous system. The autonomic nervous system expresses the astral or feeling nature, in turn conditioning those metabolic processes not under the control of the central nervous system, for example, digestive processes, hormone secretions and circulation.

The solar plexus is tremendously active in the majority of mankind, and this is because most of us are focused in the world of desire — the astral plane. The solar plexus responds to every desire no matter how subtle. Apart from desires related to our possessions and more material needs, subtle desires include things like the need for recognition or promotion in various ways. Even desire for spiritual experience or for a spiritual teacher is an outcome of solar plexus activity. The solar plexus acts as a clearing house for the major and minor centres below the diaphragm. These energies can then be transmuted through the developing aspirations of the personality towards the centres above the diaphragm. Aspiration develops gradually from desire, and slowly our aims, ambitions, and goals are transmuted by the heart centre which is the higher counterpart of the solar plexus.

It is of interest to note the emphasis by many therapists on unblocking the emotions, de-armouring muscles which have developed tensions through emotional blocks, and of encouraging feelings to flow freely. These therapies seem to symbolise the move of humanity to control and redirect the energies of the solar plexus. Many people suffer from a cramp in the solar plexus and the consequent spasm and pain often remains undiagnosed as no organic cause can be found. In sensitive children the problem is labelled abdominal migraine.

The control of the solar plexus, and closing of the door to any negative influence from the astral plane, coincides with the awakening of the heart *chakra* — the organ for expression of true love, empathy and real service. The solar plexus in a psychological sense is more related to sympathy, but this attribute often has many strings attached. Solar plexus friendship is fraught with envies, possession and jealousy. At best it gives the type of instinctive caring of the mother for the child, and expresses loyalty and devotion.

The heart *chakra* is the gateway to our higher spiritual self as it manifests on the Buddhic plane — the plane of enlightenment. This plane is understood to be the home or focus of enlightened beings and to emit energies of love/wisdom and pure reason. The heart centre is eventually able to receive and distribute these energies into the environment. The associated endocrine gland is the thymus gland which relates to physical immunity through the production of cells called T-lymphocytes.

Physical immunity may be concurrent with the more subjective developments of inclusive, magnetic and radiatory love, the characteristic energy flowing through this centre giving protection and immunity in a deeper sense at both physical and psychic levels. Psychic protection results from the repelling of negative forces by the outgoing radiatory streams of energy from the heart centre. At the physical level, these streams of energy are the stimulating factor in the production of thymus secretions, resulting finally in development of protective lymphocytes. Physical problems involving the heart *chakra* may cause lack of physical immunity to serious disorders such as cancer, multiple sclerosis and other immune deficiency diseases, and more commonly to heart and circulatory problems.

The keynote of the heart centre is inclusive and dispassionate love. The heart in this sense is the organ of fusion. In secular life, an expression of such energy will be found manifesting through an individual or group of people who are the heart of an organisation — not necessarily a spiritual organisation in the usual sense of the word. This inclusiveness expresses itself through group work and indicates a responsibility or rather the ability to respond to a sensed need. The phrase 'ability to think in the heart' is often used in speaking of the developed heart consciousness and expresses the concept of pure reason as the quality of the Buddhic plane.

The heart centre is intimately concerned with service based on need rather than service for any selfish motive. As the organ for the distribution of spiritual energy from the Buddhic plane, when awakened it gives the ability to understand another being and to enter fully into their consciousness through empathy. The energy of the heart centre transmutes the desire-life centred in the personality at the solar plexus into love/wisdom. The wisdom aspect is a marriage of discriminating intelligence and love resulting in the ability to think in the heart.

Energy from the sacral centre should pass through the heart before reaching the throat. In this way our creative work is planned in relation to group need. It is significant that humanity is witnessing as never before groups who are working for the welfare of mankind and the animal and plant kingdoms. These many networks devoted to alleviating suffering and promoting global health give an indication of the unfolding heart centre in humanity.

The last pair to consider is that of the base and crown *chakra*. The associated endocrine glands connected to the base centre are the adrenal glands. These are situated on top of the kidneys. They are intimately related to coping with various stresses in life, including biochemical, nervous and environmental problems. Adrenalin is the hormone from the medulla (inside part) of the gland, and cortisone is secreted from the cortex or outside part. Adrenalin is associated with the famous flight and fight mechanism of the threatened individual. Cortisone is needed to treat various biochemical stresses and is prescribed for patients in various serious medical conditions which are life threatening.

High and low blood pressures sometimes relate to an excess or deficiency of energy flowing through the base centre. Our basic animation or will to live comes from this energy and can vary enormously between individuals. Spiritual will is likewise connected with this last pair of centres. The fire which animates this quality dwells in the base centre and is known in the East as Kundalini. When all the chakras are perfectly developed and balanced, the fire from the base chakra can safely rise through the three esoteric spinal channels and activate the crown centre. This fire develops momentum in three stages as each of the pairs are activated and perfectly related.

Not a great deal can be said about this last pair of centres as they are activated only when we have fully developed our spiritual potential. The pineal gland is the endocrine gland which is related to the crown chakra, and is the organ for the reception of both physical and spiritual light. Medical science has found that the pineal is stimulated by light to control all the other endocrines.[13] A relationship is finally created between the crown chakra and the Ajna chakra. This magnetic field provides the traditional halo of light seen around the head of enlightened persons.

The relation between the two head centres is established through meditation and spiritual living, when the magnetic field created draws up the Kundalini fire in a safe and proper manner. The crown centre is the final point of synthesis for all the centres and registers spiritual purpose. It is in keeping with our general ignorance about this state of being that we still do not understand fully the health implications of the pineal gland.

For further study and reading in this area, the works of Bailey, Karagulla and Tansley are suggested.[14] The real understanding of the chakras and their relation to health comes from the personal experience which follows reflective thought, meditation and right service.

CHAPTER 3

The Cornerstones
of Treatment

Clinical nutrition, herbal medicine and homoeopathy are the internal therapies most widely used by natural therapists throughout the world. Training in these areas of internal medicine features strongly in all colleges of natural therapies except those which specialise in the physical remedial therapies, such as massage, reflexology, manipulation of the spine, kinesiology and acupuncture.

The clinical nutritional approach which has developed in the natural therapy profession today results from factors peculiar to the twentieth century. In the early days of the naturopathic movement nearly two hundred years ago, emphasis was placed mainly on rest, fasting, water treatments and good diet. A different approach is required in clinical practice today, although the basic naturopathic principles of improving vitality and enhancing elimination of toxins continue to be observed. Modern farming methods produce fruit, vegetables and grains which are found to be deficient in vitamins and minerals when compared with food values documented early in this century.[1] Water fasting is now inappropriate unless people have access to unpolluted supplies. The stress of modern life brings about the need for supplementation of particular vitamins and minerals.

For these reasons the practice of clinical nutrition has changed greatly. Natural therapists now find it necessary to use supplements for some months, after which time patients continue to maintain their improvement provided their diet is well planned.

Other main internal therapies are herbalism or botanic medicine, and homoeopathy. Herbalism has a very ancient background and goes back centuries in many cultures. Each civilisation has specialists who were trained in the art of collecting, preparing and administering herbal concoctions. Herbal medicines developing from these ancient cultures are still prescribed in a traditional manner. Modern manufacturing methods have, however, simplified the preparation, storage and keeping of herbs.

Homoeopathy is another traditional therapy, although it was developed by Samuel Hahnemann around the year 1790. This therapy had support by medical doctors on a moderately large scale at the end of the nineteenth century and the beginning of the twentieth century. As many homoeopathic medicines are developed from plants, herbal medicine and homoeopathy are related in some important respects.

Minerals

Minerals are the basic building blocks of the body tissues. The key minerals include iron, calcium, phosphorous, zinc, magnesium, potassium, sulphur, sodium and less commonly known trace elements such as selenium and vanadium. They must be supplied in varying small amounts via the diet throughout life or the individual may suffer from a deficiency. Natural therapists and some medical scientists contend that due to the refining of foods in the twentieth century, and to the deficiency of soils in which foods are grown, many people are now deficient in these essential elements.[2] Many of these elements such as magnesium have a synergistic action in the body and are responsible for a number of biochemical chains. Magnesium, for example, is involved in over fifty biochemical chains in the body.[3] The prevention of anaemia is not only related to iron but to an adequate placing of copper which in turn is antagonised or removed by zinc.[4]

One of the problems associated with the indiscriminate self-dosing of vitamins and minerals arises from this complexity of synergistic actions. Vitamins are often useless without the presence of associated minerals and vice versa. A simple example is the increased passage of iron across the cell membrane in the presence of vitamin C.[5]

In Part 2 of this book, the reader will note that particular mineral salts are mentioned repeatedly. Many naturopaths use the twelve tissue salts and these are prepared by a number of manufacturers. These salts were pioneered by Schussler around the middle of the last century.[6] It is essential to note that when iron phosphate or potassium chloride is mentioned, these supplements are specially prepared and they have a different clinical effect from the usual pharmaceutical dose and preparation. These work in a homoeopathic manner to regulate the molecular balance within the cell, and as a consequence assist in assimilation. This is the reason why comparatively small amounts of mineral salts prepared in this manner can remove deficiencies.

Generally speaking, mineral deficiencies are removed in three to six months of treatment. The natural therapist assesses this mainly in terms of clinical improvement, although evaluation using blood tests or hair analysis is possible. It is worth mentioning that a lot of information on mineral status can be gauged by taking a careful case history and by analysis of improvements in the clinical status as treatment progresses. In this way time can be saved and expensive pathology avoided.

Vitamins

Most vitamin research and identification has taken place during this century. For vitamin therapy to be significant, the synergistic effect of vitamins and minerals needs to be considered. It is true that many people dose themselves indiscriminately with vitamins, as some opponents of vitamin therapy claim. While there are very few recorded instances of vitamin toxicity a lot of money and time can be wasted if vitamins and minerals are not carefully selected.[7]

Vitamins are catalysts which provide the energy for many reactions in the body. Vitamin C, for instance, is directly related to electron transfer within the cell and is therefore associated with energy reactions.[8] As mentioned, many biochemical processes involving vitamins are also linked to trace minerals. It has been found that both vitamin C and vitamin E are anti-oxidants in the body and that they prevent certain ageing and destructive processes to which cells are subjected as we go through life.[9] It has also been established that the vitamins themselves are synergistic and thus work together, for example, vitamin A and vitamin E, both fat-soluble vitamins, need each other to work satisfactorily. [10]

As with the minerals, the body can easily become deficient in vitamins through inadequate nutrition and poor cooking techniques. Some vitamins are destroyed by the various chemicals which we contact in our modern environment. The use of pharmaceutical products, such as the contraceptive pill used on a regular basis, is also acknowledged by medical scientists to deplete the body of particular vitamins. [11]

There is a great deal of evidence from reputable sources to suggest that vitamin deficiencies are widespread in the community today. [12] Unless medical doctors have done extra training, they do not have adequate expertise in this area. Consulting well-trained natural therapists, however, ensures correct selection and dosage of vitamin supplementation.

Herbs

Herbs have been used since time immemorial for restoration of health. They are able to restore the function of disordered organs and thus have a toning effect on tissues. Individual herbs have been found to have an affinity with a particular organ or system. Thus dandelion and centaury have a tonic effect on the liver, while parsley and berberis have a toning action on the kidneys, and red clover and violet leaves cleanse the lymphatic system. [13] Herbs are considered to be essential to the process of eliminating the toxins which build up in the body as a result of poor diet, weak digestion and stress. They may be used as teas, infusions, liquid extracts, tinctures and solid extracts. Some of the efficacy of herbs is attributed to their vitamin and mineral content.

Many medical drugs are synthetic versions of active herbal principles. Medical scientists use this fact to decry the need for herbal medicine. The natural therapist would argue that nature has provided a balance of ingredients in the complete herb which protects against the possibility of side-effects. Indeed, the majority of herbs have few side-effects and the well-trained practitioner knows which herbs to handle with care. Side-effects may result from isolating and concentrating particular active ingredients. This problem occurs in modern orthodox medicine as a result of isolating and concentrating the active principles in herbs.

In clinical practice herbs are so useful to tone organs and assist in the elimination of toxic waste that it is hard to imagine them ever losing favour with the natural therapist. They can exert a very rapid action especially in their liquid preparations such as teas and infusions. Recent research into the impressionability of water by chemical substances may give us a clue to the apparent magic of both herbs and homoeopathy.

Herbs should only be administered by a person thoroughly trained in their use. It is not wise for an untrained person to gather or to prepare herbs as there are many closely related herbs which look similar but which may have different actions. It is also important to select suitable combinations of herbs due to their synergistic action. Dosage and frequency of dosage is critical for optimum efficacy although overdosage is rarely dangerous, unlike the use of the concentrated synthetic versions of herbs used in orthodox medicine.

Herbal medicine can be described as the most universal medicine for mankind. Herbs contain concentrated amounts of vitamins, minerals, and enzymes plus an extra special factor which according to the nature of each plant renders them applicable to a wide range of illnesses.

Homoeopathy

The science and art of homoeopathy is even more specialised than the practice of herbal medicine. Although developed by Samuel Hahnemann late in the eighteenth century, there are hints in ancient philosophies that the practice of giving the minimum dose dates back many centuries.[14]

Homoeopathic therapy is based on the premise of 'like cures like'. The doctrine of similars has been echoed to some extent in the practice of immunisation whereby the immune system is stimulated by the introduction of small amounts of the disease entity. To stimulate the production of antibodies against polio, small amounts of the live virus are given in the Sabin vaccine.

In the practice of homoeopathy minute amounts of animal, vegetable or mineral matter is given to stimulate immunity, and to enhance the body energy so that toxic matter is eliminated and organ function restored. Unlike immunisation, there are no side-effects apart from the transitory aggravation which indicates that the correct remedy has been given. The natural therapist treats the individual as a unique entity who must be given the exact remedy which matches his or her total condition. In this fact lies the difference between the practice of homoeopathy and that of immunisation programmes, where everyone receives the same substance.

To summarise the homoeopathic approach to disease, a substance is given which matches the disease pattern. Given to a healthy subject, this substance would produce the disease. This is how the phrase 'like cures like' originated. As the homoeopathic remedy is given in a very minute dose, very little aggravation occurs even if the wrong remedy is chosen. Only a skilled person is able to select the correct remedy from the many possible choices.

There are other facets of homoeopathic prescribing which indicate both its enormous range of action and its complexity. The best role for homoeopathy is the treatment of the whole constitution. This means that all aspects of the case and the whole patient are taken into consideration. Heredity, life-style, environment, present symptoms, past illnesses, psychological attributes and life goals are all considered in selecting the remedy.

Treating in a symptomatic way with homoeopathy is considered to be superficial prescribing, although it can give good short-term results which may become permanent if there is not a complicating inherited factor. In such cases, the homoeopathic prescribing is known as organ drainage and is similar to the practice of herbal medicine.

To gain all the necessary material for homoeopathic prescribing entails the need for a very detailed life picture of the patient. Time is needed for the first interview with each patient, during which the therapist records the complete history. Some homoeopaths have the patients draw up a detailed life history which is sent to the therapist before the first interview. Any gaps can then be filled after the therapist has reflected on the contents. The skilled homoeopath becomes adept in time at assessing particular constitutional types fairly quickly.

As well as the selection of the constitutional remedy, organ drainage remedies, and acute remedies will be prescribed according to each case. This further illustrates the beauty of homoeopathic prescribing, as the acute remedy for an individual person will always be found to have a relationship to their constitutional remedy. The therapist must know when to give the acute remedy, when to give remedies to antidote any inherited problems such as the tubercular taint, and when to give the constitutional remedy. Furthermore, each of these is selected from many possible potencies and may need to be given at widely varying time intervals.

In Part 2, the reader will note that sometimes a specific homoeopathic remedy is mentioned in cases where symptomatic prescribing is indicated. At other times, the requirement for the constitutional remedy is stressed, and in still other situations, more emphasis is placed on removing inherited taints or miasms. I have also indicated how natural therapists increase the potency of particular remedies as treatment progresses.

Over the years in clinical practice, it has been found essential to remove gross vitamin and mineral deficiencies before the constitutional homoeopathic remedy becomes readily apparent. These deficiencies mask the underlying constitution, whilst at the same time they contribute to the constitutional type. Improving organ tone, especially of liver and kidneys, and enhancing elimination with herbs provides a foundation for the homoeopathic remedy to work more efficiently.

In the case of babies and children, homoeopathic remedies are usually successful without the need of other supplements. This is due to the high vitality of the young body, and because there has been less time for waste of various types to accumulate. As many young children will not take tablets and herbs, the use of a few homoeopathic drops in water or fruit juice is very convenient.

Bach Flowers

This safe and effective treatment was pioneered by a Harley Street specialist named Edward Bach. He gave up a flourishing orthodox medical practice to seek a more subtle form of treatment. Searching in the woods of the United Kingdom, he found thirty-eight flowers which had remarkable properties for removing the various ailments suffered by his clientele.[15] The Bach flower remedies are particularly suited to those individuals whose disease is largely related to emotional causes.

The flowers are prepared by soaking in distilled or uncontaminated water and using the filtrate which is preserved by an addition of brandy. As the remedy is selected by matching the known qualities of the flower to the emotional state which needs treatment, one could say that the Bach flower therapy is homoeopathic in effect. The Bach flowers rarely produce any side-effect or aggravation and being fairly simple to select and apply, can be used by lay people with good results.

Recently, a further selection of Flower Essences has been researched and these are also giving excellent results in emotional states for which there was not previously a specific Bach flower. Several months of treatment are usually needed for the full results of either Bach or Flower Essences to be established.

If we consider that the flower is the most ethereal and special part of the plant, it is logical to assume that therapy using this part of the plant will have a very subtle effect on health and well-being. The claim that flower remedies can affect the emotions may be valid in terms of a resonance from the flower invoking a response from the patient through a corresponding harmonic frequency. The dramatic effect of homoeopathic remedies on emotional states will no doubt relate to the same principle of harmonics.

Clinical nutrition, embracing the application of minerals and vitamins, herbal medicine, and homoeopathy are the basic traditional pillars of natural medicine. Massage, zone therapy, acupressure, and acupuncture can all be used as adjuncts to promoting blood and nerve supply, lymphatic drainage, and toning organs. These four therapies are all based on the relation of certain points on the body to particular organs and tissues.

Vivaxis is in a category of its own and was pioneered by a Canadian named Frances Nixon. Training in this sphere and the use of Vivaxis techniques have been found most useful for fine tuning of the electromagnetic field, provided deficiencies of minerals and vitamins have been removed, a balanced life-style established and after basic psychological integration has been achieved. The techniques of Vivaxis are a means of using energy flows found on the surface of the earth to recharge and balance our own etheric energies. This form of therapy is also useful for removing the negative effects of heavy metals and other toxins from the body.[16]

Synthesis in Prescribing

Synthesis in prescribing is the most intriguing aspect of natural therapies. There are many ways of approaching health and disease using the therapies previously covered. It will be noted in

Part 2 that in most cases a selection of vitamins, minerals and herbs are used, plus at some stage, homoeopathic remedies. There are very important reasons for using these main internal therapies of clinical nutrition, herbs and homoeopathy as the cornerstones of naturopathic prescribing.

Minerals are considered as the basic building blocks of the cell, and as such form the foundation of any healing work at the physical level. To assist their incorporation in the many biochemical chains, vitamins are included as needed. A typical example of this was mentioned in relation to the effect of iron absorption in the presence of vitamin C.[17] Natural therapists usually find that basic mineral deficiencies require a time-span of up to six months for the homoeostatic mechanisms to be re-established. Vitamins do not usually need such a long time for application unless there is an ongoing need due to poor diet or extra stress.

Herbs are used in conjunction with the minerals and vitamins to improve organ function. The time needed for their application will vary according to the duration of the complaint, the inherited constitution and general life-style. They may be used as fluid extracts, solid extracts and tinctures or in homoeopathic form. A number of therapists tend to go to extremes. Either they fill the client up with many supplements of vitamins and minerals, totally ignoring the fact that a clogged system cannot absorb and adequately assimilate nutrients, or they have an almost mystical belief that for ideal therapy only a few specially selected homoeopathic remedies are needed. The middle path is always best but should involve the capacity to be very selective and discriminating with vitamins, minerals and herbs plus the specific homoeopathic remedy.

Following the use of, or in conjunction with vitamins, minerals and herbs, homoeopathic remedies can be used for toning and draining organs, for eliminating both inherited and acquired toxins, and as constitutional remedies which are particularly and specifically selected for the individual. I have found the constitutional remedy to be of most use once initial toning and elimination of waste has proceeded to a certain degree. In many cases there is insufficient vitality in the client at the beginning of treatment for any registration of the constitutional remedy. To give a homoeopathic 'bullet' in such a case would be like shooting peas through a huge net.

Of recent years, in keeping with the growing popularity of

natural therapies, some manufacturers have brought out a number of products which contain up to twenty ingredients. These are quite often a mixture of vitamins, minerals and herbs but have such small quantities of each that at best they could be considered as a general tonic. A therapist who chiefly uses these kinds of medication for their clients on a regular basis is not really practising the art of natural medicine.

The most successful graduates in the field of natural therapies are those who can cover the needs of most people in the community, either by their own skills and resources, or by referring to other appropriate persons. A synthesis of the main three internal therapies will cover most needs and can be followed later by specialised treatment in areas as needed, such as acupuncture, massage, counselling or meditation. As most clients come by recommendation from other people, it is not surprising that therapists with the largest and most self-supporting practices tend to use vitamins, minerals, herbs and homoeopathy as a baseline from which to move into various specialties.

The Patient/Therapist Relationship

It has been stated that the natural therapist endeavours to treat the whole person. This means that there is a totally different approach to the patient from that generally found in orthodox medicine, where specialisation rules. For a start, the initial interview may need to be much longer so the therapist can gather all the necessary information about the patient as a whole. But an experienced natural therapist does not necessarily need even half an hour to gather enough information for the first prescription. Fifteen or twenty minutes may be quite sufficient. Therapists who have observed clinical signs of vitamin and mineral deficiencies over a number of years will pick up vital diagnostic information from the clients at first encounter, noticing shape, colour, sounds and posture. A few well chosen questions once the patient has finished relating their story will complete the data needed.

There is always a limit to what can be achieved in the first month's treatment; further data for homoeopathic prescribing can be obtained on the second and third visit. Like all small businesses, natural therapists have high costs and overheads, and unless working from a private home it is impractical to plan to spend one hour with each patient. While spending an hour with the patient may indicate a thorough and caring approach, it may just as readily be attributed to incompetence.

Critics of natural therapists may claim that the popularity for the treatment stems from a placebo effect produced by spending so much time with each person. This assessment underestimates the intelligence of natural therapy clients. The placebo effect is important and should not be undervalued, and possibly needs to be emphasised more in orthodox medical practice. The average person is prepared to pay up to sixty dollars each month because their health is improving significantly, and not from a placebo effect alone. An interesting evaluation of placebo effect as compared to the homoeopathic effect has been explored by R. M. Morris-Owen of the United Kingdom.[18]

The value of this health insurance which takes account of natural therapy cannot be overestimated in terms of quality of life and savings in sick leave. When the government is able to provide health rebates it will certainly be easier for families to cope financially with the cost of natural treatment.

All these factors influence the relation of the patient to the natural therapist. Work in this area is very creative and the role of the therapist becomes more of an educator as the therapist helps the client with overall life-style including diet, work, exercise, recreation and relaxation. Flexibility is the keynote in our approach to the relationship between client and therapist. Some people need more time than others due to their particular case and needs. Weekly, twice-weekly, monthly or twice-monthly visits may be necessary for a particular case. To be flexible according to perceived needs is to develop a creative way of working with people.

Natural therapists are now more likely to refer patients to other natural therapists who specialise in particular areas and to orthodox medical colleagues. This is a healthy sign and is another measure that the profession has come of age.

In Part 2 of this book, space prevents describing in detail how and why each remedy was selected, or many details of the diagnosis. Sufficient information is given to allow for an understanding of the approach used for each particular disorder in terms of remedies used. The reason why particular homoeopathic remedies in specific potencies are chosen is not generally described because it would require a great deal of detail. The main aim of this part of the book is to give an understanding of synthesis in prescribing although it is necessary to point out that not all the suggested remedies for each condition are necessarily prescribed or needed.

Part 2

Disorders Treated by Natural Therapists

This section is arranged in alphabetical order. A brief explanation of each condition will include the symptoms, causes from both a medical and naturopathic viewpoint, the treatment, and wherever possible one or two case histories follow each type of disorder. Some of the case histories are recent and some date back a number of years, but in nearly every case, the patient was contacted to check on their current health status before inclusion in the book. A few difficult cases with only partial improvement have been deliberately included to indicate that natural therapies cannot completely cure everyone, and to indicate the need for co-operation between the orthodox and naturopathic profession.

The listed conditions are those most commonly treated by natural therapists, and not all medical conditions are included. It will be observed that most of the common disorders for which the average person visits their local orthodox doctor are covered.

Each heading is expressed as the usual common term for several reasons. Firstly, these are the terms which both professional and lay people have learnt to apply to various symptoms and syndromes. Secondly, if there is to be co-operation between the various health professions there must be a common language. Finally, it would be impossible for someone wishing to find out information quickly from this compendium to do so if we grouped the disorders in a more naturopathic sequence.

In some areas, the finding of suitable case histories has been difficult. From the naturopathic viewpoint, the patient is often treated for a completely different problem than that diagnosed by orthodox medicine. By treating the whole person, the causal chain is more prominent in naturopathic medicine, and this may stretch back through several generations. Some conditions will be mentioned for which no case histories have been included, either because they are conditions rarely treated by natural therapists or because no clear-cut case involving the particular ailment was documented in my existing files. A difficulty occurs in dealing with cardiac patients. Natural therapists rarely have the opportunity of treating these individuals in the early stages. Cardiac patients must take their medical drugs at the same time as natural therapy treatment which may be by this stage only palliative, as is the current medical treatment. It is difficult to find a clear-cut case where natural therapists are able to demonstrate conclusively the effect of naturopathic treatment on cardiovascular problems, although some patients improve significantly in their general health while on natural therapy treatment.

Sufficient cases have been included to give the reader a very good idea of the full naturopathic approach, and to indicate the breadth of conditions for which natural medicine is applicable.

The reader will note that some remedies appear to be listed repeatedly for many conditions. These include vitamin C, the mineral combination iron phosphate and potassium chloride, and herbs for the lymphatic system and liver. This may give the impression that naturopathic prescribing is not an individual matter after all. The real reason rests on the great need for detoxification in the average client, no matter what the ailment. These particular supplements tone the liver, cleanse the lymphatic system, improve immunity, and thus allow the more constitutional and individual prescribing to be effective. In the future, when a healthy life-style and natural diet is more universally accepted, this initial cleansing will not be necessary, and clinical practice will become even more interesting for the natural therapist and client.

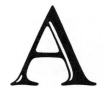

Acne

This condition of the skin is characterised by raised red blemishes which may or may not be pustular. Although there are different kinds of acne, it commonly manifests at puberty, and unfortunately in some cases the situation continues until the individual is in the late thirties. In these more stubborn cases, the blemishes frequently manifest as cysts and result in pronounced scarring once the initial inflammation has subsided.

Causes

A common cause is found to be congestion of the lymphatic system. This in turn may result from a sluggish liver which does not adequately detoxify pollutants, drugs, and the end products of metabolism or digestion. Nutrition may not have an immediate causal connection with the problem, but over a period of years, if the individual repeatedly indulges in refined and devitalised food — 'junk food' — the result will be a sluggish liver and congested lymphatic system.

Another important factor to consider in relation to the toxic condition of the body relates to the capacity to eliminate waste through the channels of bowel, skin, lungs and kidney. Any of these organs may be constitutionally weak and will need toning to improve elimination processes. A child may start life with a congested lymphatic system and this results from a lack of health on the part of the mother during pregnancy. In such a case, we are not concerned with a particular clinical disease or pathology in the mother, but with sub-clinical states like constant tiredness, poor elimination, irritability and a general lack of well-being.

Another contributing factor to acne is comparatively recent and comes from allergy to the air pollution which occurs in most large towns and cities. Air conditioning systems have also been cited as reasons for skin problems. This factor of pollution in relation to our skin is significant in proportion to the ability of the body to eliminate waste adequately.

Other causative reasons for acne are stress in the nervous system from work, the home, or general life-style, and hormonal changes such as those which occur during puberty. The more severe forms of acne are considered to be androgen-dependent conditions.[1] In these cases androgen excess, either locally or systemically, is a causative factor. This is most relevant when considering the deeper subjective causes of acne, as androgen excess can only happen if the glands are out of balance. The glands are influenced in their secretion by the *chakras* or energy centres and these are intimately related to our psyche and psychological processes. Severe forms of acne may therefore be conditions which have their bases in subtle psychological states.

A subtle explanation for skin blemishes may be described as follows. The skin is that organ which connects us with the outer world in a physical sense. The electromagnetic energy which forms the etheric body as it underlies the physical organs and tissues extends for a few centimetres beyond the skin. In a subtle sense, the etheric connects our inner nature, feelings and thoughts with the physical body — our outer instrument for perception in the world. The skin is the outer symbol for the etheric body. Blocked feelings and suppressed emotions can be held at the boundary of the skin instead of flowing into the outer world. For example, one client who had a long history of boils was relieved from this troublesome expression on the skin during a period when she was able to vent her anger at the world through 'primal screaming'. Before this therapy (which is only undertaken with a trained therapist), all manner of physical detoxifying herbs, minerals, and homoeopathics had been used with limited success.

Hence, eruptions on the skin can correspond to negative emotional states which need resolution. The therapist soon becomes aware as to whether the client is responding sufficiently to physical treatment. This topic will be explored further when discussing skin rashes. As a result of studies in connection with the autonomic part of the nervous system, medical science accepts that the nerves affect the skin profoundly.

It is not a very big step to see the possibility of acne, boils and carbuncles resulting from unexpressed negative emotions such as hatred and anger. These emotions will disturb the glandular balance and then the biochemistry involving normal bacterial colonies on the skin will be disturbed. Physical toxins will accumulate and the bacteria will multiply and provide the final expression in the pustule or boil. If this chain of events is valid, giving antibiotics for acne will be understood to touch only the final expression and not the cause.

We need to remember that not everyone with skin eruptions has a psychological problem, and even if they do, only a few psychological procedures may give lasting results. I remember with some embarrassment extolling the virtues of 'primal screaming' in my first book, explaining the parallel to the naturopathic healing crisis, only to find that many people after some years of regular 'screaming' seem no further towards personality integration and wholeness.

Evidence for the causes of the acne condition may be found in diagnosis of the iris, tongue, hand, or from hair analysis if heavy industrial pollutants are suspected, and from taking a careful history of the patient including details of diet, patterns of elimination, and general life-style.[2] In some cases examination of the parents reveals correspondences of constitutional weaknesses.[3]

Treatment

Emphasis is on cleansing the lymphatics, toning the liver and other relevant organs and tissues, dealing with any constitutional problems, and replacing deficient vitamins and minerals which have occurred through poor nutrition, and faulty assimilation. Effort is made on the part of the therapist to re-educate the client into a healthy life-style and to deal with psychological problems.

A typical treatment for one month may include:

1 Liver herbs such as dandelion, centaury and wahoo, and lymphatic cleansers which may include violet leaves, red clover, and burdock.[4]
2 Mineral compounds iron phosphate and potassium chloride for the inflammation and lymphatic congestion respectively.[5]
3 A zinc preparation to resolve and prevent scarring, promote the immune system and to activate normal hormone functioning.[6]

4 Vitamin C to boost the immune system and to help in the detoxification process.[7]

5 Vitamin B as a nerve tonic — there are thousands of nerve endings in the skin.

6 The minerals potassium phosphate and magnesium phosphate to tone and relax respectively nerves involved with the skin.

7 Vitamin A may also be needed to reduce the amount of fatty substance or sebum which can commonly clog up the skin causing whiteheads, and also for its effect on promoting the health of the epithelial tissue which includes our skin.[8]

This prescription may need to be repeated with various minor variations such as the addition of homoeopathic remedies for a period of six months or more.

Case Histories

Greg, now twenty years old, was brought to our clinic aged sixteen with severe cystic-type acne on face and chest. He also suffered allergies which congested his nose most of the time. He had been medically treated with the antibiotic, tetracycline, for five months previously with no real improvement. His only other problem was a nervous restlessness which is characteristic of a zinc deficiency.[9] He was already taking B-complex vitamins. Over a period of eighteen months, skin on his face cleared completely, with the acne on the torso clearing up more slowly, and needing another year of treatment in reduced quantities. His nose also became clear. It is now two years since he finished the main treatment and his face remains clear according to his mother who visits the clinic intermittently.

Improvement was not dramatic but it was consistent over a period of months. Greg was on a fairly good diet when he first attended, although his appetite was poor. This also improved as treatment progressed. Unlike many young people, Greg took his supplements very regularly.

His treatment included the following supplements. The minerals needed were zinc, iron phosphate, potassium chloride, and calcium sulphate. The herbs used were trifolium, burdock, violet leaves, echinacea, dandelion, fringe tree, centaury and wahoo. These are herbs for cleansing lymphatic glands and toning the liver. Vitamins B-complex and C were used throughout the treatment and homoeopathic remedies included Hepar sulphuricus, Sulphur, and Pulsatilla. These latter items were included for both nasal congestion and the skin problem.

Pam, aged twenty-eight, came about her acne which had been present since puberty. The iris revealed that toxins under the skin had mainly originated in the digestive processes. Her present diet was fair. She was encouraged to eat more salad and fruit and treatment included liver and lymphatic herbs, potassium chloride and iron phosphate, sodium phosphate for the acidity of the tissues, a zinc compound, and homoeopathic Kali bromide.

Older readers may be amused to recall that Australian soldiers in the Second World War were sometimes given large doses of Kali bromide in the crude form to dampen their sexual desires. One of the worst side effects was severe acne. A homoeopathic dose of Kali bromide has the reverse effect on skin and therefore helps remove acne. (Fortunately the homoeopathic dose does not appear to have the reverse effect in terms of sexual desires!) In the case of Pam, her acne cleared within six months.

Abdominal Migraine

This is a term used commonly at present for a condition which presents to our clinic in the form of children with pain around the umbilical area. Sometimes there are associated digestive disturbances such as diarrhoea or constipation. I have observed that these children appear to be sensitive and intelligent.

Causes

As there is no logical orthodox medical explanation, I am offering only my own conclusions, especially in the light of a simple and effective treatment for this problem. These are children with a very sensitive solar plexus energy centre which as yet they have not learnt to control. In other words they are wide open to all astral or feeling influence in their environment, and this overpowers them and causes the energy centre to go into a spasm.

This in turn can affect all the digestive processes via the autonomic part of the nervous system.

Treatment

1   Magnesium phosphate to prevent spasm of nerves, muscles, and bowel.[1]
2   Vitamin B-complex as a general nerve tonic and to improve appetite.
3   Homoeopathic doses of liver herbs as a tonic to the digestive tract.
4   Bach flower remedies to balance the solar plexus energy centre. These are selected individually for the emotional state of the child. The Bach flowers are the most specific form of treatment I have found for healing and balancing the etheric energy centres.

Case Histories

Kaine, aged seven years, presented a typical picture of this problem. In his case, the bowel had been affected to some extent so that an aperient was necessary each day. The pain was directly around the navel and spread further at times. His first month's treatment consisted of magnesium phosphate to relieve spasm, and calcium phosphate in the ratio of 2:1. Vitamin B-complex was given to improve appetite, and a liver herbal tablet to improve bowel motility without the use of laxatives. Bach flower remedies stabilised his solar plexus *chakra*. He was soon able to go without his laxative, pains became less severe and further apart, and appetite improved.

Michelle, aged seven, had a similar problem but with a different mixture of symptoms. The main disturbing factor was projectile vomiting which appeared to me to be of nervous origin. She was picky with her food, had cramps in the legs, and generally suffered from anticipatory anxiety. Other minor considerations involved conditions of the skin and nails.

The cramps and the vomiting pointed to a magnesium deficiency, and magnesium phosphate was the most important ingredient of her treatment. This was supplemented by Bach flower remedies for her solar plexus centre, homoeopathic liver drops as a digestive tonic, and vitamin B-complex for appetite. There were no further cramps or attacks of vomiting after treatment commenced, and appetite gradually improved over the next few months. Her mother still experiences Michelle as a nervy child, and so she has been kept on small doses of magnesium, but the other remedies were discontinued after a few months.

Addison's Disease

This is an uncommon insidious disease involving destruction of the adrenal glands. It is more common in men than women and although possible at any age, generally takes place between the ages of twenty and forty. Early symptoms include languor, debility, nausea and vomiting.[1] The hormonal secretions of the adrenal glands are essential for life, and one literally cannot live without these hormones.

Causes

The main cause in the past from the medical point of view was found to be tuberculosis. Increasingly, the problem is considered to be an auto-immune disorder involving destructive antibodies which are found circulating in these patients. As this is a rare disorder, natural therapists have not a great deal of clinical experience in the area. It is of interest, however, to consider those ailments which are related to the endocrine glands, as they reflect more subtle causes in the psyche from the inner point of view.

The function of the base *chakra* which relates to the adrenal glands and the will to live has been discussed in chapter 2. The very low blood pressure associated with atrophy of these glands would seem to reflect a basic lack of will and life-force in the condition known as Addison's disease. In anthroposophical medicine, the energy radiation of the kidney is considered to be excessively weak in Addison's disease as a result of lack of correct engagement of the astral body in the physical.[2] This reasoning concurs with the lack of life or animation previously mentioned in relation to hypo activity of the base *chakra*.

When considering sub-clinical states which have been mentioned as the main field for naturopathic medicine, low blood pressure, while not a clinical disease of the adrenal glands, may well be a sub-clinical state reflecting an energy imbalance at the level of the base *chakra*; this condition is discussed under the heading Blood Pressure.

Treatment

Natural therapists have little clinical experience with the disorder. The main aim would be to improve the general health of the patient, stimulate the immune system, and attend to the more subtle energy problems through counselling.

Alcoholism

No definition of this problem is needed, except perhaps to remind the reader that people often forget an addiction covers any compulsive habit, and is not necessarily related to the consumption of large amounts of alcohol.

Causes

Recently, medical groups have become more interested in vitamin and mineral deficiencies in relation to alcoholism.[1] It has been found that the status of the B group of vitamins, magnesium, and zinc, may be affected in alcoholics.[2] This does not mean that general life-style, stresses, and psychological problems are relegated to the background, as it may be a case of which comes first: the poor life-style or the alcoholism.

Deficiencies in essential nutrients produce nervous tensions in the individual which can predispose people to seek alcohol to relieve stress. A lack of zinc through genetic factors in the Aboriginal people has been found to inhibit the detoxification of alcohol in the liver, resulting in an effect on the brain which produces violent behaviour.[3] Another factor which has been considered relates to the hypoglycaemic problem in these patients. As a very complex carbohydrate, alcohol can be craved by people who have low blood sugar.

Treatment

This involves attention to life-style and the regulation of the diet to remove hypoglycaemic conditions, and the administration of those supplements mentioned, and possibly others, to re-establish homoeostasis or biochemical balance. Specific remedies will therefore include:

1 Magnesium and zinc compounds to relax the nervous system, and to help remove the hypoglycaemic factor.
2 The B-complex group to supplement the above minerals.
3 Herbal nerve tonics, and most importantly, liver herbs to help restore that organ following abuse from alcohol.
4 Bach flower remedies selected to act on various emotional problems.
5 Vitamin C for its detoxifying properties.[4]
6 The anti-oxidants, vitamin E and selenium, to deal with the disturbed fat metabolism which is found in alcoholics.[5]

Allergies

The naturopathic approach to allergies is to discover and treat the cause. Hence deletion of particular items of food, or removal of the subject from specific triggering factors in the environment is understood as a temporary measure only.

Allergies can manifest in many ways in the body; as diarrhoea, sneezing and catarrh, less commonly as constipation, as swellings of any part of the body, as pain and spasm, as nausea and vomiting, and as many kinds of headache. It is almost as if the cells, organs or tissues concerned are shrieking to alert us to their discomfort and the possible harm which may eventuate from a particular substance.

Causes

Basic causes must be distinguished from the immediate triggering factor which may be grass, pollen, insecticides, food additives, drugs, particular foods, and any of the enormous range of chemicals found in air, water and environment. A new branch of medicine is developing in this area called Clinical Ecology.[1]

When the body is in good health, with all the balancing or homoeostatic factors in working order, it is surprising how tolerant body tissues can be to a temporary invasion of a chemical or foreign protein, as occurs for instance with a bee sting. If the liver (one of the main factories producing anti-bodies) is indisposed, or if the lymphatic system is already congested from previous unsuccessful attempts to clear waste from the tissues, an allergic reaction can manifest.

We must consider yet again the inherited tendency. Some persons are genetically predisposed to release large amounts of histamine. No doubt the reader can think of examples where both parents and children have experienced hay fever at the same time of the year. Causes therefore precede birth in many cases.

Stress will play its part as with most conditions. When the body is in a relaxed state, many potentially inflammatory conditions can be avoided. This encourages us to reflect on the possible causes for allergies in the psyche of the individual. There is a large body of clinical evidence to suggest that emotional conflict can give rise to allergies. A number of popular books by clinical psychologists, psychiatrists, and other therapists attest to spectacular successes in this field using a variety of approaches including bio-feedback.[2]

In Eastern philosophy, that part of our nature which is related to the emotions is described by the term *rajas*, meaning fiery. Anxiety states, suppressed anger, hostility or resentment, may give rise to hot or inflammatory processes in the body. Some relatively minor external influence via food or touch may trigger the allergic reaction. This in no way contradicts the scientific observation of the biochemical processes which take place in the reaction.

In one branch of medicine pioneered by Rudolf Steiner — anthroposophical medicine — the term hysteria is used to cover allergic processes. In this usage of the term, hysteria is not only related to emotional states, but to the total state of the body.

The anthroposophical teaching points to the need for the digestive organs to 'denature' our food from foreign etheric and astral influences. If this is not achieved properly by the strength of the energies flowing through the digestive organs, the food acts as a foreign substance and an allergic reaction takes place.[3]

The human mind loves to categorise and specialise, and hence one group of therapists claims that all allergies are psychological in nature, while another sees only physical causes. Each group can produce spectacular success stories with their particular approach. Imagine, however, the breadth of our success when we can acknowledge all possible causes and factors, and treat both the inner and the outer situation.

Treatment

1 Liver herbs — dandelion, St. Mary's thistle, centaury, fringe tree.
2 Lymphatic cleansers — red clover, violet leaves, burdock, phytolacca.
3 Vitamin C — invaluable to boost immune system in allergic reactions.
4 Vitamin B6 — produces antihistamine reaction without drowsiness.[4]
5 Mineral combination with iron phosphate and potassium chloride — reduces inflammation and mucus formation.
6 Calcium phosphate is often indicated according to constitutional type.
7 Homoeopathic remedies can be very spectacular in reducing swelling and inflammation. Examples are Apis mellifica, Arsenicum, Rhus tox, Urtica urens. They must be selected by a therapist skilled in this area.
8 Appropriate counselling about diet, life-style and any emotional problems.

Nutrition must be eliminative and therefore based on salads, vegetables, fruit and a moderate protein intake. Any chemicals found to be allergenic are removed from the diet. In the acute stage, a severe allergy will often respond to the medication more quickly if the person goes on a juice fast, usually vegetable juice, for two days. Such a regime must be supervised by a trained person. This programme of juices relieves the organs such as liver and kidneys which can then get on with the job of metabolising and eliminating the toxins.

Case History

Amy, a seven-year-old, came to see me for itching skin lesions on legs and back which she had suffered for nine months. They commenced while her home was being extended and disappeared temporarily during the acute infectious fevers of chicken-pox and whooping-cough. Natural therapists find that chronic conditions clear up temporarily during an acute illness. She was given iron phosphate for the inflammation, calcium phosphate due to the nature of the eruption, lymphatic and liver herbs to cleanse and increase immunity, vitamin B for its effect on the skin and nerves, and vitamin C to boost the immune system. Pulsatilla was given in homoeopathic potency as the acute remedy needed immediately for the skin. During the month there was considerable clearing although eyes and lips swelled at times. The first month's treatment was repeated with a change to homoeopathic Apis (honey bee) instead of Pulsatilla for swelling of the lips. She had no further swellings for the next two months.

Five months after treatment began, Amy suffered a bad relapse with severe allergic reaction to both skin and gastro-intestinal tract following drinks of commercial orange juice on a plane flight. Cocktail sausages at a children's party had also been consumed with a very bad effect. Her medication had to be changed to deal with this crisis. For the next eight months, treatment was continued with a change from the acute homoeopathic remedy to her constitutional remedy which is Natrum muriaticum. The allergic reactions gradually lessened.

Treatment was gradually tapered off after two years, and the most important finale is that Amy can now indulge occasionally in those foods which originally caused her allergy. This is the aim of naturopathic treatment for allergies — to restore the person to biochemical balance so that the real cause of the allergy is removed, and the person can live a normal life with a healthy but not overly restricted diet. It was of interest that the allergy in Amy's case appeared to be of chemical origin through ingestion of food additives, and in these cases the person may be deficient in the trace element selenium. It was decided that the best way for Amy to take this supplement was in brewers yeast, and indeed, after commencing daily yeast tablets, there were no further severe attacks.

Alzheimer's Disease

see Senile Dementia

Amenorrhoea

Causes

Absence of menstrual periods can be either a primary or second-ary condition. There are many causes including hormonal fac-tors, reaction to drugs, stress, malnutrition, and lactation. The problem is also quite common amongst women who undertake a lot of sport. Recent exposure of the extent of hormone supple-mentation in the sport industry may explain many cases!

In relation to possible disturbances at the level of the energy centres, the sacral centre, which relates to all reproductive func-tions, will be underactive or there will be some kind of energy blockage here. This energy centre in turn stimulates the ovaries. The endocrine system is not quite this simple, however, and there may be complicating factors involving the thyroid and pituitary gland. These relate respectively to the throat and Ajna *chakras*.

Treatment

This will of course depend on the causes. Basic mineral salts such as iron phosphate and calcium phosphate may be needed. The use of herbs and homoeopathic preparations to stimulate the ovaries will be given, plus general nerve tonics such as vitamin B-complex, and potassium phosphate. The overall approach will be to balance the nervous system and the endocrine glands, with attention to any particular deficiencies of nutrition. Examina-tion of any stresses in the life-style is essential .

Case History

Jane, aged twenty-five, arrived at the clinic with a history of primary amenorrhoea. She first attended specialists at the age of eighteen and at twenty-five had never had a period. She is a physiotherapist, and a ballet dancer in her spare time. At the time of her first visit, the specialist had found that both pituitary and ovarian hormones were deficient and he recommended her to take oestrogen. Jane was not happy about having artificial periods with the 'pill'.

Apart from the absence of periods, Jane was full of life and vigour, although probably as a result of her low hormone levels and ballet activity, there was dryness and clicking of hip joints. The only other physical problem was haemorrhoids. There was one family member who had experienced an endocrine imbalance.

Supplements in this case included herbs which are rich in oestrogenic compounds. These included angelica, sarsaparilla, liquorice, fennel; other tonic herbs prescribed were avena sativa and motherwort.[1] The main mineral used was calcium phosphate and this was continued for several years. Homoeopathic gland toners, zinc, kelp and fresh royal jelly were used as regular supplements over several years to stimulate the endocrine glands.

After six months' treatment, Jane had her first period and had gained a bit of weight. A second period did not arrive for several more months, but during the second year of treatment there were four more periods at irregular intervals. During the third year of treatment, periods became more regular, and during the fourth year cycles were between twenty-six and thirty days, a great improvement on her earlier history. Further hormonal examination revealed improvement in glandular balance.

This case reveals the need to persevere for long periods of time with natural therapies in cases where an inherited factor is present, and at the same time reveals the very deep acting effect of consistent treatment. After the third year, treatment was considerably tapered off, and yet improvement continued. Jane now only takes small doses of two calcium salts, a herbal liver tonic for general cleansing, and homoeopathic drops for the glands. She attends the clinic about twice-yearly for a general check-up.

Anaemia

A lack of iron in the blood may come from many causes and is chiefly experienced as tiredness in mild cases and exhaustion and breathlessness on exertion in serious cases. A blood test is necessary to establish the degree and type of anaemia. Pale skin and lips are no sure indication.

Causes

Apart from the many rare forms which may be diagnosed through pathology tests, the main type is the simple iron deficiency anaemia. This may occur from haemorrhage, or recurrent blood loss as suffered by women with heavy periods, or it may result from poor diet and malabsorption of iron.

An interesting reflection has been thrown on the subject by Victor Bott, an exponent of anthroposophical medicine. According to Rudolph Steiner, the founder of this medical group, anaemia tends to manifest in people who are not sufficiently incarnated in their physical form. Remedies suggested by these medical doctors are chosen therefore to help unite the physical body with the higher levels of consciousness.[1] These remedies include iron, silica and phosphorous in homoeopathic doses.

Treatment

1 The diet obviously must include articles rich in iron such as leaf greens, and eggs or meat if the person is not vegetarian.
2 Iron phosphate has been found the most suitable preparation.[2]
3 Vitamin C helps transport iron across the cell membrane.[3]
4 Many herbs are rich in iron, parsley being the most common example.
5 Constitutional homoeopathy could be very valuable for the more subtle factor mentioned in the Causes section.

Angina

see Atherosclerosis

Angio-neurotic Oedema

Natural therapists frequently encounter varieties of allergic type swellings associated with the skin and mucus membranes. The problem can be very frightening if it occurs on the throat or tongue, and temporarily very embarrassing if it involves the lips or face. The swelling may last hours, days or weeks according to the type. Generally speaking, swelling of the mucus membranes lasts only a short time.

Causes

Triggering factors include pollens, grasses, food chemicals, food allergies, and stress. The natural therapist is usually concerned with underlying causes and these often relate to poor digestion, the inability of the body to deal with foreign protein, and with various chemicals which are taken into the body through food and drink.

The inflammatory process, with consequent release of histamine, causes the swelling of membranes in certain physical constitutional types. Nevertheless, there is always the need to resolve emotional conflicts which are often related to the problem.

Under the section dealing with Allergies, an unusual approach to allergies was mentioned in relation to anthroposophical medicine.[1] Likewise in the case of angio-neurotic oedema, these clients are classed constitutionally as metabolic types by anthroposophical doctors and as histamine types by orthomolecular medical doctors. An inflammatory swelling is classed by both these medical groups as a reaction of the body to cope with undigested foreign substances.

Treatment

Apart from individual variations, the treatment is very similar as for allergies. Therefore the reader is referred to that section for a typical selection of supplements.

Case History

Beth, in her seventies, had suffered attacks of swelling on her tongue and lips since her early forties. She had a nervous breakdown at the age of forty-six following a severe bout of pneumonia. She also suffered excessive anxiety over an epileptic son. Insomnia had featured in her life for many years and she took the usual medication for this problem. At the time of commencing treatment for her angio-neurotic oedema, she was on small doses of Valium when needed for attacks. She also had a history of migraines and arthritis involving hands and shoulders. These latter problems underline the metabolic aspects of the case.

There were many indications that the liver was intimately connected with most of the conditions suffered by Beth. The migraines, arthritis, allergic type swellings, and previous bout of pneumonia all gave indication of metabolic disturbances involving the liver. The nervous system obviously also needed considerable attention.

Beth had treatment for several years; this included liver herbs and homoeopathic mixtures for the liver, rheumatic herbs, magnesium and potassium phosphate for the nerves. Vitamin B-complex was also given for this factor. Vitamin C is always included for conditions involving allergic swellings. Homoeopathic Apis was added as a specific for the swellings and in the 30th potency this was usually found to be effective in cutting attacks short if a few drops were placed on the tongue at the first sign of tingling and swelling.[2]

Ankylosing Spondylitis

This is a fairly uncommon disorder in which hereditary factors play an important part. It chiefly affects men between the ages of fifteen and forty years and is characterised by low back pain and stiffness, which may resemble sciatica. There can be progressive ankylosing or fusion of the spinal joints and sacro-iliac or hip joints. There may be a simultaneous development of peripheral arthritis.[1]

Causes

From the naturopathic viewpoint, this condition must be seen in the light of faulty immune response and the general parameters which were discussed in relation to rheumatoid arthritis.

Treatment

Treatment will be very similar to that for rheumatoid arthritis, with the particular individual differences which characterise all naturopathic work. As this is not a common condition, I have no case from my files to relate.

Anorexia Nervosa

The popular press has drawn attention to the fact that this is no longer a rare disease. Individuals, usually teenage girls, suffering from this condition have an obsession with becoming thin. They either refuse to eat to the point of starvation or they eat and make themselves vomit immediately afterwards. There are a number of documented cases who have starved themselves to death. I had one client who had established such a habit of vomiting that even after the obsession with becoming thin disappeared, she was unable to stop vomiting. The slightest amount of stress in the environment caused her to lose the last meal.

Causes

At first it was considered to be a disorder chiefly of psychological origin, but in the last few years there are indications from medical scientists and nutritionists that these individuals may be severely depleted of the mineral zinc.[1] From the point of view of the natural therapist, there can be both psychological and physical causes. The latter may not only include zinc but all those elements which have an effect on the nervous system.

It is quite likely that anorexia nervosa is associated at the subtle level with an imbalance of the sacral *chakra* as this relates to appetite in general. The associated menstrual disturbance of these girls, while expressing a biochemical imbalance, may also relate to diminished energy flowing through the sacral *chakra*. It is of significance that the problem often commences during puberty, a time when distinct changes are taking place in the energies which govern the sacral centre, and consequently in the endocrine glands.

Treatment

As this is a disorder where the overlap between psychological and physical states is very marked, one cannot give very specific guidelines except to list those elements which are important for energising and relaxing the nervous system.

1 Minerals — zinc, magnesium and potassium compounds.
2 Vitamin B-complex as a general nerve tonic.
3 Antispasmodic and relaxing herbs: valerian, vervain, passiflora, hops, avena sativa, and motherwort.
4 Bach flower remedies such as mimulus, white chestnut, hornbeam, star of Bethlehem, cherry plum, and rock rose.
5 Homoeopathic constitutional prescribing.

Case History

The most outstanding case encountered in this area was early in my practice and unfortunately the file is not available. The essential components of the case are however well remembered and are presented here.

Helen was aged about seventeen when her mother first brought her for treatment. She had been hospitalised for anorexia nervosa some months earlier and was still under medical supervision. The iris indicated gross mineral deficiencies of calcium, potassium and magnesium, heavy lymphatic congestion was present, and the pupil of the eye was larger than normal indicating nerve exhaustion from our point of view. Associated problems with the aftermath of the condition were a lack of menstrual periods and in addition there was a bad sinus condition which was related to the lymphatic congestion.

Helen had just begun to want to eat again due to the very

caring supervision and influence of the resident medical officer who looked after her case in hospital. She came to our clinic for nutritional advice and treatment for the various associated problems. She had been away from school for a long time and wished to get back to her studies as soon as her health permitted. I managed to change her mind about the strictly puritanical vegan diet she was about to embark on and which perhaps illustrated her remaining psychological disturbance in the area of appetite.

In all, Helen was treated for about two and a half years and it was a long slow haul back to health again. At one stage she developed glandular fever due to her weak condition and this interfered with her resumed study. The main treatment consisted of calcium, potassium and magnesium phosphate to improve nerve tone and energy levels, potassium chloride and iron phosphate as the minerals needed for lymphatic congestion, lymphatic and liver herbs for cleansing, vitamin B-complex in the form of yeast tablets, vitamin C for increased immunity, and various supplements to start the menstrual cycle.

In the days when Helen was treated, the connection between zinc deficiency and anorexia nervosa had not been made. Yeast, however, is rich in zinc and she received this over a period of time. Perhaps the menstrual cycle would have been more easily established if we had given comparatively large doses of zinc. Helen regained energy and weight slowly and surely and went back to her studies. From memory, I think menstruation was still not established when I last saw Helen and this may indicate the severity of her problem occurring as it did during puberty, plus indicating the need for larger doses of zinc.

Anxiety

see also Neuroses

Some years ago the naturopathic profession did a fairly informal survey of illnesses treated by its members. Nervous complaints were on top of the list. Natural therapists have many clients coming with marked symptoms of anxiety; some openly discuss this as their main problem, others are unaware that anxiety is the problem. They may present with palpitations, excessive sweating of hands, insomnia, inability to cope with crowds, or excessive worrying over trivia. There are other symptoms both overt and subtle.

Causes

Here natural therapists diverge from contemporary medical thought, as we find that many anxieties are largely removed by using mineral, vitamin and homoeopathic supplements including the Bach flower remedies. Natural therapy understanding therefore is conditioned by the clinical experience that anxiety is enhanced by certain deficiencies, and that many negative and conflicting emotions appear to be diminished by skilled homoeopathic treatment.

Anxieties have many psychological causes as contributing factors. The effect of negative and conflicting emotions on the etheric body and energy centres provides the psychosomatic effect in many disorders. As the bridge between psychological states and the physical body, the etheric vehicle is likely to develop blockages in anxiety states. The excellent results of various therapeutic groups who do body work which they call de-armouring, rolfing, and other terms illustrates this effect.[1] When therapists from these schools are able to release muscle tensions in their clients, there is often an accompanying dramatic expression of emotional energy. The popular art of re-birthing works with the same principles.

Meditation involving creative visualisation is a very positive psychological approach to anxiety and involves less risk than those approaches which may suddenly release a lot of negative emotion. Meditation has the effect of gradually stabilising the etheric vehicle and of balancing the *chakras*. Blockages are removed in a gentle manner by substitution of positive thoughts for negative emotions, and through resolution of blocks by taking the personality focus off problems. This is almost the opposite approach from the old schools of psychoanalysis, whereby the problem was explored *ad nauseam*.

Treatment

1 Potassium phosphate and magnesium phosphate for toning and relaxing the nervous system.[2]

2 Vitamin B-complex as a general nerve tonic. [3]
3 Selected Bach flowers and homoeopathic remedies. These work on the emotional gateway known as the solar plexus centre.
4 Herbal sedatives such as valerian, passaflora, vervain, and scullcap.
5 A herbal liver tonic is usually needed in long standing cases to eliminate acids which have accumulated through stress.

Case History

Nancy, aged twenty-five, had symptoms including, in her own words, anxiety attacks. Other symptoms featured diarrhoea, headaches, gurgling and bloating of stomach, and weight loss. She was the manager of a plant nursery and had recently been married.

The first treatment included calcium, potassium and magnesium phosphates in a particular proportion to each other, B-complex vitamins, homoeopathic liver and diarrhoea drops, herbs for cleansing the lymphatic system, and Bach flower remedies to stabilise the solar plexus energy centre. After one month on treatment, Nancy was improving in all respects. Over the next few months, the number of bowel actions reduced to two per day, and she put on weight.

This may seem a very simple combination of remedies, and yet it has been found that there is a synergistic or working together of the various component parts. If any part is left off, the clinical results are not the same. For example, the magnesium slows down the gut action, but without the effect of the Bach flowers on the solar plexus *chakra* — the gateway to the emotions — the condition may well have recurred after the magnesium was discontinued.

The patient's life-style is also very important in terms of stress at work, etc. During the course of treatment Nancy made the break from being employed to going into business for herself, and this change was very beneficial to her peace of mind and general well-being. She has been able to go back to regular exercise and is feeling good in all respects.

Arthritis

This is one of the most common diseases treated by natural therapists. It is an area where we can offer positive curative therapies even in fairly advanced cases. A particular joy is derived from restoring mobility and life to stiff and immobile limbs which have rendered the sufferer a bundle of misery. The two main forms encountered are Osteoarthritis and Rheumatoid Arthritis.

Osteoarthritis

Osteoarthritis is the most common type and usually manifests from middle-age onwards. The condition is characterised by the gradual development of swelling, inflammation, enlargement and stiffness of joints. Joints most commonly affected include the terminal phalanges or joints of fingers, and the large joints such as hip, shoulder, and knee. The spine can also be afflicted.

Causes

The most obvious causes from the point of view of the natural therapist relate to faulty nutrition, and especially to over-indulgence in refined foods. Contributing factors are a sluggish liver resulting in accumulation of acid waste in the tissues (bio-chemical imbalances), poor elimination through bowel, kidney and skin, and stress. As regards stress, the hormonal changes which occur at menopause may put too much strain on the endocrine glands of some women. The natural supply of corti-sone may be inadequate in these cases. When the ovaries cease to function at menopause, other glands which should readjust may manifest imbalances.

More subtle factors related to the problem can be the lack of energies flowing through the sacral and throat *chakras*. Thus when changes occur in the energy pattern when a person is in their late forties, instead of the energies flowing through the throat *chakra* into creative pathways which are not associated with childbirth and rearing, a crystallisation takes place. This hardening literally ossifies the joints, preventing movement. In the case of males, the psychic crystallisation may manifest, but as there is no obvious climacteric change as in women, the gland changes are not so obvious or sudden.

There are also inherited factors manifesting in arthritis. These may result in conditioning factors from problems which were not resolved in previous lives. People interested in the concept of reincarnation and karma sometimes take the view that there is nothing that can be done to change illness which has its causes in past lives. This is a negative view of the meaning of karma. There is nothing to stop karma being worked upon in a creative way so that resulting health problems are resolved. If the underlying psychic problem is resolved, and this may have its origin in a previous life, skilled homoeopathic treatment can heal the physical part of the inherited problem.

Treatment

Nutritional changes must be developed to remove those acid wastes which cause inflammation of joint structures. The client needs alkaline foods such as salads and leafy green vegetables in particular, and ripe fruits, preferably those in season. Proteins and refined carbohydrates are kept to a minimum.[1] It has been found helpful to eradicate the deadly nightshade family from the diet, these are mainly tomatoes, peppers, eggplant and potatoes. Elimination through the skin can be encouraged through daily brushing for five minutes with a dry pure bristle brush. The lifestyle must be reorganised to allow for adequate relaxation and most importantly, for creative activities to get the energies flowing through the body again.

A typical treatment programme for one month may include the following:

1 Liver herbs such as centaury and dandelion to stimulate the liver, plus kidney herbs such as parsley and nettle. Rheumatic herbs to reduce inflammation of joints include guaiacum, manaca, yellow dock and burdock.[2]

2 Mineral combination of potassium chloride and iron phosphate to reduce inflammation and exudate in the joint capsule.

3 Vitamin C to improve function of adrenal glands and to supplement the raw ingredients for the collagen in tissues.[3]

4 Vitamin B-complex for general nerve tone and energy.

5 Potassium phosphate and magnesium phosphate to improve energy, assist relaxation, and in this case, to balance excess calcium around joints.

6 Sodium phosphate compound may be needed to balance the acidity of body tissues; this buffering effect is related to urinary excretion of acid.[4]

7 Silica is the most specific mineral administered for gradually breaking up joint adhesions, but this must be introduced slowly after detoxification has been commenced, otherwise excessive discomfort may ensue.[5]

8 Specific homoeopathic remedies to cover constitutional problems.

As arthritis is a condition which develops over a long period, treatment may be needed for up to two years.

Case Histories

Edna, aged sixty-six, attended the clinic six years ago with a typical type of osteoarthritis which was affecting the cervical joints in the spine and the right shoulder. It was interesting that six months previously I had treated her for cystitis which is often accompanied by a lowered pH in the urine (acid urine). This can relate to a basic problem of acid/alkaline balance in the body which often precedes the calcium imbalance occuring in osteo-arthritis. The fairly typical Australian diet is more acid than alkaline, and is hard to change in people over sixty.

Over this period of six years, Edna had intermittent treatment which has been largely successful in relieving her arthritic condition. Natural therapists find many people in this age group regard naturopathic treatment as a health insurance, and although they are not prepared to radically change their life-style, good health is maintained for many years with intermittent treatment.

Remedies for Edna included rheumatic and liver herbs, the minerals potassium and magnesium phosphate for nerve tone, potassium chloride and iron phosphate for inflamed joints, vita-min C in a buffered form, and vitamin E to improve circulation around joints. When her bladder developed cystitis from time to time, she was given sodium phosphate, bladder herbs, and homoeopathic remedies for the bladder such as Cantharis.

Winifred, aged fifty-six, attended the clinic for aches and pains in various joints throughout her body. She had suffered a minor stroke five years ago, but had no blood pressure problems. Tiredness was a problem, and perhaps this is why she enjoyed ten cups of strong tea daily.

The first month's treatment consisted of magnesium and potassium phosphate for nerve tone, liver and rheumatic herbs, and sodium phosphate to give more alkalinity to the tissues. She was encouraged to reduce her intake of tea which was contributing to the acid state of her tissues. She made significant improvement after the first two months of treatment but suffered a few aches and pains after neglecting treatment for a few weeks. Two months is not sufficient time for the body biochemistry to be balanced.

After another few weeks of treatment she improved again and stayed on a maintenance dose for some time without needing to see me each month. This is a fairly familiar pattern with osteoarthritis. A recent phone call to ask permission to include her case confirmed her continuing health.

Rheumatoid Arthritis

Rheumatoid arthritis is a more serious disorder, being in the category which is known as auto-immune disease. The body immunity is severely affected and it is thought that destructive antibodies are produced which attack the body tissues. It is therefore a systemic disease, meaning that the whole body is affected. This state is reflected in specific blood tests.[6]

Rheumatoid arthritis affects all the joints of the body and they become grossly deformed much more rapidly and from a much earlier age than happens in osteoarthritis. Young children can be affected. There is an inherited factor operating and the natural therapist pays particular attention to this aspect, otherwise there can at best be only remission and palliation. In addition, anaemia, weight loss, exhaustion and depression can occur.

Causes

Apart from the inherited factor already mentioned, the lymphatic system is often found by iris diagnosis and palpation to be very congested. Constitutional weaknesses of liver and kidneys may be noticed, and this is observed to give rise to a very sluggish elimination via the skin as this organ becomes overburdened. Poor nutrition in some cases has certainly aggravated the condition.

The psychic causes for rheumatoid arthritis are more complex than those of osteoarthritis. An auto-immune disease is a self-destructive process and consequently we often find in the client a corresponding self-destructive attitude. I have certainly observed this, and a great bitterness and resentment has been noted in some patients who are slow to make progress on the physical remedies.

Sometimes one finds a case where the psychological resolution seems to have been largely resolved or accomplished, and these people progress comparatively quickly on the physical natural therapies. The cases listed in this section all have a positive approach to life.

Treatment

Rheumatoid arthritis, being a chronic disease, needs treatment over some years. In the early stages, efforts will be made to tone up the basic organs of elimination, improve energy and vitality. Later, work on the inherited factor will be undertaken. Nutrition will be supervised, with the same emphasis on alkaline foods as for osteoarthritis. A treatment regime may include the following:

1 Similar herbs as for osteoarthritis.
2 Mineral combination of iron phosphate and potassium chloride for inflammation and adhesions around joints.
3 Potassium phosphate for energy.
4 Calcium phosphate to help restore demineralisation of joints.
5 Zinc compound for improvement of immune system.[7]
6 Vitamin B-complex for energy and vitamin C for immunity and improvement of collagen in tissues.[8]
7 Homoeopathics to stimulate elimination, the endocrine system, and immunity.[9]
8 Individual homoeopathic constitutional prescribing.

As rheumatoid arthritis is a chronic disease, it is obvious that treatment may span several years. In cases of successful naturopathic treatment, the phenomenon of retracing will occur, so that once the joints have improved, a more sub-acute condition may occur such as continual mucus from the respiratory passages. The following case of a six-year-old girl who was brought to me by her mother illustrates this basic principle.

Case Histories

Michelle is now a vivacious child who has been attending our clinic for treatment at lengthening intervals for two years. She had previously been treated with the standard procedures of cortisone and anti-inflammatory drugs, but was in an active stage of the disease with swollen painful knees when first seen.

Her iris indicated heavy lymphatic engorgement and pronounced acidity throughout the tissues of the body. The skin action was very sluggish as also indicated by the iris. Over the first couple of months she was treated with liver, kidney and rheumatic herbs to promote elimination of acid and with iron phosphate to reduce inflammation of joints. Potassium chloride was given to reduce serous swelling of the knees. The general nerve tone was improved with B-complex, and another mineral combination involving phosphates. Her mother already gave her vitamin C on a regular basis.

There was not much improvement until during the third month when a deep acting homoeopathic was given to begin working on the inherited tendency of the problem. A dramatic improvement then resulted which was sustained for over eighteen months, after which time this constitutional treatment needed repeating. Michelle is now able to run about normally and there is very little swelling. Some muscle wasting which occurred in the initial stages of the disease still remains on the thigh which was most affected.

It was of great interest to observe the classical retracing which occurred in this case. Some time after the initial pains and swelling disappeared from the legs, Michelle suffered from a continual series of heavy colds. The reader is reminded that this relates to the sub-acute stage of disease which often manifests as the chronic stage diminishes. Extra remedies were brought in to hurry this process through its expression.

Valerie is thirty-five years old. She was diagnosed as having rheumatoid arthritis at the age of twenty-one. Gold injections were administered at this time, followed by penacillamine which helped for one year. When she visited me in 1985 she was suffering stomach problems caused by anti-inflammatory drugs. She had undergone extensive surgery on hands and feet with some joint replacement in the hands. Skin rashes had become a problem, and pain and nausea accompanied her menstrual periods. Severe headaches occurred regularly with neuralgia down the side of the face.

After a month on supplements, headaches were less. After nine months' treatment she has no headaches, and is largely free from pain and discomfort. She also feels very well generally. Remedies include liver, rheumatic and lymphatic cleansing herbs, vitamins B and C, sodium phosphate to reduce acidity in the tissues and potassium chloride and iron phosphate to reduce inflammation.

Constitutional treatment was commenced in the second month and consisted of two different homoeopathics in varying potencies. The greatest improvement occurred after the administration of sodium sulphate in a high homoeopathic potency which was given as her main constitutional remedy.

It is of note that Valerie has an excellent psychological outlook which distinguishes her from many cases of rheumatoid arthritis wherein the self-destructive processes which develop in the immune system often appear to arise from the psyche. She is ready to get well. Perhaps any basic underlying cause of her problem at the psychological level has been resolved; or maybe the disease represents the final physical working out of a previous incarnation. Thus, as also in the previous case of the small girl, the remedies are able to carry out healing work without obstruction.

A third case involves the female principal of a country girls' school. Judith was aged thirty-four when she came to visit me four years ago after having been diagnosed with rheumatoid arthritis. She had a history of swollen ankles, painful heels, thrombosis in one leg, constipation, and night sweats.

After one month's treatment, pain and swelling were reduced and night sweats eliminated, but she was still very tired. She began to go through the classical retracing process and developed a series of severe sore throats similar to those suffered earlier at the age of eighteen. A persistent sore in the nose also became troublesome. The night sweats, and respiratory infections in the case of Judith, remind the natural therapist that rheumatoid arthritis may have a tubercular basis in the family genetic tree. A tubercular homoeopathic nosode is therefore included as part of the treatment regime.

After one year of treatment, the retracing through the respiratory symptoms was almost completed. The joints had been good through most of this period, indicating that the chronic part of the disease process had given way to the sub-acute as manifested in the respiratory symptoms. The reader will see the parallel with the case of Michelle.

During the last three years, although Judith's professional duties have been very demanding, her health has been very stable with very little trouble from joints, and hardly any sore throats. She also has a positive approach to life.

Her treatment has consisted of a zinc compound and vitamin C to increase immunity, potassium and magnesium phosphate plus vitamin B-complex for increasing nerve tone; lymphatic, rheumatic and liver herbs; potassium chloride and iron phosphate for reducing inflammation first of joints and then of respiratory passages, and selected homoeopathic constitutional remedies. Most of us know that it is common to have remissions in rheumatoid arthritis, but two of the cases mentioned have now been observed over a period of years and are virtually symptom-free.

Asthma

This condition is distressingly common in young children growing up in the 1980s. Most pre-school patients with the problem are diagnosed by the medical profession as having bronchial asthma. Their disease pattern starts with a respiratory infection and rapidly develops through the coughing to the wheezing stage. The main characteristics of the problem are bronchospasm, mucosal swelling, and secretion of sticky mucus in the bronchial tubes.

Causes

Consumption of refined foods with chemical additives has taken place on a large scale in the second half of this century. Increasing air pollution on our globe, and the high levels of individual stress have also contributed to the increase of asthma cases. Perhaps the most obvious biochemical causes are a diet of devitalised and refined foods, allergies to dairy products and chemicals in foods and to environmental pollution.[1] Vitamin and mineral deficiencies are intimately related to the biochemical imbalances which cause mucus development and bronchospasm.

Asthma is classed as a sub-acute disease process, and frequently occurs in families where some members suffer from the acute skin condition called eczema. This skin problem will be covered later in the text. Many natural therapists consider that the suppression of eczema in one generation causes the likelihood of asthma in subsequent generations. Mass childhood inoculations which are known as triple antigen are cited as an assault on the immune system and, given a certain genetic constitution, may precipitate asthma.[2]

Causes include nutritional factors, inherited disposition, indiscriminate inoculation, and suppression of acute skin eruptions with drugs.[3] Most skin eruptions of the itching rash type are treated with cortisone creams, thus reducing the inflammatory response of the body but at the same time weakening its natural vitality. Air pollution, chemicals in foods, and stress have been mentioned as causative factors.[4]

In relation to stress, it has been observed that asthma sufferers are poor breathers, rarely using their abdominal muscles to breathe even when not suffering a wheezing attack. This stressful condition of the body results often from emotional blocks which in turn cause tightening or armouring of the muscles enclosing the abdomen and thorax. The general weakness and tension of the chest may also be caused by an inherited factor.

Natural therapists who use iris diagnosis frequently find evidence of a constitutional respiratory weakness. A history of tuberculosis in the family, sometimes going back several generations, is often confirmed by asthma patients or their parents.

More subtle problems in the asthmatic can be related to the etheric body in the area of the throat *chakra*. This *chakra* rules respiration and in terms of consciousness is the creative organ of expression corresponding to the concrete mind in the personality. I have noted that many asthmatic children are precocious in their intellectual development. They usually do very well academically but are often mediocre in the field of physical or artistic expression. It seems likely that these individuals have suppressed their natural emotional development and expression, and subsequently there is a corresponding energy imbalance which is expressed as a tightness in the throat and chest, and in the armouring of the muscles. The physical chest is typically narrowed and underdeveloped, and the person seems to abhor the very types of exercise which would develop the chest to its normal capacity. Too much emotional energy is locked in, producing inability to breathe normally. This may have the effect of overstimulating mental development as it expresses through the throat *chakra*.

The anthroposophical branch of medicine has developed an interesting observation and theory about asthma in connection with the emotional or astral nature. They see asthma as resulting from an inability of the person to exhale adequately.[5] This breathing problem in turn is produced by a lack of rhythm between the astral and physical body. Specific herbs are applied to regulate and restore the harmonious action between the astral and physical levels of being. This explanation fits with the previous comments about the locking-in of emotional energy.

Treatment

General treatment will cover the nutritional needs and especially the reduction of dairy produce to an absolute minimum, as these foods have been found to foster mucus production.[6] Relaxation techniques include biofeedback, meditation, and suitable breathing exercises. Some children are particularly allergic to chemicals in foods and hence the emphasis will be on fresh vegetables, salads, and fruit, with a moderate selection of suitable proteins.

Specific supplements may include the following:

1 Mineral combination of iron phosphate and potassium chloride to reduce inflammation and mucus respectively.
2 Vitamin C to reduce mucus and to improve immunity to chest infection.[7]
3 Vitamin B6 has been found to correct biochemical imbalance associated with neurotransmittors (nerve pathways) and B12 for sulphite sensitivity.[8]
4 Codliver oil capsules to help absorption of calcium especially during winter.
5 Bio-flavanoids for their anti-histamine activity.[9] Usually combined with vitamin C.

6 Calcium phosphate or magnesium phosphate according to the particular constitution of the person.[10]
7 Potassium phosphate and vitamin B-complex for energy.
8 Herbs for strengthening the lungs, eliminating mucus, and cleansing the lymphatics. These may include red clover, horehound, coltsfoot, lobelia, liquorice, and elderblossom. Liver herbs will also be included such as dandelion, or maybe St Mary's thistle.
9 Selected homoeopathics to tone the lungs, remove mucus, correct constitutional weaknesses, and to dilate the bronchial passages to their normal capacity.[11] Tincture of Ammi visnagi is excellent in this respect.

Case Histories

Norma had suffered asthma for thirty years and had been on standard bronchodilators. Since a bout of pneumonia six years earlier, she had experienced recurrent bronchitis. In her own words the condition improved 100 per cent during the first month's treatment, and when contacted recently, some eighteen months since treatment ceased, she had not relapsed.

Her supplements included iron phosphate and potassium chloride to reduce inflammation and mucus secretion, magnesium phosphate, potassium phosphate and the herb Ammi visnagi to reduce spasm, lymphatic cleansing and liver herbs, sodium sulphate and vitamin C. Sodium sulphate was also given as a constitutional remedy in ascending homoeopathic potencies.

Norma was a long-standing case of asthma and improvement was maintained after treatment was discontinued. This continuing freedom from asthma was most likely due to the constitutional remedy of homoeopathic Natrum sulphate which was given alongside the herbs, minerals and vitamins. It is the homoeopathic treatment which works deeply into the constitution and gives lasting results.[12]

Mark was a fairly typical asthma case and commenced treatment at the age of seven in 1978. His father and uncle had both suffered asthma. His asthma usually developed following a cold. As with many asthmatics, he was a picky eater and associated problems were tiredness and bed wetting. His first month of treatment included the mineral combination iron phosphate and potassium chloride, vitamin C, calcium phosphate, codliver oil capsules, a herbal liver tablet, and a herbal lymphatic cleanser.

After this first month of treatment, there were no asthma attacks and eating improved. The prescription was repeated for two more months and during this time there was some slight wheezing and a partial relapse during the third month. It is important for clients to understand that improvement often features the phenomenon of two steps forward and one backward. At this stage of Mark's treatment, Ammi visnagi drops for wheezing were added.

Improvement was then steady and there was no full relapse, just some slight wheezing occurring when the family were away. After nine months of treatment, Mark was able to do without his medical prescription of Intal. Treatment was continued another five months. Then during May of the following year, four bad attacks occurred. The prescription was changed to include one of the homoeopathic tubercular remedies, plus a homoeopathic mixture of Kali iodatum, Kali sulphuricum, and Antimonium tartrate, all in the 6th decimal potency. These latter remedies were for mucus formation in the chest. Sodium sulphate was added as the mineral salt applicable for a manifestation of asthma occurring at the change of seasons.

The prescription was repeated for another month and Mark has remained free from asthma without treatment in the intervening years. In all, he had about fourteen months treatment. His mother has sent several asthmatic children to the clinic, so we hear from time to time of Mark's continuing health.

Shane is another young asthmatic who needs periodic treatment for asthma. As the result of naturopathic treatment, he has gone nearly four years without drugs. His wheezing would usually commence with a cold. The only other problem was recurrent mouth ulcers. After a year of good health he was brought recently for a consultation. He was exhibiting signs of chest wheezing and it was noticed via iris diagnosis that he still has signs of the chest weakness which runs through the family tree.

His original prescription contained calcium phosphate to strengthen the lung tissue, iron phosphate and potassium phosphate to reduce inflammation and mucus in the bronchials, and homoeopathic drops for toning the liver and cleansing the lymphatic system. In the winter months codliver oil was added to help calcium absorption. Vitamin C is always a basis for the enhancing of natural immunity. Once these children have stopped growing and have stabilised their mineral metabolism, the asthma problem is often resolved without further treatment.

On reviewing our many asthma cases, a familiar pattern is noted in many instances. Clients need to continue treatment for up to two years if recurrences are to be avoided. Hence the average asthma case is helped by natural therapies, and is usually able to dispense with pharmaceutical asthma drugs after the first few months' treatment, but recurrent bouts of asthma can occur at certain times during the year until treatment has been established consistently over a long period.

Rosa is a sixty-four-year-old lady of Greek nationality who came to me two years ago with wheezing chest, recurrent duodenal ulcer, constipation, extreme tiredness and haemorrhoids. Her diet was good but the iris revealed a number of digestive and constitutional problems. Nevertheless, in spite of all these symptoms and her age, after one month's treatment all areas had improved. She then had a break from the treatment and after a few months the asthma relapsed.

Treatment was resumed; it included herbs for liver and stomach and magnesium phosphate for the bronchial spasm which was much worse with emotional disturbance, B-complex as a nerve tonic, and the herbal asthma drops mentioned in the previous cases — Ammi visnagi. Vitamin C in moderately large doses of 2g daily was given together with iron phosphate and potassium chloride to reduce inflammation and mucus. She also had a mineral combination for the haemorrhoids.

Relief from all chest symptoms has been maintained for many months without any medical drugs. Rosa comes periodically for a review of her maintenance supplements.

Atherosclerosis

see also Blood Pressure

Angina, coronary artery disease, and cerebral ischaemia or hardening of the cerebral and other arteries are discussed under this heading. The treatment may be individual to some extent in terms of the constitutional homoeopathic prescribing, but certain basic approaches will be similar. High blood pressure resulting from atherosclerosis and angina resulting from coronary artery disease are probably the most common expressions of arterial disease.

Causes

The causes are similar whether the aorta, cerebral or coronary arteries are involved. There is a gradual accumulation of lipids (fat) and the chief ingredient of this deposition is cholesterol. The atheroma or atherosclerotic plaque which gradually hardens the artery involved results in blockages which have become the leading cause of death in the Western world. Perhaps this is the one area of disease where there is agreement on a number of causes of the disease by the naturopathic profession and the orthodox school of medicine.

One of the most widely accepted theories for this disorder is that the atheroma develops as a result of injury to the arterial endothelium. Causes for this injury include immunological, viral and chemical factors. Lipoproteins from plasma, platelets, and a migration of smooth muscle cells all conglomerate to form a fibrous cap to the injury, upon which further fats accumulate. Our approach explains that this particular reaction to injury only occurs in a biochemical situation resulting from deficiencies and imbalances of particular substances needed for health.

Life-style factors are accepted as causative factors by both orthodox medicine and natural therapists. It has been demonstrated that exercise reduces cholesterol and increases the protective lipoproteins known as HDL.[1] Inclusion of fatty fish in the diet has also been found to increase this HDL factor.[2] Cigarette smoking has been proved as an important contributing cause; apart from other effects, smoking increases platelet aggregation.[3] Diets deficient in fibre and high in animal fats and sucrose are another obvious cause over which there is little disagreement.[4]

Deficiencies which concern the natural therapist include magnesium, vitamin C, vitamin E, and vitamin B6. Other minerals which may be out of balance are chromium, which is related to triglyceride levels, selenium and zinc. The more subtle causes of circulatory disorders will be discussed under the headings of angina and coronary artery disease. These factors result from problems with the energy centre known as the heart *chakra*.

Treatment

1 Nutritional changes involving increase of vegetables, salads, fibre as in whole grain cereals, soy beans, fish such as salmon, mackerel and herring, and deletion of refined flour and sugar products and coffee.[5] The addition of alfalfa sprouts to the diet has been found to reduce cholesterol.[6]

2 Suitable exercise programme under supervision.

3 Attention to life-style factors involving stress, and instruction in meditation to reduce tension and to promote creative living.

4 Magnesium orotate or phosphate to reduce arterial spasm and influence health of nervous system and heart muscle.[7]

5 Vitamin C to reduce cholesterol and to improve health of collagen of artery walls.[8]

6 Garlic in diet and in capsules to reduce fibrin.[9]

7 Herbs for the liver to help prevent excess of cholesterol.

8 Vitamin E for its ability to reduce tendency to thrombus and platelet aggregation and to reduce damage of cell membranes.[10]

9 Lecithin — increases solubility of cholesterol.[11]

10 Bromelain, a pineapple enzyme which inhibits platelet clumping.[12]

11 Specific homoeopathic remedies which reduce arterial spasm and which have an effect on arterial disease.

12 Constitutional homoeopathic remedies prescribed on an individual basis.

Particular ailments stemming from atherosclerosis will now be examined together with case histories. The treatment in each division will contain a number of elements from those just examined and will not be duplicated under each division. As arterial disease develops over a number of years, patients often need lengthy periods of treatment. Their medical drugs are reduced very slowly and only in conjunction with medical supervision.

Angina

Angina is characterised by a sensation of pain, tightness, or heaviness in the centre of the chest. Typically it is aggravated by physical exertion and eases off with rest. The pain may radiate down the left arm, and occasionally go up into the jaw on that side. It can be aggravated by a heavy meal or emotional state. Onset of the condition may be gradual or sudden.

Causes

The condition usually results from hardening and narrowing of the arteries which supply the heart muscle, following plaque formation. The plaque develops often in relation to high cholesterol levels in the blood, and this is caused by the dietary and metabolic factors already discussed. Some of the metabolic factors appear to be inherited. Thus a person may have very little fat in their diet and yet the body tends to make an excess of cholesterol.

Inner or subjective factors which may relate to the development of circulatory disease relate to imbalances in the energy flowing through the heart *chakra*.[1] This energy centre in the etheric body relates to group work, and during the last hundred years in particular, we have witnessed the development of groups large and small in all departments of living. Group consciousness has developed and on the positive side, this has emerged as a tendency to inclusiveness and is part of a growing sensitivity to life as a whole. We are very much in an interim stage between responding to group needs on the one hand, while continuing to desire more and more for the personal self. Hence we swing violently in many cases between the consciousness centred in the solar plexus which expresses self-centred needs, and that of the heart — the organ of fusion which expresses love for the whole.

These fluctuations in energy flows at the psychic and etheric level can place strain on the related organs. Usually, for disease to develop, there will be an inner and an outer cause. In the case of coronary heart disease there may be physical factors relating to diet, lack of exercise, and poor working habits, and on the psychic side, an erratic flow of psychic energy through the heart centre which in turn affects the physical heart.

Treatment

Re-education about life-style is all-important with adequate periods of rest, relaxation, nutritional training, and exercise all playing their part in the rehabilitation programme. Biofeedback techniques have been found valuable to reduce angina attacks.[2]

The specific supplements for angina have been covered under the previous section. It is of interest to look at one other approach to angina which can replace the need for bypass surgery, even in quite advanced cases of disease. Chelation therapy may be undertaken either orally or intravenously. The latter approach is only undertaken by a registered doctor and is a technique whereby a chelating chemical is used intravenously to strip the plaque gradually from the arterial wall. There are few side-effects from this treatment provided the patient has healthy kidneys.

An alternative approach provided by natural therapists consists of capsules which act as chelating agents by virtue of a synthesis of many substances. Some have been mentioned in the list of supplements for Atherosclerosis; others include homoeopathic doses of specific agents for removing plaque and balancing the cholesterol metabolism.

Case Histories

'Kenneth' was a retired public servant who attended the clinic for angina in 1980. He had suffered from this problem for ten years and it first accompanied high blood pressure. On his first visit to me his systolic blood pressure was 160 and diastolic 100. After four months treatment his blood pressure was stable at 138/90. The angina disappeared fairly early in the treatment.

His treatment emphasised use of magnesium orotate to reduce tension in all parts of his physiology — nervous system, arteries, and muscles. A herbal sedative which featured antispasmodics was included along with liver herbs to cleanse the body of accumulated toxins, and potassium phosphate was added as a nerve tonic. A Bach flower remedy to work on the emotions and nerves consisted of agrimony, gorse, gentian, wild oat and vervain. B-complex was used as a general nerve tonic.

The reader will notice from the treatment described in this particular case an emphasis towards relaxing and toning the nervous system. Another person may need more emphasis on cleansing of the arteries. As the blood pressure responded well to the treatment, we can conclude that the approach to treatment was correct in this case.

Mary, a sixty-three-year-old dressmaking teacher, developed the same problem following the loss of her husband. She came to the clinic in 1979 and was on a common drug for angina plus tranquillisers. By the second visit, and following natural treatment, she was off medical drugs and feeling much better. It should be stressed that natural therapists usually reduce medical drugs very slowly in the case of circulatory disorders and usually only under medical supervision. Mary, however, was determined to use natural therapies alone.

Her treatment consisted of magnesium phosphate, a different magnesium compound from that given to the previous client. She was also given a herbal sedative and tonic, plus liver herbs and vitamin C for cleansing. In the third month's treatment, a herbal rheumatic remedy was added for aches in the back. Her treatment progressed without problems.

Anne, aged eighty-three, had previously been treated by my husband some years ago. Her case is a good example of how helpful natural therapies can be in old people. She had been a fairly severe case of atherosclerosis and the carotid arteries were involved. When she visited me in 1983 her main complaint was loss of balance and her blood pressure was a dangerous 200/95.

Her first month's prescription consisted of herbs for the arteries including mistletoe, garlic to help cleanse the arteries, herbs to tone the liver and reduce cholesterol formation, magnesium phosphate to balance and relax the nervous system, and homoeopathic Cocculus indicus for the vertigo. There was a slight improvement to the condition and blood pressure by her second visit.

During the second month, the dose of blood pressure herbs was doubled, and herbs to relax the nervous system were added. Instead of the Cocculus indicus a homoeopathic mixture of vervain and magnesium phosphate was given twice daily. After this prescription, the blood pressure reduced to 168/80 over the next three months. Given her age, this is a very satisfactory reduction.

Coronary Artery Disease

Unfortunately, this is one condition which the natural therapists find themselves called upon to treat after the event of a coronary occlusion or blockage. In many cases there will be a history of angina either before or after the coronary occlusion. As the latter often results in death (infarct) to some of the heart muscle, natural therapists would prefer to be dealing earlier with the situation.

Some researchers claim that symptoms of blockage do not arise until the artery is clogged up by over three-quarters. This is one area where iris diagnosis may help a great deal. Although the findings in the iris should always be cross-checked with other forms of diagnosis and evaluation, clogging of the arteries can usually be seen at a very early stage. This would alert people to the need for blood tests for cholesterol and for urgent review of their diet and life-style.[1] Arterial changes can also be seen very early in the blood vessels of the retina, yet this simple form of evaluation is rarely performed by the average medical doctor.

Causes

The causes have been explored under the heading of Atherosclerosis and Blood Pressure. In relation to the heart at the physical level, natural therapists would stress the acknowledgement of medical scientists that a deficiency of magnesium is a key factor in coronary artery disease.[2]

The inner subjective factors involving energies flowing through the heart *chakra* will have a particular relevance for diseases of the heart itself. The relationship which exists between the energies of the heart *chakra* or energy centre and the health of the heart and circulation has already been explored in the discussion on Angina. We need to remind ourselves that in most diseases there is an inner and an outer cause. The inner cause in coronary artery disease may well relate to an imbalance of energies flowing through the heart. The energies may be disturbed by stress, grief, isolation, or by a situation where too many people are 'pulling on our heart strings'.

Treatment

This will be very similar to that listed under atherosclerosis, except for more emphasis in the case of angina on magnesium phosphate or orotate to relax spasm in the arteries.[3] A number of homoeopathic remedies are applicable in a specific and constitutional sense for heart disease.[4]

Case History

Dennis, aged forty-six, is a businessman and first attended the clinic in 1976 with high blood pressure and bouts of asthma. He was treated for one year during which time his blood pressure normalised. He then discontinued treatment, taking up a position which involved a great deal of pressure. More than two years later, he returned following a coronary occlusion, and benefited by a further course of treatment. A year later further treatment was undertaken for a number of months.

The main constituents in this treatment consisted of magnesium phosphate to help the heart muscle and reduce spasm of coronary arteries, herbal sedatives, liver herbs to help regulate cholesterol manufacture, potassium phosphate (also for nerves and heart muscle), vitamin B-complex, and Bach flower remedies for nerves. In this particular case of arterial trouble, the main ingredient for illness was understood to be stress and tension in the life-style.

Recently, Dennis returned for another check-up following a problem with gout. Otherwise he has been keeping in good health and taking a maintenance dose of supplements to keep his circulatory system in good health. It is of interest that very often gout is related to a sluggishness of the liver which we also understand plays an important part in cholesterol regulation.

Auto-immune Disorders

These disorders appear to be on the increase. In *Harrison's Principles of Internal Medicine*, this problem is described as involving the breakdown or circumvention of self-tolerance.[1] In layman's language, the diseases thus engendered are said to result from the body's defences attacking its own tissues. Disorders included in this category are rheumatoid arthritis, multiple sclerosis, glomerulonephritis, haemolytic anaemia, and Acquired Immune

Deficiency Syndrome (AIDS). Cancer may also be related to this problem.

Causes

In many of these cases, white blood cells known as lymphocytes are involved. In particular, there appears to be a problem with the T-lymphocytes which are produced in the thymus gland. In immune disorders, T-lymphocytes are often found to be deficient and a corresponding excess of B-lymphocytes is identified.

In terms of first causes, the thymus gland is traditionally linked to the energy centre in the body known as the heart centre. It seems logical to assume that the thymus secretions and activities will be stimulated by the right kind of meditation as this would stimulate the heart *chakra*. Perhaps this is the explanation for the very positive influence which meditation can have on many serious disorders including cancer, and for the miraculous remissions of such disorders following meditation.[2]

The more immediate physical causes relate to accumulation of toxins which congest the lymphatic system (see Rheumatoid Arthritis), and serious deficiencies in minerals and vitamins, especially vitamin C which has a very profound effect on the immune system.[3] Causes must therefore be traced to poor diet, lack of exercise, stress, and possibly to inherited factors.

Treatment

Treatment of immune disorders emphasises the cleansing of the lymphatic system and promotion of immunity.

1 Herbs to cleanse the lymphatic system, and to tone the liver.
2 Vitamin C in doses up to 10g daily. Some patients would be referred to medical associates for intravenous C in doses up to 50g daily.
3 Toning of the nervous system with vitamin B-complex, magnesium and potassium phosphates.
4 Constitutional homoeopathic prescribing.

Case History

Lyn, who is now aged forty, was referred by another practitioner of natural therapies for a serious glandular condition which had been variously diagnosed by medical specialists first as a malignant condition known as lymphoma, then as glandular fever, then as toxoplasmosis — a viral disease transmitted by cats. She had enlargement of spleen and liver, nausea, and a very acute form of dermatitis totally covering her face.

The iris revealed moderate lymphatic problems and the lymphatic glands in the neck were found to be considerably enlarged on palpation. The iris also showed moderate toxaemia of the gastro-intestinal tract from the naturopathic viewpoint although her present diet was good. On examination of the hands, a typical manifestation of toxins was found in the dermatoglyphics or skin pattern. She had lost five kilograms over a period of two years.

The main treatment was directed towards cleansing the lymphatic system and thus towards improving the natural immunity of the body. A mixture, given four times daily, included dandelion, centaury, violet leaves, red clover, parsley and echinacea. Homoeopathic drops for the liver and spleen, vitamin C, and a mineral combination of iron phosphate and potassium chloride to reduce inflammation and enlargement of the lymphatic glands completed her first two weeks' medication.

In dramatic cases which involve the immune system and elimination through the skin in the form of severe rashes, the client is prepared to expect that the remedies will produce a 'healing crisis'. This is heralded as a good sign. Lyn suffered a sudden flare-up of her rash during this period as expected, and was treated for this stage with the homoeopathic remedy Arsenicum album in the 30th potency for three days. The rash responded immediately. After one month's treatment there was still some enlargement and soreness of glands.

By the end of two months' treatment there were no palpable glands, no headaches, and less acid waste showing through the skin patterns on the hand. She still felt very tired and nervy. This was not helped by her specialist who, in spite of Lyn's improvement, encouraged her to think that lymphoma remained a strong possibility, although pathology tests revealed no abnormality.

Improvement was maintained and continued over the next few months on a diminishing number of medications, and Lyn is now off treatment and maintaining her health and well-being. A few months after the first draft of this book was prepared, she had a small temporary relapse of exhaustion and skin problems after eating a lot of chocolate at Easter!

Bell's Palsy

This paralysis of the seventh cranial nerve which supplies the muscles of the face can manifest quite suddenly on one side of the face. The paralysis causes a characteristic grimace involving the mouth and eye on the affected side. The nerve is believed to become oedematous or swollen within the facial canal. Without natural treatment the improvement is very slow and may take up to a year with some cases remaining permanently affected.

Causes

From the naturopathic viewpoint, the cause results directly from a deficiency of those nutrients necessary for the healthy functioning of the nervous system. Causes are therefore (a) dietary, either directly or indirectly, when there is an inability to assimilate adequately certain essential nutrients or (b) profound nervous stress which would in turn deplete the system of factors such as B-complex and potassium phosphate.

Treatment

Using natural therapies for this condition usually gives spectacular results in a few days. The following are aids in restoring nerve function although it is quite likely the B6 is the most specific ingredient. This supplement reduces the oedema of the nerve.[1]

1 B-complex in large doses, that is, 50mg of each component twice daily.
2 Vitamin C to reduce inflammation, and to reduce associated toxic waste.
3 Magnesium and potassium phosphates to reduce spasm and reintroduce healthy nerve function.[2]
4 Bach flower remedies for shock to the nerve.
5 Appropriate homoeopathic remedies.

Case History

The following brief description involving Gary, a plumber aged thirty-seven years, comes from the files of my husband. Gary had already been under treatment for stress and rheumatic ailments when he developed a very severe bout of Bell's palsy following extra strain with his trade. It was one of the worst cases seen by Alf in his thirty-five years of practice.

Gary was already on the mineral combination potassium and magnesium phosphate, liver and rheumatic herbs, plus a second mineral combination involving potassium chloride and iron phosphate. At the time of his attack, the potassium phosphate component was increased and given also in homoeopathic form as Kali phosphate. In five days, the worst of the paralysis had abated, and in one month there was no trace of the problem. In this case there was no vitamin B given although two of the mineral combinations were in a base of yeast. The main improvement here was attributed to the inclusion of homoeopathic doses of potassium phosphate every few hours.

Blood Pressure

see also Atherosclerosis

In keeping with the holistic approach, this section covers both high and low blood pressure. It would be inappropriate in this book to list high blood pressure separately from hypotension (low blood pressure), as the inner cause of circulatory imbalance is related in terms of the energy centres.

At our clinics practitioners are often presented with cases of both high and low blood pressure. High blood pressure is obviously the most dangerous of the two conditions and is often associated with atherosclerosis. There are basically two categories of high blood pressure. Essential hypertension is the most common and accounts for over 90 per cent of cases. Presumably, medicine has so named the condition because its cause is unknown. The remaining cases are allied with kidney or endocrine disorders.

Causes of Hypertension

These are considered to be both genetic, dietetic, and involving other life-style factors. Caffeine, alcohol, and smoking are all well recognised and accepted factors contributing to hypertension.[1] Stress is also accepted as being a cause, and is locked in to the inner causes for hypertension.

In many cases of high blood pressure natural therapists find the liver is sluggish and they therefore regard liver toning as an essential component of treatment for circulatory disorders. Obesity is another obvious cause and is often found in the type of patient who over-indulges in refined foods and fats and whose liver is consequently sluggish.

Other causes not discussed earlier under atherosclerosis involve arterial disease from pollutants such as aluminium,[2] fluorine, lead and cadmium. Many stomach powders contain aluminium, and tea has a high level of fluoride. Sodium chloride or common table salt is perhaps the most common dietary indiscretion which may lead to this problem of arterial disease.[3]

At the more subtle level, all problems of the circulation are related to the flow of energy through the heart *chakra* and more specifically in the case of blood pressure, to the balance of the base *chakra* which governs the will to be.

Energy blocks involving the heart *chakra* will express as circulatory dysfunction. The development of the quality known as wisdom is considered to be intimately related to the healthy function of the heart *chakra* and its associated streams of energy. This innate wisdom no doubt protects us from dietary indiscretions, and produces a rhythmic life-style involving work, rest, relaxation and exercise — a life-style which protects against circulatory disorders.

In the case of high blood pressure, there is probably also an imbalance with the base centre; the 'will to be' has become too strong and threatens to burst through the channels (arteries) carrying its impulse. In low blood pressure the reverse takes place and the 'will to be' at the physical level is not strong enough.

Treatment

The first consideration at the physical level is nutrition. It has been found that items like garlic, sprouts, and green leafy vegetables inhibit cholesterol formation.[4] A diet high in fibre has been found useful in assisting prevention of atherosclerosis. Unsaturated oils rich in linoleic acid are found to have a hypotensive action and are encouraged together with vitamin E in moderate amounts to prevent atherosclerosis.[5]

The following specific remedies are often prescribed.

1 Vitamin E in small amounts to prevent clots: it is important that vitamin E is increased slowly in cases of high blood pressure due to its stimulating action on the heart muscle.
2 Vitamin C; plasma levels of C are lower in hypertensives.
3 Herbs such as dandelion, centaury, and burdock to tone the liver.
4 Herbs which have been found specific for lowering blood pressure; some are crataegus, garlic, and mistletoe.[6]
5 Magnesium compounds have been shown to lower blood pressure.[7]
6 Indicated homoeopathic remedies such as Aurum metallicum and magnesium phosphate.

Case Histories

The following case involves high blood pressure in a young woman with no apparent arterial degeneration. It appeared to be a case of essential hypertension which had its main cause in stress.

Susan, aged thirty-four, first attended the clinic in 1981 and now attends infrequently for 'maintenance' therapy. Her presenting symptoms were an insecure feeling in the head with associated giddiness, recurrent colds, and a history of high blood pressure. On the day she presented, systolic blood pressure was 180 which is certainly high.

During the first month she was prescribed magnesium phosphate to relax and balance her nervous system, potassium phosphate and vitamin B-complex for their nerve toning properties, herbs for relaxing the nervous system, minerals for recurrent colds, and liver herbs. She felt no improvement after this prescription but it was explained that a few months may be necessary to make up basic deficiencies before improvement would be profound. The blood pressure had dropped, however, by thirty points.

During the next two months she experienced improvement and the same treatment was continued. Blood pressure improved generally but would sometimes elevate for emotional reasons. It was decided to use the standard herbs for arterial disorders although atherosclerosis was not evident. A much larger dose of magnesium in the orotate form was used in an endeavour to stabilise the nervous system. Susan was encouraged to undertake relaxation classes.

A year after treatment began there was stabilisation, but Susan relapsed when her mother underwent breast surgery. Bach flowers were added for stress. A few months later, after a moderately stable period, it was decided that the homoeopathic constitutional should be selected. Treatment could then be accelerated following the basic work which had been completed. There was still some problem of over-reaction to stress with dizziness and blood pressure increase. Accordingly, one of the senior naturopathic students helping in the clinic spent several hours researching the case in terms of homoeopathic repertorisation. Pulsatilla in a high potency was administered at the next visit and continued intermittently thereafter. There was a great improvement from this time onwards with complete stabilisation of the blood pressure, and no further dizziness even when under stress. Susan moved further towards health. She has continued the relaxation techniques, and a maintenance dose of the various supplements is continued.

This case illustrates the profound improvement which can be effected by treatment with the constitutional remedy. It also indicates that perseverance is necessary to achieve maximum gains with naturopathic treatment. As Susan has attended for over two years, we have also been able to observe fairly marked positive changes in the iris.

Elisabeth, aged fifty-four, had suffered high blood pressure for one year and she suffered from chest pains and felt strain on her left side. She had been nursing but was off work at the time of treatment. Her blood pressure had been as high as 230/135. At the time of her first visit it was 160/108. Iris diagnosis indicated impaired circulation particularly in the head area, and weakness in the heart area. She had taken herself off medical hypertensive drugs and was taking only a diuretic at the time of her first visit. Fluid retention was a constant problem.

Elisabeth was already taking vitamin B, B6, C, E and a calcium compound. Her treatment included magnesium orotate, a diuretic herbal mixture containing pellitory, parsley, burdock, dandelion, centaury and trifolium, a herbal blood pressure tablet, sodium sulphate for regulating fluid balance, and a herbal sedative for sleep. After a month on this regime her blood pressure was 120/90 and she was feeling generally better. The prescription was repeated.

At her next visit, Elisabeth expressed concern over ribbon-like stools and some bleeding per vagina following a stabbing pain. The prescription was repeated with the addition of potassium chloride and iron phosphate for these new symptoms, although it was considered that the main prescription already covered most aspects of her concern. The blood pressure was by this time down to 120/80. The following month found her still concerned with the shape of the stools and she was suffering from wind and gurgling. It was considered by me that these symptoms were of nervous and psychic origin and Bach flower remedies were added to her basic prescription.

Over the next seven months, blood pressure was stabilised except for a few weeks when she left off tablets during a bout of influenza. Fluid retention continued to be a problem from time to time with swollen breasts and hands on occasions. A diuretic herbal tablet was introduced to replace the mixture and this was found to be suitable. Rheumatic herbs were introduced when a knee became stiff and sore. Hot flushes needed homoeopathic treatment for a few months. During her fifteen months' treatment, the blood pressure remained stable without medical drugs and when last seen, Elisabeth was improved in all respects.

Low Blood Pressure

This condition sometimes seems more difficult to treat than high blood pressure, although it is far less dangerous. Symptoms of low blood pressure often include exhaustion, a tendency to faint and a general lack of energy and vitality. These symptoms result partly from lack of blood to the brain. Low blood pressure is not dangerous except in the extreme form which manifests in Addison's Disease.

Causes

The average patient presenting with this problem is a young woman of slight build. The nervous system is generally run down. The medical profession does not have much to say about the aetiology of low blood pressure. There must be a connection between low blood pressure and the endocrine system, although this may be too subtle to register in our present range of pathology tests.

Subtle causes were mentioned earlier in connection with insufficient energy flowing through the base *chakra*. This 'basic' energy flow literally provides the will to live. European medical doctors in the anthroposophical branch of medicine have made an observation with which I agree. They suggest that some females are not sufficiently physically grounded. There is a lack of alignment between the physical and astral body especially following sleep. Remedies which help this alignment after sleep are phosphorous and iron in homoeopathic potencies. Although low blood pressure may not be accompanied by specific disease of the adrenal glands as in Addison's Disease, nevertheless it can often take all the lustre out of life due to feelings of exhaustion.

Treatment

Natural therapists find that basic life-style changes including diet will improve mild cases. Exercise should be encouraged as part of life-style changes which may also need to be directed to any debilitating factors in the environment. Acupuncture can be helpful, working by redirecting the energy flows of the body and thus stimulating the nervous system and adrenal glands.

Specific remedies are as follows:

1 Vitamin C and B5 to tone the adrenal glands — there is more vitamin C found in the adrenal glands than in any other part of the body.
2 Vitamin B-complex in large doses as a nerve tonic.
3 Potassium phosphate in small doses to tone the nervous system.
4 Iron phosphate which can raise blood pressure as a result of a tonic effect on blood vessels.
5 Vitamin E to strengthen the heart action.
6 Tonic herbs such as hops, avena sativa, and gentian plus herbal endocrine tonics like fennel, angelica, liquorice and sarsaparilla.

Case History

Sharron, aged twenty-five, had a very responsible and busy

office job with a firm of accountants. She visited our clinic with problems of fainting, headache, nausea and lack of appetite. She was unable to eat breakfast or dinner and her only meal was muesli at lunch time. Her periods were very painful. Sharron smokes about twenty-five cigarettes daily. Her systolic blood pressure at the first visit was 100. This is definitely on the low side.

This case is included because of the fact that improvements in general well-being occurred without the blood pressure changing. In other words, the fainting, nausea, headaches and periods all improved, with only very marginal raising of the blood pressure. The objective analysis is not perhaps so important as the patient's experience of well-being which resulted from treatment.

Treatment included a calcium compound for the painful periods, herbal liver treatment for the nausea, magnesium and potassium phosphate and B-complex for improved nerve tone, and vitamin C to help counteract toxicity caused by smoking. A herbal nerve compound was also given. Improvement in all respects took place after the first month's treatment, but as there was continuing pressure at work there was some recurrence of headaches; homoeopathic doses of magnesium phosphate were given for this problem.

In a case where the life-style is a great strain such as the work in which Sharron is involved, the problems are likely to recur unless change can be made. I sometimes explain to clients that we are pouring our supplements into a bottomless pit if healthy rhythms of work, rest, recreation and diet cannot be developed. A recent phone call to Sharron, however, informed me that she had no further problem with fainting and other symptoms.

Bronchiectasis

This condition invariably follows an earlier history of bronchitis or pneumonia and sometimes follows childhood fevers such as measles. It is rare to have a patient with this condition who has not had some previous history of chest problems. Chest infection is very common, as is the accumulation of yellow and green sputum which the patient finds very difficult to expectorate.

Recurrent bouts of pneumonia following a respiratory virus is common in these clients. The most characteristic symptom is a chronic cough with yellow or green sputum.

Causes

The immediate cause is a chronic dilation of the bronchi caused by loss of elastic and muscular tissue in those structures. This destruction of the bronchial wall is considered to take place through the agency of bacteria in association with chronic bronchitis, or following pneumonia. In some cases there are inherited factors such as occur in cystic fibrosis. It is my opinion that the long term use of bronchodilators for conditions of recurrent bronchitis and asthma must also have a very weakening condition on the bronchial tissues. Other contributing factors are air pollution and smoking.

Treatment

Although it is considered that the dilation of the bronchi is irreversible, natural therapists have had considerable success in preventing chest infections which occur often in bronchiectasis. With the use of natural therapies to improve the health of the chest, the mucus problem is partly resolved, and immunity increased. It does appear in some cases that the use of minute amounts of calcium fluoride can restore elastic tissue in the body. In the area of the bronchus, elasticity can therefore be partially restored by a long period of treatment.[1]

It should be noted that the fluoride compounds added to city water supplies do not have the same effect as those occurring naturally or in this form of medication. Specific treatment is as follows.

1 Vitamin C in large amounts to improve immunity and to reduce mucus levels.[2]
2 Calcium phosphate which is usually needed to strengthen bronchial tissue.
3 Vitamin A which helps prevent infection due to its effect on the epithelial tissue lining the bronchial tree.[3]
4 Calcium fluoride in suitable amounts to help restore elastic tissue.

5 Herbs to enhance expectoration, tone the bronchi, and to cleanse the lymphatic glands; trifolium, horehound, colts-foot, violet leaves, elderblossom, and marshmallow would be a typical mixture for the chest.
6 Liver herbs, essential to the detoxification process.
7 Codliver oil, useful during the winter months to help calcium absorption.

Case History

Some cases are of such a nature that an actual cure cannot be envisaged. Nevertheless, the client receives great benefit while on treatment compared to the general state of health when not taking supplements. Such was the case of Rita who had a very long history of bronchitis which later developed into bronchi-ectasis. She came at intervals for treatment and during this time, general energy improved and the chest improved to some extent.

Rita had suffered respiratory failure twice during the 1970s. Mucus from the chest appeared infected at the time of her visit in December 1979. Lymph glands were enlarged, and palpitations were experienced on occasions. At the time of her first visit, Rita was already taking vitamin B-complex, vitamin C, potassium, magnesium and calcium, lecithin and kelp. Our main contribution involved cleansing the lymphatic system and attempting to reduce the mucus production. To this end, a herbal mixture was given which contained horehound, coltsfoot, yellow dock, wood sanicle, liquorice and marshmallow. Liver herbs were given in tablet form, and the mineral salt potassium sulphate was administered for the green mucus. This salt was later used in a high potency with some good effect.

After some initial cleansing, a calcium fluoride combination was introduced to attempt to restore elastic tissue. The herb Ammi visnagi was used for wheezing attacks, and a tubercular nosode was given for a few weeks to try to combat the inherited factor. Rita has an amazingly positive approach to life and achieved an extraordinary amount of daily work on a country property in spite of her respiratory limitations.

Bronchitis

In winter, more children are treated in my practice for bronchitis than for any other condition. Twenty-five years ago, one was considered unlucky to have children with this problem. Now it is considered almost the norm. Bronchitis simply means inflammation of the bronchi or breathing tubes which lead to the lungs. The inflammation is characterised by incessant coughing due to the irritation present, and is followed by a build-up of mucus in the area. Combined with some spasm, the condition often leads to asthma-type wheezing and the child is then diagnosed as suffering from bronchial asthma.

Causes

In particular, congestion of the lymphatic system is found; this is often illustrated, via iris diagnosis, as white flecks through the area of the iris corresponding to the chest.[1] Spasm in the area is typically seen as cramp rings in the iris. This form of diagnosis is particularly valuable in the assessment of children as one can see at a glance any inherited weakness of the respiratory apparatus which may be predisposing towards the problem.

As in asthma, there may be a tubercular history known or unknown in the family and homoeopathic treatment is essential to eradicate this basic constitutional trait or miasm. It will be realised that the natural therapist does not regard the infective virus or bacteria as the primary cause, but as a secondary manifestation taking place in the presence of the previously mentioned factors.

Treatment

Nutritional considerations are very important as many of these children are allergic to dairy produce and some are very sensitive to chemicals in food.[2] The restriction of refined sugar and white flour products is important as these often leave residues of 'acid' waste in the system. Ironically, asthmatic children are notoriously picky and poor eaters and often with the best good will in the world, the parents are simply unable to get them to eat a good diet.

As treatment progresses, children do often improve in their eating habits, which appear to have been partly distorted by the biochemical imbalance in their bodies. Specific treatment for recurrent bronchitis is similar to asthma in many respects and may include the following:

1 Vitamin C to boost the immunity and to help dissipate mucus.[3]

2 Mineral combination of iron phosphate and potassium chloride for the inflammation and mucus formation respectively.

3 Liver homoeopathics for toning of that organ so that metabolism and breakdown of waste is more efficient.

4 Zinc, sometimes needed to improve immunity if warranted by the signs.

5 Calcium; signs of deficiency are often found.

6 Homoeopathic remedies, especially chosen to deal with inherited factors and to eradicate any negative effect of immunisation.

7 Codliver oil which is beneficial in the winter months to help absorption of calcium and for the vitamin A content which improves immunity.[4]

Case History

John is a typical case and fits into the above category. At the age of eleven he attended me with a history of bronchitis and wheezing which started when he was eighteen months old. As with many 'bronchial' children, he was excessively picky with his food, and ate no fruit or vegetables. His diet virtually consisted of white bread and toast, milk, potatoes and meat. He also suffered congestion of the nose and headaches.

By taking a thorough case history, and making certain observations including iris diagnosis, it was noted that John suffered deficiencies in calcium, magnesium and potassium phosphates, vitamin B-complex and vitamin C. These items were included in the first prescription in carefully arranged balance, plus herbs to tone the liver and cleanse the lymphatic system. Thyme and Ammi visnaga were given in a homoeopathic potency for any wheezing.

During the first month's treatment the nose and headaches cleared, but he had two attacks of bronchitis. The second attack came when remedies had not been taken for a week. Improvement continued and there were no attacks during the third and fourth month.

Discussions were held with John about the importance of his diet and it was realised that he had a real fear about eating and trying new foods. Bach flower remedies were added during the third month and from that time John began attempting to include more vegetables and other healthy foods. His improvement has now been established and he has now been through his first winter without antibiotics.

Cancer

Natural therapists agree with the orthodox medical profession that this is a very complex disease, although possibly we see it as complex for different reasons. In this book, I will not deal separately with the many different forms of cancer, such as melanoma, carcinoma, leukaemia, multiple myeloma and lymphoma. Of all diseases, cancer is one which must be treated in a most holistic fashion, and our treatment does not usually vary a great deal according to the type of cancer, but rather according to the individual.

Although cancer is a disease which natural therapists are not able to treat legally in some countries, a natural therapist can feel free to assist the case with natural medication, provided a registered medical doctor is also monitoring the patient.

Causes

It is of great interest that the medical profession is paying more attention to the role of the immune system, and coming close to the naturopathic viewpoint that lack of immunity may be the one real cause of cancer. We see this lack of immunity resulting firstly from inherited factors, and from deep within the psyche of the patient. We find that emphasis is now placed on finding the deep-seated destructive tendencies which in turn may be affecting the physical immune system.[1] Cancer can now almost be classed as an auto-immune disorder. A severe emotional shock or period of emotional stress is often found to precede the development of cancer by a period of two years.

An important contribution to understanding the cancer problem has been made by Rudolf Steiner. Medical doctors in Europe who follow his suggestions about cancer understand health as the state resulting from the balancing of two sets of energy which are associated with the two physical poles of our being — the nerve or sensory pole and the metabolic pole. People are found to gravitate generally to one of these extremes.

In the cancer process, the nerve or consciousness pole takes a wrong direction and an abnormal sclerosis takes place, often occurring after a deep-seated grief or shock. This sclerosis is the opposite of the inflammatory process.[2] It is certainly true that spontaneous remission of cancer has been shown to take place after a severe inflammatory condition manifests. This also accounts for the common finding that cancer patients often have a medical history showing no evidence of even such minor inflammatory conditions as the common cold.

The aim of this approach to cancer is to balance up the 'poles' again through counselling, nutrition, general life style, herbs, and through the use of mistletoe injections.[3]

It is not possible to understand the cancer process fully without recognising the role which the etheric body plays in keeping the 'pattern' or mould intact for the physical cells and tissues. The function of this life field has been extensively explored by medical researcher, Harold Saxton Burr.[4] As the mediator between our psychological states and the physical body, the etheric body is affected by both outer problems involving diet and environment, and inner subjective factors from the astral or feeling nature.[5] Recently, controversy has arisen over electronic pollution which may cause cancer in people living near power lines, and other sources of man-made magnetic fields. As our etheric nature is closely related to electromagnetic energy, the possible effect of strong magnetic or electric fields is understandable.

If the etheric field is electromagnetic, and if it loses its pattern through either emotional or physical causes, cells and tissues can grow in a random fashion. The extraordinarily positive effect on the cancer process through meditation is no doubt due to the re-establishing of the correct pattern in our life-field or etheric. The mistletoe injections used near the site of the tumour are likewise an important aid in restoring the etheric balance and strength, apart from the cytostatic effect of this herbal preparation.[6]

Physical causes arise from poor diet, as for instance in deficiency of anti-oxidants — vitamin C, E. selenium, and of vitamin A which is needed for resistance of all the epithelial tissue.[7] In the absence of these protective nutrients, industrial chemicals ingested in food, air and water can cause foci for cancer development. Other contributing causes are poor lymphatic drainage which may be an inherited tendency or produced by poor diet and lack of exercise.

Treatment

Treatment for cancer can be discussed only briefly in this book as it is a very large and complex area, dealt with in some detail in a number of excellent books.[8]

The main areas to be covered are as follows:

1 Psychological counselling to remove deep-seated negative tendencies in the psyche and to enable the client to undertake self-fulfilling, creative activities.

2 Teaching the patient to meditate so that deep-seated tensions may be resolved and to release healing energies from within the self. Some therapists use creative visualisation so that the patient consciously directs healing to deal with diseased cells and tissues.[9]

3 Diet is usually radically changed with emphasis on raw foods for purposes of detoxification of the lymph system and the gastro-intestinal tract. Raw vegetable juices, and the use of coffee enemas may be included for detoxification.[10]

4 Herbs for cleansing the lymph system may include violet leaves, trifolium, burdock, echinacea, and blue flag. Dandelion, centaury, and wahoo may be used to tone the liver so that waste may be more adequately metabolised. This process is extremely important as the tumour breaks up and toxins are released.

5 Anti-oxidants such as vitamins A, C, E, and the trace element selenium, are included, as well as the mineral zinc to improve immunity.

6 Homoeopathy both for drainage, immunity and for removing inherited taints is invaluable. It also has an important role in neutralising industrial toxins.

7 Potassium phosphate, magnesium phosphate and vitamin B-complex are added to provide energy and nerve tone.

8 Mistletoe injections. The mistletoe was discovered by Rudolf Steiner to be an appropriate medication for cancer. The plant has no root system of its own and its leaves and berries are not dependent on the seasons for their development. Steiner taught that because of the unusual properties of this plant it is perfectly balanced within itself and able to

balance the nerve sense pole and the blood metabolic pole in cancer patients. Medical research in Europe indicates the great value of this type of therapy.[11] Mistletoe increases immunity and also has a cytostatic action on cancer.

Case Histories

Marika was ten years old at her first visit to the clinic six years ago. It was explained that a brain tumour was diagnosed four years earlier, and since then she had undergone surgery, radiation, and chemotherapy. She had a permanent shunt to drain away fluid from the brain, and it was expected the tumour would grow again. Since undergoing naturopathic treatment her general health has improved considerably, and the last time the shunt had to be replaced, the specialist reported no further growth in the tumour. Due to some permanent damage to the brain, Marika does not have the normal development of the average girl of her age, but she enjoys attending a special school, and does not have any serious physical problems at the moment.

Her treatment was aimed particularly at cleansing the lymphatic system as this was observed via iris diagnosis to be very congested. In this respect she has improved greatly. She also has much more energy, and has been noticed to cope better at school. Specific supplements include vitamin B-complex and vitamin C, lymphatic cleansing herbs, iron phosphate, potassium phosphate, potassium chloride, brewers yeast tablets for their selenium content, and homoeopathic drops for the endocrine glands. Kelp has been used to stimulate the thyroid.

This is a good example of how orthodox treatment can be combined with natural supplements, thus enabling a state of remission and good general health to prevail.

Judith, aged fifty-six when she first visited me, has multiple myeloma, this condition being first diagnosed fourteen years ago. She had undergone chemotherapy and her blood becomes affected from time to time with a low haemoglobin, and lessening of white blood cells. She had suffered a lot of aching in the left hip and right knee. Nervous diarrhoea was also a problem.

Treatment commenced with lymphatic and blood toning herbs, rheumatic herbs, vitamin C, kelp, magnesium and potassium phosphate, plus sodium phosphate. Improvement in the haemoglobin took place after the addition of homoeopathic doses of Ferrum picrum. After a few months, the aches and pains gradually disappeared. After more than two years' treatment, her condition has been fairly stable. A recent phone call confirmed her continued remission.

One more study is included to indicate how a terminal case can be restored to complete health, given a positive approach to life and natural therapies. Frances, aged fifty-two, came to my husband for treatment in October 1985. Three years prior to her visit, she underwent a total hysterectomy followed by radiation for cancer to the uterus. Just before commmencing naturopathic treatment she had a portion of the large bowel removed for secondary carcinoma in that organ. It was noted by the surgeon that there were malignant growths in the liver.

Frances decided to explore every avenue to improve her condition. She followed the Gerson diet and regime including the coffee enemas for detoxification of the liver, and attended my husband once per month.[12] Her remedies included lymphatic cleansing and liver herbs, potassium, magnesium and zinc compounds, homoeopathic mixtures for organ drainage and nerve toning, plus homoeopathic Thuja in a high potency. In August 1986, Frances advised my husband that a recent medical 'scan' showed the liver and all other organs completely clear of malignant growth.

Cervical Dysplasia

It is now standard practice for women to have regular smear tests to check that the cells of the cervix are healthy. This is an area where natural medicine can be of great assistance, and one where there can be co-operation between orthodox practitioners and natural therapists. On a number of occasions, our clients have been given the all-clear after six months on the naturopathic treatment following a previous finding of cell changes to the cervix.

Causes

As discussed under the heading of Cancer, the general life-style, psychological state, and nutrition are all paramount factors in the development of those cell changes which lead to cancer. The causes of cervical cancer are no doubt quite complex. By treating clients at the stage when erosion first occurs, tissues can be regenerated in a healthy manner.

Recently, medical scientists have considered that venereal herpes and warts are causes of cervical cancer. Promiscuity from an early age has also been cited. It would appear that any irritation to the cervical cells can be a contributing factor. For cells to withstand the various provocations of our environment, good nutrition is essential.

Treatment

1 Lymphatic cleansing and liver herbs for detoxification of the body.
2 Vitamin C to improve immunity.[13]
3 Vitamin A to improve resistance of cervix to dysplasia.[14]
4 Zinc compound to enhance healing and prevent scarring.
5 Specific homoeopathic prescriptions.

Case Histories

Dorothy, aged forty-five, had a dilation and curette for menstrual problems and cell changes were found. A later smear test also revealed problems. She had a history of heavy periods, and pain in the left ovary for some time. There were also recurrent digestive and sinus problems. After three months of treatment most of her symptoms had disappeared except for a continuing intermittent tiredness. After six months of treatment, the smear test was negative.

Her treatment consisted of a herbal mixture containing mainly lymphatic cleansing herbs, a liver herbal tablet, potassium chloride and iron phosphate (which is the mineral combination to work on lymph glands), vitamin C for the immune system, and a high potency B-complex for energy. Later additions and changes included vitamin P for the bleeding tendency, homoeopathic drops to regulate menstruation, and vitamin A to work on producing healthy epithelial tissue. Included also was the mineral combination mentioned many times in this book to improve energy — potassium and magnesium phosphate compound. Individual homoeopathic prescribing was also used for constitutional aspects.

In this case, as with others which have been described, when the more chronic dangerous problems disappear a fairly long period of retracing through the sub-acute phase then ensues. This took place in Dorothy's situation over a long time, involving the digestive problems and sinus. The menstrual problems and cervical erosion did not recur.

It is understandable that with the majority of malignancies, treatment with supplements would need to be an ongoing procedure to maintain the general health. Many cancer patients tend to give up natural therapies if they have any kind of relapse because of the high cost of this unsubsidised branch of medicine.

Susan, aged forty-six, was diagnosed as having cervical dysplasia; three cervical smear tests showed a problem. The last two reports made mention of carcinoma of the cervix with a note about the likely origin as being the papilloma virus associated with venereal warts. Susan decided not to go ahead with standard medical treatment and preferred to try natural medicines. Her iris revealed a basically good constitution although there was emphasis on nerve tension and instability, plus a lack of digestive enzymes.

Associated problems were tiredness, grief over her father's death, insomnia and hypoglycaemia. Susan was already taking vitamins A, B-complex and C. Her first month of treatment included a herbal mixture of lymphatic and liver herbs, magnesium and potassium phosphate for energy, and Bach flower remedies to balance her *chakras* and to help with the emotional states she often experienced. She was also advised to attend another physician who specialises in mistletoe therapy.

On her first return visit, Susan reported that her sleep had improved and she felt she was coping with life quite well. She had commenced the mistletoe injections. Her treatment continued over many months; one of the main hurdles was the exhaustion she experienced from coping with her mother and other relatives. She had begun to meditate regularly and certain suggestions were made in this respect. Magnesium phosphate in homoeopathic potency was given to resolve bowel spasms. The physician handling the mistletoe therapy arranged for blood crystallisation tests to be done to monitor progress of the etheric energies.[15] This was undertaken about seven months after treatment started. The tests did not find any problem in the area of cervix or uterus, but problems of potential malignancy appeared in the bowel area.

Susan was encouraged to work much more resolutely on the

psychological problems and this was the turning point in her progress. She coped very well with terminating a difficult personal relationship, and also began dealing more easily with relatives. Energy began to improve more consistently. The basic cleansing, nerve toning and mistletoe therapy continued. Magnesium phosphate was increased in potency to the 200th dilution. At her last visit, Susan joyfully produced the report of her recent smear test which reported all-clear.

Economic savings to the government could be significant if serious thought and consideration were given to assess the role of natural therapies in assisting the rehabilitation and maintenance of people with chronic diseases such as cancer. The cost of natural therapies and their role in preventive medicine needs to be compared with the far greater cost of orthodox procedures and maintenance for persons with chronic diseases.

Carpal Tunnel Syndrome

This condition is quite common in women and is not always related to constant use of the hands. It manifests as pain in the wrist caused by compression of the median nerve. Often the first symptom is nocturnal tingling of the fingers, usually in the hand most used. The tingling may be accompanied by pain in the hand, elbow or more rarely the shoulder. As the condition progresses, the patient may wake with fingers numb and swollen. Symptoms are aggravated by using the hands.

Causes

Arthritis, ganglion of the wrist joint, and less commonly endocrine disturbances may all be precipitating factors. From the naturopathic point of view, causes are more basic and relate to a calcium, magnesium or silica imbalance, often accompanied by a vitamin B6 deficiency. The latter supplement alone has completely cleared a number of cases.[1]

Treatment

As this condition is closely related to the rheumatic and arthritic constitution, treatment will include that outlined under arthritis and will also emphasise whichever minerals are needed plus large doses of B6. The following would be a typical example treatment schedule:

1 Iron phosphate for inflammation of the nerve.
2 Calcium phosphate for the numbness and tingling.
3 Rheumatic herbs.
4 Liver herbs.
5 Vitamin B6.

Cataracts

This is a condition which causes gradual deterioration of the sight mechanism from a developing opacity in the crystalline lens of the eye. The problem generally occurs after middle age, but may occur earlier in diabetics or from the use of particular medical drugs.

Causes

In the average case which develops in late life, the natural therapist is concerned with the biochemistry. Why has the lens become opaque and what natural therapies can reverse the biochemical changes? The balance of calcium and silica is critical from the natural therapist's point of view. It is very easy for this balance to become disturbed because of Western dietary patterns.

Treatment

Nellie, aged sixty-six, is a good case to explain the treatment. Her case is typical of many observed during fifteen years in practice. She did not come originally for cataracts, although these must have been developing already. Her problems included a very sore tongue, exhaustion, sluggish bowels, haemorrhoids, sinusitis and vertigo. These conditions were all successfully resolved and she returned intermittently for further maintenance treatment over a period of several years. Natural therapies were also used to restore health after surgery to her thyroid gland.

Treatment for the cataracts was started in 1985. The chief ingredients to dissolve the opacity of the lens in most people are homoeopathic silica and calcium fluoride, both in the 30th potency. In some cases this must be continued over several years. Nellie was pronounced free of her cataracts by the specialist about eighteen months after treatment commenced.

The basic naturopathic treatment which she had taken over a period of years would have accelerated the treatment of the cataracts. Supplements during this time included liver herbs, magnesium and potassium phosphate, vitamin C and vitamin B-complex. Magnesium, vitamin B2, and vitamin C, have all been shown to influence the health of the crystalline lens of the eye.[1] Without these supplements, the homoeopathic remedies would probably not be very effective. The synergistic activity of natural therapies is again obvious.

Cerebral Vascular Disease

see also Atherosclerosis

From the naturopathic point of view it is most useful to discuss stroke (sub-arachnoid haemorrhage), hardened cerebral arteries (cerebral ischaemia) strokes caused by clots or embolism, and aneurisms (weakness of cerebral arteries), all in the one section. In each case, natural therapists find that there are basic disturbances of circulation to the cerebral area caused by mineral deficiencies, waste material clogging up the areas, or inherited weaknesses of the arteries in the cerebral areas.

In the case of haemorrhages and clots, the main symptoms include headache, progressive loss of consciousness, and/or one-sided paralysis according to which side of the brain is affected. The more gradual symptoms which often precede this dramatic stage, and which are the result of a gradual clogging of the arteries with cholesterol, include progressive loss of memory and concentration, exhaustion through lack of blood to the brain, high blood pressure, and senility.

Causes and Treatment

The same parameters will apply in naturopathic practice as those for atherosclerosis and the reader is referred to that section. The section on blood pressure should also be examined as 'stroke' often follows a condition of hypertension.

Chicken-pox

(Varicella)

This is a common childhood infection which usually runs a mild course. It begins with general malaise such as fever and headache, with the rash often the first sign to appear. Vesicles appear initially in the mouth and then the rash appears mostly on the trunk rather than the extremities. The rash appears as a succession of crops so that there are papules, vesicles, pustules and crusts all at the same time.

Cause

It is interesting to compare the orthodox and naturopathic viewpoint here. The natural therapist can predict by observing the state of the lymph system through iris diagnosis whether or not a child is likely to have a severe bout of the infection. Although it is accepted that the immediate cause is the infecting virus, the severity of the illness will be in keeping with the need for the body to eliminate toxins through the skin. This will vary in accordance with the degree of lymphatic congestion. In orthodox medicine, a virus is considered as being 'caught' and although it is accepted that people are immune to a greater or lesser degree, no causal connection is made between the severity of the disease and the state of the lymphatic system.

Treatment

It is handy to know some simple remedies especially for those cases where the rash is very heavy and where secondary infection could take place. Remedies may include:

1 Iron phospate for the fever and inflammation of the skin lesions.
2 Potassium chloride to dry up the vesicles as quickly as possible.

3 Liver and lymphatic herbs in homoeopathic doses to cleanse the system.
4 Vitamin B-complex for the irritation of the many nerve endings in the skin.
5 Zinc compound if it appears likely that there will be scarring.
6 Vitamin C to promote immunity and healing and to prevent secondary infection.[1]

Chilblains

Although not given much space in medical books, chilblains are a distressing and common ailment which responds well to natural therapies. It is a vasospastic disorder which may be either acute or chronic. Symptoms include vasoconstriction and blueness of the skin on the extremities. Slight swelling, intense itching and blistering may occur in severe cases.

Causes

The immediate cause is exposure to cold. From clinical experience, natural therapists have found that the real cause is a circulatory disturbance connected with mineral imbalances involving calcium and magnesium salts in the body. A lack of magnesium causes the vasoconstrictive action of the skin on contact with cold. A lack of calcium gives a general sensitivity to cold.[1] Natural therapists have found a relationship between the autonomic nervous system and the calcium/magnesium levels and their ratio in the tissues.

Treatment

1 Calcium phosphate supplementation for at least three months before winter.
2 Codliver oil capsules during winter to assist absorption of calcium phosphate.
3 Vitamin E to promote circulation.
4 Magnesium phosphate or orotate if indicated by the general constitution.
5 Advice about exercise and relaxation techniques.

Case History

Robyn, a twenty-seven-year-old nurse, suffered from very bad chilblains during each winter. The circulation was also bad in summer with aching feet as a result of her hospital work, and swelling of fingers and toes in the heat. As she visited us in spring, her first prescription included attention to the heat problem which was likely to develop in the next few months.

The first month's treatment consisted of a herbal mixture to tone the liver and kidneys in relation to the fluid problem, magnesium, potassium and calcium phosphates, and vitamin B-complex for general energy and nerve tone. She returned after five weeks and reported less swelling in her feet. The same treatment was continued for the next two months and on the fourth visit, Robyn reported some problem with the swelling but it was not as bad as in the previous summer.

A slight rearrangement of treatment was continued through the autumn and winter The mineral salt sodium sulphate was introduced to work on fluid balance in the whole body, and the herbal ingredients for the kidneys were changed. Codliver oil capsules were added during the cold months to help the absorption of calcium phosphate.

Robyn went throughout the winter without any chilblains although there was still some swelling if the feet became hot.

Climacteric

see Menopause

Coeliac Disease

This is not a common disorder although, as the severity varies considerably, it is apparently hard to find any accurate incidence in the population. The disorder is characterised by malabsorption in the small intestine and common symptoms are weight loss, abdominal distention and bloating. Diarrhoea may or may not be present, and steatorrhoea (fatty stools) frequently feature in the problem. Seventy per cent of cases in any series are women and there appears to be an inherited factor as the incidence in siblings is higher than in the general population.[1]

Evidence of anaemia and other deficiencies can be present without any apparent malabsorption, as many cases do not manifest diarrhoea. Likewise, puzzling metabolic bone diseases with considerable demineralisation can sometimes be found to have their cause in coeliac disease.

Causes

This disease is of particular interest to naturopaths because we see so many ailments resulting from deficiencies and with causative factors in the poor state of the digestive tract. In coeliac disease there is an abnormal flattening and blunting of the villi of the small intestines. As these are microscopic finger-like projections, which by projecting into the lumen of the intestine are responsible for food absorption, any flattening will diminish the rate and amount of absorption. As a result, mineral and vitamin deficiencies are common in this condition. An immunological factor is strongly suspected as a contributing factor to the damaged mucosa.[2]

The main and obvious cause has been found in an allergy to wheat gluten. By placing the patient on a gluten-free diet, symptoms disappear and absorption improves in many cases. Natural therapists are interested that many people with allergies are intolerant to wheat apart from those diagnosed as having coeliac disease. Is it possible that we have hundreds of potential coeliac cases coming to our clinics, or is there just no hard and fast division between people who have difficulty digesting wheat and that group with small intestine pathology?

Patients with this condition are found to have a number of enzyme alterations in their mucosa. Natural therapists find that many conditions involving the digestive tract result from enzyme deficiencies. Bloating, diarrhoea, inflammation and malabsorption characterises these problems and this is why it is hard to isolate coeliac disease from the many digestive disturbances encountered which respond to wheat-free diets.

Weakness in the digestive process of the small intestine is found so commonly in natural therapy clinics that natural therapists are inclined to broaden the causes of coeliac disease to include biochemical imbalances and digestive organs which are functionally weak. In such a state, given the notorious difficulty in digesting wheat, is it any wonder that the intestinal mucosa develops pathological changes.

As with all digestive disturbances, subtle causes which in turn influence biochemical and physiological function may be attributed to an imbalance of energy flowing through the solar plexus *chakra*, and to associated etheric or astral blockages or congestion.

Treatment

This will include the standard approach of removing gluten from the diet, but natural therapists are also concerned to correct the biochemistry and function of organs which perhaps initially exacerbated an inherited tendency to gluten allergy. To start the corrective process in motion, raw vegetable juices will be included in the form of carrot, apple, celery, beetroot, cabbage and lettuce. At least three glasses per day on an empty stomach will be suggested.

Millet meal is the most allergy-free cereal and this will be ideal for a breakfast cereal. Unpolished rice is another suitable starch which could be used for breakfast or instead of bread at lunchtime.[3] Rice cakes and gluten free bread are other alternatives to wheat and rye. All refined and adulterated foods are removed from the diet as being inimical to the health of the digestive tract. Specific supplements will be as follows:

1 Iron phosphate for the inflammation and iron deficiency tendency.
2 Vitamins B-complex and C as water soluble vitamins most likely to be deficient.
3 Vitamin A for its effect on epithelial tissue.
4 Liver and digestive herbs such as melissa, angelica, dandelion, centaury, wahoo, and marshmallow, plus trifolium as a lymphatic cleanser.
5 Sodium sulphate as the tissue salt with most affinity for liver and pancreas.
6 Selected homoeopathic digestive remedies.

Case History

Yvonne, aged thirty-three, attended me in 1975; and she had

been diagnosed as having coeliac disease nine months earlier. Symptoms included diarrhoea and wind with intolerance to fats and carbohydrates. Her daughter was also diagnosed as having the same condition. The first month of treatment included a herbal mixture for the digestion, iron phosphate for inflammation, magnesium and potassium phosphate as a general nerve tonic, papaya enzyme tablets, rosehip tablets and homoeopathic Hydrastis as a further tonic for the intestinal epithelium.

On the first return visit, Yvonne reported spasmodic diarrhoea and had suffered a bad reaction after eating fat at one stage during the month. The treatment was repeated with the addition of sodium sulphate tablets for liver and pancreas plus vitamin B-complex.

Yvonne was not seen again until nine months later. She was then seven months' pregnant. She was at the time suffering from pale bulky motions and colic. The last prescription was repeated over the next three months and the digestion improved almost immediately. She had a fairly good labour and breast-fed the baby. The digestion remained good while on treatment. Yvonne was next seen two years later after a severe pelvic infection and had just become pregnant again. She responded well to treatment and I would have liked her to continue treatment for some time but we lost touch with her at this stage.

Colic

see also Abdominal Migraine

Colic is caused by a spasm to the bowel and gives abdominal pain which can be mild or severe.

Causes

This is one condition where natural therapists are able to point to a specific deficiency causing a recurrent and acute disorder. I have used magnesium compounds more than any other remedy to help colic cases of all ages from babies to old people. Doses have varied from 400mg of magnesium orotate daily to minute homoeopathic doses of magnesium phosphate.

In spite of this successful application of magnesium, one must not gloss over the causes because here we have a condition which from my point of view is intimately connected with emotional states.

Colic is related to a spasm in the solar plexus *chakra* or energy centre and this is usually triggered by an imbalance, even if temporary, in the feeling or astral nature. It is especially common in young children who are very sensitive and who have not learnt to control the energies flowing through their small psyches. In such cases the term abdominal migraine is often used. The child or adult may have associated spasticity of the bowel with either constipation or diarrhoea, or these may alternate.

In speaking of the more esoteric causes, it is not intended to deny the role of the autonomic nervous system and the associated nerve plexi with problems of the colon. Rather the intention is, once again, to pinpoint first causes. From my point of view, the state of the solar plexus *chakra* is the main conditioning factor for the autonomic nervous system.

Treatment

1 Magnesium phosphate in varying doses and potencies.
2 The B-complex vitamins as needed for all nervous disorders.
3 The Bach flower remedies for the emotional states involved.
4 Liver herbs or homoeopathics to regulate the digestive processes.

Common Cold

Contrary to popular medical opinion, there is a great deal that can be done both to prevent and to relieve the common cold. Many of our clients have reported with glee after a particularly bad season for colds that they were the only one in the office who did not succumb. Another plus for natural treatment in those suffering from colds is the ability to cut short the duration so that infection does not progress into the chest.

Causes

Here again, natural therapists have to diverge from medical opinion, which speaks authoritatively about immunity and the common cold, yet does not really offer anything specific for treatment or enhancement of immunity. The cause, apart from the immediate infection with a virus, relates to our biochemical and emotional balance and to the state of our immunity as the result of such balance or imbalance.

Natural therapists are concerned with the nutritional status of the individual. So we may include in the diet an emphasis on unprocessed food, and a minimum of those foods contributing to waste which clogs up the lymphatic system. The lymphatic system must be healthy for the immune system to work adequately. Vitamin C status in the body is important but is not the only factor in preventing or helping colds. Zinc, calcium salts and iron status are all significant in relation to respiratory infections, as is vitamin A.

Treatment

Treatment is related to reforming the life-style in terms of nutrition, rest, and exercise, and to improving the air purity in work situations by preventing smoking, etc. Specific supplements may include the following,

1 Vitamin C for immunity. [1]
2 Vitamin A to improve immunity through its effect on epithelial tissue lining nose and bronchial tree. [2]
3 Codliver oil capsules which are useful instead of vitamin A during winter.
4 Mineral combination of iron phosphate and potassium chloride for the inflammation and to clear mucus discharge respectively.
5 Potassium sulphate for green discharge or calcium sulphate for yellow discharge.
6 Any one of a number of homoeopathic remedies according to the individual case concerned.
7 Homoeopathic remedies for the underlying inherited taint or miasm which may be predisposing to recurrent colds.
8 Herbal mixture with pectorals or chest herbs such as coltsfoot, liquorice, horehound, and marshmallow, if a cough has developed.

Case History

Very often recurrent colds form part of the general patient history. In the case of Adam, he was losing time away from school with recurrent viruses, and also suffered from hay fever in season. His first prescription included vitamin C, iron phosphate and potassium phosphate, lymphatic cleansing herbs, liver herbs, and homoeopathic sinus drops.

During the first month's treatment he had another heavy cold, and a further during the second month but this was less severe than usual and he did not need to miss school. He then had longer periods without colds and when they did manifest, he felt well enough not to miss school. Hay fever drops were added as needed in the spring season and these helped his seasonal nose problem.

Constipation

The medical profession has become more conscious of the need for high fibre diets to prevent diseases of the colon, including diverticulitis, cancer and colitis.[1] There is now not such a gap between natural therapists and the orthodox medical practitioner on the subject. Naturopaths have always been very conscious of the need for the major part of the diet to consist of unprocessed foods with particular emphasis on vegetables, salads, whole grain cereals, and the use of seeds or nuts.[2]

It should be mentioned that many clients are under the impression that constipation does not relate to how many days one goes without a bowel action, but rather to whether the contents of the bowel are difficult to expel. Logic dictates that if we are even having one meal only per day, there should be an elimination through the bowel on a daily basis. The fact that some people use the bowels only every four days but without any discomfort does not mean that waste is not accumulated and re-absorbed.

Causes

It is simplistic to assume that all cases of constipation are related to lack of roughage. I have encountered many cases where the diet was excellent and yet chronic constipation prevailed. Other causes can relate to imbalance in the autonomic nervous system so that nerve impulses governing the bowel movement are insufficient. A sluggish liver is a major cause of a sluggish bowel.

More subtle factors relate to an imbalance of the energy flow through the solar plexus energy centre. This may be caused by emotional suppression or to blockages of feelings. The solar plexus *chakra* is related to all digestive functions and is psychologically related to the desire for possession, and to acquisition. A concentration of feeling and emotion in this area can cause a blockage in the energy flow which in turn inhibits flow of digestive secretions and normal nerve impulses to the bowel. The rectum or last part of the bowel is more under the control of the sacral centre.

Treatment

1 Digestive herbs.
2 Magnesium phosphate and potassium phosphate to regulate nerve impulse to the bowel.
3 Vitamin B-complex for its tonic action on the nervous system.
4 Calcium fluoride compounds if tone in the bowel is deficient such as occurs in diverticulitis.
5 The use of linseeds as a dietary supplement to produce the normal mucus secretion of the bowel. This measure is far more effective in constipation than the use of a roughage like bran.

Case Histories

Nancy, aged fifteen, came for naturopathic treatment with problems of constipation, and painful periods which were accompanied by vomiting. She was able to use her bowels only every three days. The diet was poor and included a lot of white bread. Her constitution by iris diagnosis was found to be generally good and rapid improvement was expected with dietary changes and a few supplements. Bioenergetic diagnosis using the Vega instrument indicated a sluggish thyroid and liver, plus a biological index in excess of her chronological age.

The treatment for the first month included liver herbs in crude and homoeopathic form, vitamin B-complex, and kelp which was given to stimulate the thyroid gland. This treatment covered the sluggishness of liver and bowel. In addition she received calcium phosphate and homoeopathic drops for the uterine cramps. On her return visit, Nancy reported using the bowels every one or two days and there had been no problems with the period. The treatment was repeated and after another month the bowel was working every day. Freedom from period problems continued. The Vega diagnosis indicated considerable improvement with thyroid, liver and bowel function.

Another two months of treatment were given and then treatment was tapered off. Provided Nancy maintains her good diet, there is no reason why her condition should relapse. It is of interest that from the subjective point of view, the uterus and large bowel are both under the control of the sacral *chakra*. This is often temporarily disturbed during or following puberty.

Alice, aged twelve, visited me one month after she was hospitalised for a blocked bowel. In addition to her chronic constipation, she slept badly and had catarrhal problems, tiredness and headaches. All these symptoms can be related to a toxic load in the system as a result of poor elimination. Alice was able to empty her bowel only every second day and then only with the assistance of laxatives.

It was observed via iris diagnosis that nerve stimulation to the digestive system was poor and there were indications of poor tone and distension in various parts of the bowel. The food regime which Alice followed was not giving her much raw fruit and salad, nor any whole grain cereal.

Her first month's treatment consisted of calcium phosphate for general signs of deficiency observed in the iris, magnesium phosphate for bowel spasm, potassium phosphate to improve nerve tone to the bowel, vitamin B-complex as a general nerve tonic, liver herbs to increase digestive ability by stimulating the liver, and homoeopathic drops with both digestive remedies and Bach flower remedies to work on the solar plexus *chakra*.

After one month's treatment, the bowel was much more regular but sleeping was still poor. Alice explained this was because she could hear the television through the timber wall next to her bed. I mention this fact because, in my opinion, the electromagnetic radiation constantly next to Alice as she tried to sleep each night was definitely a predisposing factor in her problem. I tried to explain the significance of research in this area to her father, but no effort was made to move the television from near the bed.[3]

On the third visit Alice reported using her bowel every day and she was sleeping better. On the fourth visit, it was reported that sleep was good but the bowel still needed a laxative as well as our treatment. At least the two forms of treatment together produced a bowel action every day and not just every second day as with the laxative alone. Further improvement was attempted with the addition of magnesium phosphate in a high potency. The aim with this remedy was to give a more deep acting and lasting effect.

Alice did not return again; this sometimes happens when improvement continues and the family see no need for further treatment.

Corneal Ulcer

This condition is not commonly handled alone by natural therapists, although it is an area where natural therapies can greatly hasten and aid the healing process. The cornea is the covering of the eyeball and therefore the main complication, from lack of healing and consequent scarring, is interference to the vision.

Causes

Natural therapists find that some persons are predisposed to this condition and they need all possible nutrients to promote quick and adequate healing. Industrial accidents, chemicals, and particular infectious disorders which affect the eye are some of the causes of corneal ulceration.

Treatment

1 Iron phosphate to reduce inflammation, and zinc compounds to prevent scarring. Silica, especially in homoeopathic preparation, may be constitutionally indicated.
2 Vitamins A and E, both necessary to promote healing of the cornea.

3 Specific homoeopathic remedies as indicated, for example, Mercurius corrosivus.
4 Vitamin C for its healing effect.[1]

Case History

John, in his early thirties, developed a corneal ulcer following chicken-pox. His main accompanying complaint was severe dyspepsia and acidity of the stomach plus nervous tension. A fair degree of stress came from his work as a private consulting engineer. The iris revealed a very poor constitution with gross deficiencies of calcium and other minerals, a large amount of catarrhal waste, and pronounced acidity and inflammation of the stomach.

The treatment for the first month included calcium phosphate, iron phosphate, vitamin A, vitamin B-complex, liver herbs, and homoeopathic drops for the eye consisting of Hepar sulphuricum, Chelidonium and Mercurius corrosivus. He was already taking large amounts of vitamin C himself. The eye specialist reported that the ulcer was less deep whereas previously, the medical treatment had not produced any changes. The same basic treatment was continued with the addition of a zinc compound to prevent scarring and Bach flowers to counteract depression and anxiety were added to the eye drops.

Further improvement was reported at the next visit and minor changes to the treatment were made with the addition of lymphatic cleansing herbs for the catarrhal waste noted in the iris plus hay fever drops. The mercury salt for the ulceration of the cornea was also changed. After this third month of treatment, the ulcer was quite healed without scarring.

John continued treatment for his stomach acidity for a number of months. A further corneal ulcer developed after influenza about fourteen months after his first visit. The specific treatment was repeated immediately and this time the ulcer cleared up within a couple of weeks. This improved healing time is a common experience with recurrence of an ailment after someone has been on natural therapies for a period of months. Over a period of some years, he has had no recurrence of eye trouble.

John is still taking medication for his stomach, five years after his first visit. This may seem a very long time, but given the very poor constitution with which he started treatment, and his stress at work which mitigated against a speedy improvement, the length of treatment is understandable. The iris has revealed considerable strengthening of the body tissues, and gradual elimination of catarrhal waste. The stomach has been the most persistent organ to remain disturbed; this is in keeping with the retracing syndrome of naturopathic philosophy which sees most physical disease as starting in the stomach through wrong choice of food.

There is one other point of interest in relation to this case. If John had not had extensive natural treatment for the stomach, the hyperacidity would have probably developed towards stomach ulcers. The basic tendency of ulceration comes from an inherited miasm and in the case of John, this tendency was manifesting as corneal ulcers, and is still present as the stomach problem. This particular taint comes from syphilis in bygone generations and is discussed later under that heading as a tendency to ulceration.

Cramps

Cramps may be of many kinds and often involve the calf muscle. This variety of cramp often occurs during the night. Intermittent claudication occurs in cases of atherosclerosis and results from insufficient blood to the leg muscles during exertion. Cramps are characterised by fairly sharp and severe pain to whatever part of the body is concerned.

Causes and Treatment

It is of continual surprise to the natural therapist that something so simple as the basic mineral deficiencies which cause cramps have been overlooked for so long by the majority of the medical profession. The main minerals involved are calcium and magnesium. A lack of either of these minerals can cause intense excitability and contraction of muscles in different parts of the body.

As these minerals have an antagonistic action to each other in the body, the skilled therapist must decide by clinical evaluation which is needed and in what form.[1] They may be required in crude or homoeopathic form, and are also present in many herbs such as valerian, vervain, cramp bark, and skullcap.[2]

Case History

Helga, aged fifty-seven, had suffered excruciating pain in the calf muscle for four months when she visited me in 1986. She lives in a housing commission flat, and the pain first occurred after walking up twelve flights of stairs during a lift breakdown. Some inflammation and swelling was present but this occurred after a rather poorly administered series of cortisone injections, and may not have been associated with the original problem. Physiotherapy had not helped.

Other problems included diverticulitis, anal fissure and constipation. Although these may seem unrelated to the problem, a basic mineral deficiency featured in all Helga's problems. The cramping of the calf muscle occurred after climbing up flights of steps, an activity which would have strained tendons and ligaments. The associated mineral deficiency was calcium fluoride; this mineral is necessary for healthy elastic tissue. The same deficiency is present in cases of diverticulitis — a condition resulting from formation of pouches in the bowel due to weakness of elastic tissue.

Treatment for the first month included iron phosphate for the inflammation, magnesium phosphate for spasm and cramp, calcium fluoride for the ligaments, and liver herbs to speed up metabolism of waste. B-complex and potassium phosphate were given for the nervous exhaustion caused by the incessant pain, and rheumatic herbs were included because it was considered that a rheumatic process may have started in the area following injury.

Over the first two months of treatment Helga felt much better generally and was free of pain for one or two weeks at a time. This gave her confidence to continue the treatment.

At this stage, I realised the cramp condition was the main factor, even though it may have started from other causes. During the next three months this factor was treated more specifically with larger doses of the magnesium compound and vitamin E was included to improve circulation through the calf muscle. Sodium phosphate was added to deal with any build-up of uric acid in the calf tissue, plus a selection of Bach flowers to work on the nerves which she said were still 'on edge'. A low potency of copper in homoeopathic form was included with the Bach drops to reverse the cramping tendency.

During the third and fourth months' treatment, Helga had no

pain in the leg at all and improvement has continued to the present, subsequent to the winding down of treatment.

Crohn's Disease

One of the greatest challenges to the natural therapist is to control severe inflammation of the bowel. These patients can only take small amounts of medication, and react very violently to anything as strong as herbs. I have found that for the first few months all work must be achieved by carefully selected minerals, and homoeopathics, and small doses of vitamins.

The most common inflammatory conditions which cause problems with the bowel are ulcerative colitis and Crohn's disease. In the latter, the problem is characterised by inflammation, thickening and narrowing in either the large or the small bowel. The inflammation causes diarrhoea and this may be associated with fever, exhaustion, and weight loss due to malabsorption. The greatest incidence of the problem occurs between fifteen and thirty-five years. In severe cases, the narrowing of the bowel can progress towards intestinal obstruction.

Causes

The inflammation is of unknown origin from the medical point of view. It is thought possible that an auto-immune factor may be present (see Auto-immune Disease). The inflammation extends through all layers of the intestinal wall and involves the adjacent lymph nodes.

From our point of view as natural therapists, biochemical imbalance is the key. This may have resulted from incorrect nutrition, possibly preceding the disease by many years. Extraordinary improvement through a few simple supplements and dietary changes underlies this point. One study revealed increased growth in children with Crohn's disease after changes were made to nutrition.[1] The involvement of lymph nodes in this disease indicates its toxic aspect which the natural therapist will be particularly concerned to treat.

Natural therapists must also consider the more subtle aspects involving the balance of the solar plexus *chakra* which governs all digestive processes. As mentioned in the information about constipation, emotional states have a direct influence, via this energy centre, on the autonomic nervous system. Any imbalance in this part of the nervous system can affect the peristaltic action of the bowel, causing diarrhoea or constipation. The inflammatory aspect of the disease is partly caused by toxaemia and is one reason why the associated lymph nodes are enlarged.

Medicine has long recognised the relationship between certain psychological states and chronic bowel inflammation. In Part 1, chapter 2, I describe the mechanism of relationship between emotional states and the final physical problem.

Treatment

1 Magnesium compounds for spasm.
2 Vitamin B-complex for toning nerves.
3 Iron phosphate for inflammation.
4 Selected homoeopathic remedies for liver and gastro-intestinal tract. [2]
5 Zinc to prevent adhesions.
6 Bach flower remedies to balance the solar plexus *chakra*.

Case History

Cheryl, aged thirty-five, had suffered from inflammation of the bowel for six years and had undergone two surgical procedures to remove part of her seriously affected bowel. She was having a great deal of pain still, in spite of the administration of cortisone and anti-inflammatory drugs over a period of twelve months. Her bowel actions numbered ten per day.

She was advised to change to the following diet: millet meal and mashed bananas for breakfast, at least two glasses of fresh juice daily (in this case a mixture of carrot, celery and apple was chosen), salad and lightly boiled egg for lunch, and vegetables and fish or other light protein such as bean curd for dinner. Her remedies included magnesium orotate in large doses to reduce bowel spasm, magnesium phosphate in homoeopathic potency to give a deeper acting effect for pain and spasm, small doses of B-complex, iron phosphate for inflammation of the bowel, and homoeopathic liver and bowel remedies. Bach flowers were also included.

After one month on the change of diet and treatment, pain had significantly diminished, indicating reduction of inflammation and spasm, and bowel actions were reduced from ten to two or three daily. She also had more energy. Improvement was maintained over the next ten months and during this time she reduced her cortisone to a very small dose without any relapse.

Cystitis

An acute inflammation of the bladder with frequent and painful urination characterises this infection. The inflammation commonly causes both blood and pus to be found in the urine. The condition is more common in females due to the shortness of the urethra from bladder to external opening or urethral meatus.

Causes

Commonly, these persons are found to encourage bacterial growth in the bladder as a result of acid/alkali imbalance in the body. They very often have diets predisposing them to very acid urine, for example, emphasis on refined flour and sugar, and on meat and cheese, with a lack of fresh vegetables. The iris is characteristically found to illustrate this acid state.

Treatment

Apart from correction of the life-style and diet, the following treatment usually clears the problem within forty-eight hours.

1   Iron phosphate to reduce inflammation, and sodium phosphate to promote alkalinity.
2   Soothing or demulcent herbs such as cornsilk, marshmallow, and others such as nettle and buchu which are commonly used for the bladder.
3   A buffered vitamin C which assists in iron absorption and kills bacteria.[1]
4   Specifically selected homoeopathics such as Cantharis for the burning and/or constitutional homoeopathics which are chosen to meet the individual needs of the patient.[2]

Case Histories

Mavis, aged sixty-one, had suffered recurrent cystitis for years and when she visited me in 1979 she was taking antibiotics continuously. Her medical history also included high blood pressure and a bout of convulsions during menopause. She was on anti-convulsant drugs for this tendency. Hay fever was another ailment.

The first prescription included iron phosphate for inflammation of the bladder, specific herbs for toning the bladder, sodium phosphate to make the urine more alkaline, vitamin C to eliminate bacteria and raise immunity, and a homoeopathic mixture which included Cantharis for bladder irritability.

On her first return visit Mavis reported that the bladder condition had greatly improved. She had another four months' treatment and remained in excellent health. Her long term antibiotics were safely discontinued. A recent phone call confirmed her continued remission from this ailment.

Glenda, aged twenty-nine, attended our clinic during 1980. She presented with a history of recurrent headache during the past year, asthma over a period of twenty years, and an 'acid' vaginal discharge which became more severe immediately prior to her menstrual period. Cystitis had been a problem a few months earlier and she had suffered a bout of nephritis at the age of ten. Her iris indicated a weakness in the left kidney and acid waste deposits in the tissues. Intermittent sinusitis completed her medical picture.

Her first month's treatment did not specifically address the cystitis as this did not flare up until a few weeks later. The history of both cystitis and vaginal discharge indicated that the body was burdened with some kind of acid waste which it was endeavouring to eliminate.

The first prescription included vitamin B-complex and mineral combination magnesium and potassium phosphate for headaches, sodium phosphate to buffer the acid tendency in the body, liver herbs to increase metabolism of toxic waste, and a mineral combination of iron phosphate and potassium chloride. The last mentioned mineral salts are always given for the first and second stage of any infection or inflammation such as occurs in both cystitis and vaginal discharge.

On her return visit, Glenda reported a few less headaches but she was on antibiotics for a severe attack of cystitis which included the passing of blood. Asthma was no better. If we had known about the cystitis manifesting at this point of time, it would have been possible to control it without antibiotics. It is preferable if clients contact us about problems which arise between their official visits to the clinic, although this is not always possible. The need for taking a comprehensive history at the first visit is illustrated here, as in Glenda's case she did not mention cystitis at the first visit.

The second month's treatment included the addition of large amounts of vitamin C in a buffered form (alkaline), and herbs for the bladder. The mineral combination for inflammation was increased to six times daily instead of three times. At her third visit, Glenda was able to report less headaches and no cystitis or asthma. The vaginal discharge was still present before the period.

Natural therapists find it is much easier to resolve health problems if the natural treatment is allowed to run a course without the use of antibiotics such as occurred in this case. Sometimes they are necessary for a short time if infection occurs before our treatment is fully underway. During the third month, Glenda was given the addition of garlic capsules for the vaginal discharge, vitamin B-complex was increased in strength, and rheumatic herbs were added for a joint condition of one shoulder.

At the next visit, no further cystitis was reported, but headaches and sinus remained plus a worsening condition of the shoulder. Adjustments were made to the treatment for these conditions. Glenda did not return so it is hard to say whether adjustments were successful, or whether she lost heart to continue the treatment. This case is a good example of the various ways of elimination which the body will attempt to use to unburden the system of waste.

The rheumatic problem with the shoulder indicated that in spite of our attempts at treatment, deeper structures of the body were starting to become affected by the acidity. The naturopathic interpretation is that the body was attempting to eliminate acid through sinus, vagina and bladder. Any bacteria or virus involved would be understood as a secondary factor.

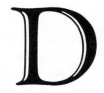

Depression

One of the most common statements made to natural therapists by clients is that they have come for a general check-up because of feeling generally low. These subclinical states are the sphere par excellence for natural remedies. Perhaps one should distinguish between the more basic insidious state known as endogenous depression, and that situation which afflicts all of us from time to time to a greater or lesser degree. The strains and stresses of modern life cause most people to suffer depression at some stage and as long as this is transient, the need for specific treatment may not arise.

Causes

These are manifold but include in particular, deficiencies of the B-complex group, a water soluble vitamin easily destroyed in cooking, and the mineral salts of potassium phosphate and magnesium phosphate. These particular nutrients are found to become depleted during times of stress, and may need to be supplemented at these periods.

Other causes can be lack of fresh air and sunshine. Recent research on the pineal gland suggests that some people are very sensitive to the lack of light which occurs during the winter months. They suffer a tangible and biochemical depression during the winter months due to a deficiency in secretion of the pineal gland.[1]

Treatment

1 B-complex vitamins especially thiamine or B1, to counteract depression.[2]

2 Potassium and magnesium phosphate as a nerve tonic.
3 Liver herbs to help metabolise toxins which may be contributing to the problem.
4 Bach flower remedies for depression; examples are gorse and mustard. Others may be needed according to the associated emotions.
5 A variety of homoeopathics depending on the constitution of the client.[3]

Case History

Claire is a trained nurse who lives and works in a country town. She suffered a severe depression and had felt suicidal at times, and she noticed an aggravation before each menstrual period. Headaches occurred nearly every day and were more severe in the second half of the menstrual cycle. There was an associated numbness down the left side of the face accompanied by deafness. Asthma had featured earlier in her life. Other problems included constipation and continual tiredness, with exhaustion exacerbated by unpleasantly vivid dreams. Her diet was fairly good by naturopathic standards.

After a month on potassium and magnesium phosphate to relax and tone the nerves, accompanied by B-complex, herbal sedatives, and liver herbs for cleansing and stimulating the bowel, Claire was less depressed, suffered less headaches, no numbness and more energy. Improvement continued over the next few months, with a setback of tiredness following gastric influenza. Some digestive symptoms came to the surface, and these were mainly treated via the solar plexus and nervous system with a repeat of the original prescription plus Bach flower remedies. The latter therapy is fairly specific for subtle problems with the energy centres.

Claire has felt very stabilised for two years now and makes occasional visits to our clinic for a check-up and repeat of maintenance doses of those supplements which keep her in balance.

Dermatitis

Dermatitis simply means inflammation of the skin. It is a term used very often for dry, red itching skin occurring in adults, commonly accompanied by flaking or peeling of the skin. The term eczema is more likely to be used in the case of a weeping eruption, especially that occurring in childhood.

Causes

The immediate causes of dermatitis are many and include reactions to contact with certain plants and chemicals. It may also be induced by ingestion of food to which the patient is allergic, and by reactions to particular bacteria.

The natural therapist searches more deeply to find why the client has reacted so violently to a particular metal such as nickel, or dyes, or particular foods.[1] In the case of reactions to foods, the health of the digestive system is examined, especially that of the pancreas, liver, and the colon or large bowel. In the case of reactions to chemicals it has been found that, for example, a deficiency of selenium may be the underlying cause for skin reaction.[2]

Therapists working in the psychological realm have examined the interesting possibility that as the skin is the organ which separates us from the external world, a chronically inflamed skin may perhaps also result from our inability to cope with the outside world. In this case we may react in a hypersensitive way to outside factors. The phrase 'thin skinned' may be applicable here, but should only be considered seriously after all physical factors have been evaluated.

Treatment

As the skin is an organ of elimination, the natural therapist is concerned to make sure that all the eliminative organs of the body are in working order. Special focus is placed on the liver for it is the organ which must handle and detoxify all chemicals which enter the body either as drugs, insecticides, or chemicals from the work environment. Herbs are the main treatment for detoxification and for toning the organs.

Minerals are given as tissue salts or in homoeopathic form to reduce inflammation and remove deficiencies which may have contributed to the problem. Homoeopathic treatment can have outstanding results for long-term skin diseases and its successful application is possibly the best test for a skilled homoeopath.

Vitamins also have an important role in skin disorders. Examples of treatment would be:

1 Liver herbs for promoting more rapid detoxification in the body.
2 Lymphatic herbs for drainage of toxins.
3 Vitamin C for detoxification and for promoting the immune system.
4 Vitamin B-complex for toning the nervous system. There are very many nerve endings in the skin.
5 Mineral salts such as iron phosphate for reducing inflammation, and potassium sulphate for flaking and scaling. Zinc, selenium, and silica may also be needed depending on the particular indications.
6 Specific homoeopathic remedies.[3]

Case Histories

Maureen, aged forty-two, visited me in 1984 with dermatitis on the hands. She had suffered this for twenty years. There were deep cracks in the skin. Her previous medical history involved a partial thyroidectomy. Diet was only fair and she was a coffee drinker. Other life-style problems included smoking twenty-five cigarettes daily. The iris revealed toxic deposits in the lymph system, kidney weakness and digestive disturbances.

In the case of Maureen, the first prescription included calcium phosphate to make up severe deficiencies of this salt which were noted in the iris. The mineral combination of iron phosphate and potassium chloride was given for the inflammation and weeping of the skin on the hands. Liver herbs were administered for improving metabolism of waste, and lymphatic herbs for cleansing. Vitamins A, B-complex and C were also included. A homoeopathic dose of Mezereum completed the month's regime.

On her second visit, Maureen reported considerable improvement after the second dose of Mezereum, but she had a pronounced crisis involving infection of the broken skin of the hands. With smokers the circulation of all extremities is impaired and this infection had to be dealt with fairly quickly as there was a danger of it worsening. The cleansing herbs were increased, as was the dose of vitamin C. Potassium sulphate was added in both crude and homoeopathic doses as this works well on infections in people suited constitutionally to this salt.

Maureen was informed that if the infection did not clear in forty-eight hours she would need medical antibiotics. She did have recourse to medical treatment, and after the infection cleared her improvement continued undisturbed. It is likely, however, that unless the life-style is changed, especially the smoking, the problem will recur.

Shirley is a law clerk. She visited me with very bad dermatitis on the hands and feet in her fifty-eighth year. She had an extremely stressful job and was a heavier smoker than the previous case as she smoked sixty per day. Her dermatitis had commenced with an allergy to rubber experienced twenty years earlier. In summer months, her feet swelled badly and she was currently taking diuretics from a medical doctor. She had been taking garlic and kelp on her own initiative.

The first prescription included 3g of vitamin C powder daily to help counteract the smoking and to detoxify the body, lymphatic draining and liver herbs, yeast tablets as a nerve tonic, herbs to relax the nervous system, iron phosphate for inflammation of the skin, potassium chloride for the weeping and oozing of the skin, and calcium phosphate.

Shirley improved after a few weeks on this regime and improvement continued over the next few months. Another mineral compound was introduced to help control cracking of the heels; this compound included calcium fluoride. The mineral compound sodium sulphate was later given to balance fluids in the body. In all, Shirley had nine months' treatment and stayed in good health and with almost complete remission of the dermatitis. Some attempt was made to give up smoking towards the end of her treatment period. As with the previous client, it is likely that a relapse will occur unless the smoking problem is resolved.

This is a good case to illustrate how, in spite of stress and inadequate life-style in terms of the smoking, considerable improvement to a distressing condition can take place with natural therapies. With dermatitis, there is not the same emphasis or need for homoeopathic prescribing as with eczema cases. This is because we find that the problem in eczema is more likely to be inherited, whereas many dermatitis cases are brought about through environmental factors such as allergy or life-style. It needs to be explained, however, that many cases which we would class as ezcema are called dermatitis, and vice versa. A careful case history is needed to distinguish between the two problems.

Diabetes

Diabetes is of two types. The description here will be confined to the common type which is called *diabetes mellitus*, usually known as sugar diabetes. This can be further subdivided into insulin-dependent diabetes which often occurs by the age of forty, and mature-onset diabetes, commonly occurring in middle age or later. The latter type is usually non-insulin dependent and develops from poor eating habits.

Heredity plays a part in most *diabetes mellitus* but is more pronounced in the heredity of mature-age diabetes. In both types the disease is characterised by an inability of the pancreas to produce insulin, the hormone which is chiefly responsible for regulating blood sugar. Diabetics develop a very abnormal blood sugar curve with high levels of blood sugar for most of the time. Mature-onset diabetes features more circulating insulin as the pancreatic cells are less likely to be destroyed.

The symptoms resulting from this excess of sugar often include great thirst, excessive urine, exhaustion, and weight loss, especially in young people. As the disease progresses, chronic infections of the extremities are common, plus circulatory problems especially in older people. Unless appropriate medical treatment is instituted, coma and death may occur.

Causes

In the insulin-dependent type, which affects the minority, destruction of the cells which produce insulin in the pancreas is taking or has taken place. It is thought that viral activity followed by destructive antibodies may be one cause. Particular chemicals which have a destructive effect on the pancreas are another cause.

The non-insulin dependent type, which comprises 90 per cent of diabetics, appears to be more associated with the typical Western diet, which is high in refined carbohydrates. Obesity is often a key factor in this type. It is estimated that 1 per cent of the population of the USA are diabetic and that cases are increasing by 6 per cent per year.[1] It has been observed that as cultures previously eating more natural diets switch to the typical Western diet, their rate of diabetes increases.[2]

One interesting chain of events has been put forward as a theory explaining mature-onset diabetes. This concept has been examined by a few of the orthomolecular medical doctors. These physicians consider that, particularly in the case of mature-age diabetes, the causative factor may be hypoglycaemia in early life caused by faulty diet. This theory is explained as an initial over-stimulation of the pancreas through the constant intake of refined sugary foods. Over a period of years this is considered to exhaust the cells of the pancreas which produce insulin. The initial reaction of the body is to produce so much insulin that the blood is actually lacking in sugar, hence the term hypoglycaemia or low blood sugar. The craving for sugar is understood to relate to deficiencies of zinc, chromium, magnesium and the B-complex group and certainly these supplements have been found useful in both hypoglycaemia and diabetes.

The following chain of events may occur: deficiencies causing craving for sugar; over-stimulation of pancreas causing low blood sugar; exhaustion of pancreas leading to diabetes. The large increase of diabetes in our society, and amongst native people when they adopt a Western diet, indicates that this chain of events is logical.[3] It may also explain why diabetes is constantly increasing amongst affluent societies.

One can then go further back in the chain and examine more subjective causes. The relation of the pancreas to the energy centre known as the solar plexus has already been discussed. The solar plexus is the most active energy centre in mankind today and is the inner organ associated with all our desires. It is intimately associated with all digestive processes in the body, and due to its constant activity, easily gets out of balance. The final physical result is over- or under-stimulation of the various digestive organs and secretions.

In the case of diabetes, there is an obvious under-secretion and this follows an imbalance of energy flowing through this particular centre. The reader may wonder how this accounts for juvenile diabetes. The concept of reincarnation may assist us to understand. Young children with serious chronic diseases can be expressing disease patterns which have been conditioned by a previous life. In the case of diabetes, there may have been a serious emotional disturbance in a previous life which was not resolved and which continues to cause an imbalance in the solar plexus centre. The incarnating soul will be attracted to parents who will give an inherited disposition suitable to the working out of the inner causes. The final expression of this situation is poor development of the pancreas early in the life, perhaps triggered by environmental factors.

The emotional suppression or repression affecting the energy centre in diabetes is often very deep-seated, and far greater than the temporary disturbance which causes a host of milder digestive disorders. There are many cases of diabetes on record following a severe emotional shock. These are the more obvious causes of changes to the solar plexus *chakra*.

Treatment

As these patients must be regularly monitored for their insulin requirements, the natural therapist can assist the general health of the patient by working with the doctor. In Australia it is illegal for natural therapists to treat diabetes. In some cases, following general improvement, the doctor has been able to reduce the amount of insulin.

The following supplements and approaches have been found useful:

1 An increase of exercise. It has been discovered that the insulin receptors on cells are improved 30 per cent by a regular exercise programme.[4]
2 Large doses of vitamin C. These have been found to reduce insulin requirements.[5]
3 A number of herbs which have a toning effect on the pancreas, for example, jambol.[6]
4 Vitamin E to reduce circulatory problems.
5 Minerals such as potassium phosphate, chromium, and zinc.[7]
6 Bach flower remedies which can work directly on the solar plexus centre.
7 Nutritional changes are enormously important and the effect of increasing fibre in the diet has been well documented.[8] Many mature-onset diabetic conditions have been resolved by removing all refined foods and replacing those foods with slow release complex carbohydrates, and a variety of vegetables. Dietary changes in diabetics must be strictly monitored by appropriately trained persons.

Case History

Sue, aged thirty-six, was diagnosed as a diabetic at the age of twenty-four. The immediate onset of the problem occurred following a uterine haemorrhage at the time of a 'miscarriage'. Her excessive thirst, weight loss, and polyuria was misdiagnosed following her curette as anaemia, in spite of the fact that her brother was also diabetic. When first treated at our clinic she was on forty units of insulin daily, thirty in the morning and ten at night. Her condition was not stable and she suffered frequent hypoglycaemic and hyperinsulin states. Other problems included vaginal monilia.

The iris indicated typical disturbances to the autonomic part of the nervous system, and fairly heavy lymphatic congestion which would account for the monilia. There were some weaknesses indicated in the digestive organs of both liver and pancreas. Of particular interest to me was the diagnosis of pancreatic weakness using the Vega instrument, and a subsequent vastly improved reading which was taken after less than one month of treatment.

Her treatment commenced with jambol tincture, one of the herbs for the pancreas. This had a fairly dramatic effect with temporary exacerbation of glucose imbalance. After two weeks, however, she was able to discontinue the evening insulin injection. She had been interested in natural therapies for some time and was already on multi-vitamin and mineral tablets, including zinc. A herbal liver tonic, chromium supplement, potassium and magnesium phosphate, and homoeopathic drops for the pancreas were added.

Initially, the liver herbs caused a temporary disturbance in glucose levels and digestion but this soon passed. The monilia disappeared, and Sue has reported feeling better and more stabilised than in years. Of great relief to her is the disappearance of sugar craving. Recently, her constitutional homoeopathic remedy was established and Natrum sulphate in the 200th potency was given twice weekly. This is clearing up a stubborn dermatitis on the hands and has also resulted in a further reduction of her daily insulin.

Diarrhoea

This condition will be discussed in the context of the more

simple forms which are generally met in clinical practice. These are usually caused by an infective organism, particularly in children, or by an imbalance of the autonomic nervous system leading to nervous diarrhoea.

The trained natural therapist is able to distinguish between or identify those dangerous gastro-intestinal infections in babies and young children whose severity may cause states of dehydration. These may need urgent medical attention with hydration therapy. More commonly, bouts of diarrhoea occur which are accompanied by nausea and vomiting, and are characterised by griping abdominal pains and repeated bowel actions. Alternatively, symptoms may be chronic, extending over a period of time with less severity.

Causes

Acute attacks of diarrhoea are usually triggered by an infective organism, either bacteria or virus, and run a short course of one to two days. As usual, the natural therapist understands the infection as a secondary factor. The primary factor is lack of immunity through low levels of vitamin C, a weakened mucosa of the gastro-intestinal tract which may result from disturbed intestinal flora or bacteria, mineral and vitamin deficiencies, and poor function of the liver and pancreas.

The primary causes explain why individuals suffer varied reactions following infection. There can be mild nausea and stomach pains, without actual vomiting or diarrhoea, while in severe cases dehydration from excessive vomiting and diarrhoea may take place. In severe cases, natural therapists would consider immunity had been in a lowered state prior to infection.

With more chronic forms of diarrhoea, the nervous system is involved and increased peristaltic action or bowel movement is closely related to an imbalance in the autonomic nervous system. This part of our nerve function, not being under the control of the brain, is more difficult to influence. It can, however, be profoundly influenced by meditation and various relaxation techniques.

The understanding of the subtle counterpart of the nervous system is of great value in chronic diarrhoea. It is worthwhile to study the relationship of the solar plexus energy centre to the whole digestive process. The reader is referred also to Crohn's Disease for relevant comments on this area. If the problem of chronic diarrhoea is not resolved, then it may move towards chronic inflammatory bowel disease.

Treatment

Considerable emphasis is placed on the diet in both acute and chronic cases. The best way to start in both situations is with freshly extracted vegetable juices or diluted fruit juices. This rests the bowel, provides plenty of vitamin C and enzymes to improve the state of the mucus membrane lining the bowel, and provides natural sugars to keep energy at reasonable levels.

In acute cases, one to two days on eight glasses of juice daily is sufficient, with a maximum of four days for more chronic cases. The juice fast must be broken very gently, especially in chronic cases, usually by taking small helpings of fresh ripe fruit and natural yoghurt. Steamed vegetables and well-cooked whole grain cereals should feature later in the day.

In chronic cases, the therapist must attempt to eliminate from the diet all foods likely to produce allergy. These may include foods which the average person considers healthy, but which are not tolerated by the person in question. Later, when the pancreas and liver have been suitably strengthened, these foods may be tolerated on a rotational basis, excepting of course, foods which are known to be generally detrimental to the body. For example, coffee, alcohol, refined sugar, salted peanuts and other foods commonly labelled junk foods, would be allowed only occasionally.

Case Histories

Diarrhoea is one of those problems which clears up quite easily with natural therapies, provided there is no deep-seated or complicating factor. Anne, aged fifty-one, had intermittent loose bowels and was suffering from nausea and lack of appetite. She also had some pain and discomfort in the bowel area, and had lost four kilograms.

After two months on magnesium phosphate to relax the nerves, potassium phosphate to tone the nerves, and a selection of homoeopathic herbs and minerals for her particular type of diarrhoea, plus B-complex as a general nerve tonic, she had no further digestive problems. She was also given treatment for insomnia, as the underlying nerve tension associated with this problem was no doubt related to the bowel condition. Hence the natural therapist is making decisions based on the underlying cause of the disease and is seeking to define the overall problem. In this case, it would not have been sufficient to treat the bowel problem in a local sense only.

The specific treatment would be similar for any inflammatory bowel disease but probably would extend over a shorter period. In the case of young children and acute cases in adults only the following few remedies are needed:

1 Iron phosphate in small amounts for the inflammation.
2 Magnesium phosphate or orotate for spasm.[1]
3 Digestive homoeopathics for liver, bowel, and stomach (fluid extracts of herbs should not be given as they are too laxative).[2]

Patricia, aged twenty-five, was another typical case who responded well to treatment over a period of seven months. She attended me for recurrent viruses of the gastro-intestinal tract. Symptoms included nausea plus a flushed feeling. She admitted to a diet lacking in raw food such as fruit or salad. Treatment for the first month included iron phosphate, vitamin C, a herbal liver tablet and homoeopathic liver drops, vitamin A and a high potency vitamin B-complex.

On her return visit she reported one virus but said it lasted only a day. The prescription was repeated with the addition of a mixture containing lymphatic herbs for a sore throat. The following month she remained well but during the fourth month she suffered a bad bout of influenza-like symptoms. This is a common occurrence during the first few months of naturopathic treatment. Treatment was continued during the next three months and Patricia remained well and free from gastric disturbances. During the treatment time she gradually reformed her diet. In this case there was no need for the magnesium supplement as although the whole gastro-intestinal tract was affected, there was not much emphasis on diarrhoea.

Diverticulitis

Many of the comments about diarrhoea and constipation also

apply in this condition. Similar dietary causes, subjective factors and stress factors are at work. There is however an added problem. A diverticulum is a small or large pouch in the bowel wall caused by loss of elastic tissue. These pouches are clearly seen in X-rays following a barium enema, and evidence may also be supplied by iris diagnosis.

Causes

Constipation may seem to be the most obvious cause, and yet it is of interest that not all lifelong sufferers of constipation suffer from diverticulitis. Of more significant concern is the mineral salt deficiency which results in loss of elastic tissue; this salt is calcium fluoride. The reader may surmise that fluoridation of water supplies will cause the condition to disappear. Unfortunately the addition of crude fluoride does not have the same effect as calcium fluoride in homoeopathic or tissue salt preparation.[1]

In clinical practice by natural therapists, the problem of adequate assimilation of the calcium salts is found to include an inherited factor. Hence treatment can be needed over a long period. The actual inflammation which occurs in the pouches is the main cause for concern in both orthodox and naturopathic disciplines. The name relates to inflammation of the diverticulum.

Treatment

The main emphasis will be on improving the diet, promoting suitable forms of exercise, promoting adequate elimination through the bowel, and reducing the inflammation present in the pouches. Long-range goals would seek to improve the elastic tissue. Specific supplements may include:

1 Liver, lymphatic, and astringent herbs.
2 Vitamin C for detoxification in conjunction with the herbs.
3 Iron phosphate with vitamin C assists in reduction of inflammation.
4 Vitamin B-complex for toning of nerves which in turn control bowel movements.
5 Calcium fluoride in various types of preparation for gradually restoring elastic tissue.
6 Magnesium and potassium phosphates to help balance autonomic nerve impulses to the bowel.

Down's Syndrome

This is a genetic condition involving an extra chromosome in the cells of the patient. It occurs more commonly in children whose parents are over forty at the time of conception. In a genetic condition involving the numbers of chromosomes, the role of the natural therapist is to improve the general health, as it is not possible to reverse the condition.

Treatment

To improve the general health, children with Down's syndrome respond to supplements which promote health of the endocrine glands and the nervous system. For some reason the lymphatic system of these children is often very congested as indicated by particular markings in the iris. Suggestions for supplements are as follows:

1 Vitamins C and B-complex.
2 Minerals such as zinc, magnesium and potassium phosphate.[1]
3 Herbs to detoxify the lymphatics.
4 Homoeopathic complexes to act as tonics for the endocrine glands.

Case History

I recollect only one case of Down's syndrome in my practice. It was of interest that his mother mentioned how medical persons had noticed prominent white flecks in the iris of these children. It is these white 'beads' around the edge of the iris which have been correlated to lymphatic congestion by iridologists.

This particular small client was given lymphatic cleansing homoeopathic drops, herbal drops for the liver, and magnesium phosphate and potassium phosphate for general nerve toning. The teacher at his special school noticed a definite improvement in his well-being while on treatment.

Ear Infections

Ear infections are very prevalent in children following upper respiratory tract infections. Repeated infections produce deafness in the child and this is a major problem today. Children often complain of pain in the ear during or following a cold, but this is not always the case, especially where the condition has become chronic. There may be sensations of blockage and catarrh in the ear, and the cervical lymph nodes are usually enlarged.

Causes

The immediate cause is an infective organism which follows a cold virus or other infectious disorder such as measles. Natural therapists believe ear infections are more common today due to faulty life-style involving diet, and to the mishandling of infectious disorders. Allergy to dairy produce is a major contributing factor to long-standing mucus problems, and an imbalanced diet with over-emphasis on refined foods causes accumulation of toxic waste.[1] This waste forms the breeding ground for bacteria which follow a virus infection.

Treatment

1 Improved nutrition includes eliminating dairy produce and refined foods and increasing the intake of vegetables, fruits, and whole grain foods.
2 Herbs in crude or homoeopathic form to cleanse the lymphatic system.

3 Herbs or homoeopathic remedies to tone the liver so metabolism is improved.
4 Iron phosphate and potassium chloride to reduce inflammation of lymph nodes and to reduce inflammation and mucus.
5 Vitamin C to improve immunity, and to reduce mucus.
6 Specific homoeopathic remedies for the ear.

Case History

Ben, aged four, was a typical example, representing dozens of children who visit our clinic with otitis media or infected middle ears. These problems usually start with a common cold, and this was the case with Ben. His treatment included calcium phosphate, iron phosphate and potassium chloride for the inflammation and for reducing mucus, vitamin C, homoeopathic lymphatic drainage remedies, and specific homoeopathic drops for the ear. These contained Hepar sulphuris, Pulsatilla, and Capsicum in suitable potencies.

The ears became rapidly resistant to infection and did not relapse during the course of subsequent colds. Treatment was continued for some months on a reduced scale, and small alterations made to meet various changes in health needs.

Eczema

A number of aspects involving this problem have been discussed already in relation to dermatitis. More children are affected with eczema, and the inherited factor features most strongly. Perhaps the main clinical variation from dermatitis is the severe itch which nearly always accompanies eczema. According to the 10th edition of *Harrison's Principles of Internal Medicine*, over 30 per cent of eczema patients develop respiratory allergic manifestations.[1]

Causes

Environmental factors such as pollution, foods, chemicals, and stress can act as triggers.[2] Other problems are poor elimination through weakness of liver and/or kidneys and sluggishness of bowel and skin. These latter problems may be inherited and often accompany a particular constitution which predisposes towards chronic skin ailments.[3] As part of this inherited tendency in cases of childhood eczemas, natural therapists often find a lack of assimilation of important minerals such as calcium.

Treatment

The treatment of skin conditions by the natural therapist varies more from the orthodox approach than in any other condition. Any form of treatment which is suppressive such as cortisone, tar ointments, or even mild anti-inflammatory agents such as calomine lotion is strictly avoided. Eczema is treated as a toxic condition which involves an inherited factor. Treatment is directed to improving elimination through bowel, kidney, and skin, and to improving detoxification by toning the liver. Constitutional homoeopathic treatment is essential in all cases, otherwise any relief gained through natural remedies may only be temporary.

Specific treatment will be predominantly the same as for dermatitis; however, as mentioned, calcium salts may be needed, especially in children. Homoeopathic treatment features more strongly than in cases of dermatitis. In keeping with the constitutional emphasis associated with eczema, treatment may be needed over a long period of time, perhaps for two years.

Case Histories

The following case is of interest because it indicates the familial incidence and manifestation of eczema plus the classical response of the skin to natural treatment. Martha, aged thirty-nine, attended the clinic with an itchy bout of dry eczema which she had suffered for three weeks and which was rapidly spreading. She has a placid temperament and her diet was fairly good. There was nothing one could pin-point in her environment to account for the outbreak of the skin condition.

Her treatment for the first two weeks included iron phosphate for the inflammation, calcium phosphate for an observed deficiency of same, lymphatic herbs for cleansing, liver herbs and vitamin C to help detoxify the body, and vitamin B-complex as a general nerve tonic. Homoeopathic sulphur was given in low potencies to help itching, and the patient was advised that the condition would temporarily worsen after ceasing cortisone creams and commencing natural medication.

By the third week, as expected, the condition was much stimulated with raw surfaces and enlargement of the affected area. Lymphatic and liver herbs were increased and homoeopathic Arsenicum in 10M potency was administered on the new indications which emerged after the basic cleansing had commenced. Her healing crisis included congestion of the kidneys with severely reduced output of urine.

On the third visit, after four weeks treatment, she reported that the rash was diminishing in cycles, and that the urinary output had been restored after one day. A bad patch of eczema remained between her thighs near some varicose veins. A number of moles on the body had begun to change and new ones were developing. This illustrates how after one inherited tendency is treated another tends to come to the surface. The same basic prescription was repeated with the addition of low potency homoeopathic remedies for the veins, and homoeopathic Thuja was found to be the most suitable remedy for the moles.

After a further two weeks, Martha reported the rash almost gone. The moles had ceased to grow further, and she was well in all respects. She then came at longer intervals on reduced treatment and this was tapered off after six months.

Martha then became pregnant and had a healthy boy whom she brought to the clinic with a condition of the scalp called cradle cap. He also had patches of eczema on the face. This is rapidly clearing under treatment. The family incidence is obviously repeating itself, but through treatment shortly following birth, this new family member will probably be saved problems in later life. Martha herself has not suffered any relapse.

Tony had a bad bout of eczema on the legs and arms which was very itchy, and which had commenced two weeks previously. He had been suffering from pressure at home and work and was feeling run down and nervous. Sleep was poor.

In his case the eczema cleared very quickly with basic remedies and without constitutional treatment. The treatment included lymphatic cleansing and liver herbs, vitamins A, C and B-complex. Magnesium phosphate and potassium phosphate were given for the nervous stress.

Emphysema

The most noticeable problem with this condition is shortness of breath particularly on exertion. This difficulty is caused by loss of elasticity and dilatation of the lung tissue so that the patient cannot exhale without using a great effort. Usually patients are elderly but the condition may begin in youth or middle-age depending on previous respiratory problems.

Causes

The more obvious causes are long-standing asthma or recurrent bouts of bronchitis. The natural therapist, however, as discussed when dealing with bronchiectasis, understands that mineral deficiencies in the calcium group predispose towards weakened bronchial and lung tissue. These deficiencies are often causes of the original tendency towards bronchitis or asthma, in addition to the more subjective factors discussed in relation to asthma.

Other contributing factors may be air pollution, smoking and a congested lymphatic system which will add to the burden of trying to drain the lungs of mucus. Poor diet further predisposes towards accumulation of mucus.

Treatment

This is a very difficult condition to reverse. Natural therapies can help prevent infection of the lungs, and can improve the general health and energy of the patient. Treatment would of necessity extend over many years, and in younger patients may restore some of the elastic tissue of the lung sacs.

Therapies used would be similar to that for bronchiectasis except for the individual homoeopathic prescribing, plus the fact that each patient is given a combination of remedies which is to some extent individual. From a naturopathic point of view, emphysema is considered to be a more deep-seated disease process than loss of elastic tissue in the bronchial tree, as in bronchiectasis.

The same basic procedures occur in each — clearing out the

lymphatic system, removing mineral deficiencies, improving the immune system, and endeavouring to replace the elasticity of bronchial or lung tissue.

Endometriosis

Of many conditions which may interfere with the quality of a woman's life, and for which medical science has not really found any satisfactory answer, endometriosis is a regular challenge to the natural therapist. The main problems are intermittent pain throughout each menstrual cycle, and infertility is common. Most clients come for treatment having already undergone a laparoscopy which has demonstrated the presence of endometriosis in various parts of the pelvic cavity.

The tissue involved develops outside the uterine wall away from where it naturally belongs, and is usually cystic and haemorrhagic.[1] Such tissue is under hormonal control and therefore bleeds into the pelvic cavity each month. This is the main reason for the pain suffered in severe cases. Adhesions can easily form and involve the bowel and fallopian tubes. The uterus itself is often involved with unhealthy endometrial tissue which includes the presence of cysts which infiltrate the uterine wall. The uterus becomes enlarged and infertile.

Causes

Medical science has not discovered why the endometrial tissue is found both within and outside the peritonial cavity in some women, nor why it develops metaplastic changes in both the uterus and organs and tissues outside the uterus. Natural therapists are mainly concerned with possible biochemical imbalances and with toxic factors involving the lymphatic system. They are also interested in the homoeopathic theory of inherited miasms. The inherited miasm for this problem involves gonorrhoea at some stage in the family tree. This chain of events has been explored in connection with vaginal discharge. In the case of the type of cystic formation occurring in endometriosis, this is attributed to the sycotic or gonorrhoeal taint. It involves inability in the person to assimilate calcium adequately, plus the formation of cysts. Treatment is directed to these problems. At the subjective level, this area is that controlled by the sacral *chakra* and there may be imbalances of energy in this centre.

Treatment

1 Lymphatic cleansing herbs over a long period of time to cleanse the pelvic area of waste.
2 Zinc compound for adhesions if present.
3 Potassium chloride and iron phosphate for bleeding and swelling of tissue.
4 Calcium phosphate is the main mineral for cystic tendency.
5 Vitamin C for its effect on producing healthy collagen tissue.
6 Homoeopathic remedies for regulating the hormones.
7 Constitutional homoeopathic prescribing for the inherited miasm.

Case History

The following case is included from the files of my husband. It is an outstanding example of the possibilities of natural therapies in re-establishing normality in cases of endometriosis. Karen, a teacher aged twenty-nine, was told by her medical specialist that she was the worst case of endometriosis he had ever seen and that she would never conceive. She first visited our clinic in March 1985.

Apart from the endometriosis and apparent infertility, problems included recurrent sore throats, enlarged lymph glands and constipation at period times. An early history of childhood eczema confirmed that lymphatic involvement and congestion had existed from an early age. Facial hairs indicated some hormonal imbalance apart from the endometriosis. It was interesting that she had suffered from plantar warts as this is a sure indication of the inherited miasm mentioned.

Over a period of nine months, Karen had the following supplements. Iron phosphate for the bleeding, potassium chloride and calcium phosphate for the cysts, magnesium and potassium phosphate for nerve toning, lymphatic cleansing and liver herbs, and homoeopathic and herbal remedies to regulate the menstrual cycle and hormones. She was also given homoeopathic Thuja for the inherited aspect of the problem.

She was overjoyed to become pregnant after nine months of treatment as she had been trying to conceive for seven years. Treatment was continued throughout the pregnancy and she continued her work as a music teacher until seven months pregnant. There were no complications and a healthy boy was born.

Epilepsy

Epilepsy is of several kinds, although causes from both the subjective and physical angle may be similar. The most famous type, 'grand-mal', is characterised by strong convulsions which occur after the patient falls unconscious. A milder form features momentary loss of concentration and awareness and is known as 'petit-mal'. There is also a variation in symptoms according to the particular part of the brain which is affected.

Epilepsy may affect people of all ages, more often than not commencing before adulthood around the age of puberty. It can also occur following a physical accident. A family history of epilepsy in first or second degree relatives is obtained in about 30 per cent of all patients. [1]

Causes

In addition to the constitutional factor mentioned, predisposing factors include pre-natal disorders, birth injuries, and neo-natal disturbances. Other precipitating causes are known to be stress, exhaustion, and hypoglycaemia.

The natural therapist would add the possibility of mineral deficiencies such as magnesium, calcium and zinc. [2] These deficiencies when present from birth may be closely linked to the constitutional metabolic problems. A deficiency of B6 in spite of a diet containing the B group is another common finding. [3]

In reflecting on the more subjective causes of epilepsy, this brief lack of consciousness is considered to result from a weakness of the etheric body in its relation to the physical body. As the more subtle part of our physical body, the etheric substands the gross physical structure, but is nevertheless an inherited component of our nature.

In esoteric teaching about the etheric constitution, two threads of energy are known to link our vehicles of consciousness and higher self with the physical body. The thread of consciousness is linked near the pineal gland in the brain, and is withdrawn temporarily during sleep, and permanently at death. The life-thread is anchored in the heart, and is only withdrawn at death. In epilepsy, the consciousness thread is considered to be periodically and abruptly withdrawn due to a weakness in the etheric. This distinguishes the process of epilepsy from that of sleep which tends to be more under our control and from which we can be aroused.

Treatment

This is one of the conditions that a natural therapist should not treat unless the patient is also under the supervision of a registered medical practitioner. Fortunately there are increasing numbers of medical doctors who are prepared to co-operate with natural therapists.

I have found that many epileptics have bad acne and this coincides with the fact that the lymphatic system in epileptics is noticed by iris diagnosis and palpation to be congested. A cleansing diet is fairly important with an emphasis on raw salad, steamed vegetables, whole grain cereals, light protein such as fat-free cheese, almonds, bean curd and white meat.

Specific remedies may include the following:

1 Magnesium or calcium salts depending on the indications.
2 Vitamin B-complex group and vitamin C.
3 Antispasmodic herbs such as valerian, vervain, passaflora, and mistletoe.
4 Liver herbs, and possibly lymphatic cleansing herbs if indicated.
5 Specific homoeopathics for the individual constitution.
6 Zinc if indicated.
7 Bach flower remedies to work on the etheric level.

Case History

Kathy, aged twenty-three, was brought by her boyfriend to the clinic after he enquired whether we could help epilepsy. His whole family had been treated by my husband on and off since he was a young boy. Kathy had been advised to have an exploratory investigation with electrodes implanted in her brain. It was expected that this would show up areas of the brain which could be amenable to surgery.

Kathy was not suffering from grand-mal, but had about four petit-mal attacks per day which lasted from one to thirty minutes. They began when she was seventeen following a skating accident. The petit-mal was also associated with panic attacks. Her memory and appetite were both poor, but this was not surprising considering her heavy medication, and she suffered from tension headaches. The proposed investigation and possible surgery seemed a drastic approach to petit-mal epilepsy, and Kathy was keen to try natural medicine first.

I would judge Kathy's general health as probably poor before the skating accident, and any mineral deficiencies would be exacerbated at that time. Our approach is to tone the general health of the patient, rather than to treat the epilepsy as such. Findings in Kathy's iris indicated considerable deficiencies in magnesium, potassium and calcium, plus an accumulation of toxic waste in the lymphatic system. The liver appeared to be in a sluggish state.

After a month on magnesium phosphate, potassium phosphate, vitamins B and C, and a homoeopathic mixture, her attacks had reduced from over one hundred per month to ten, and there had been no panic attacks. Memory and appetite had also improved.

After ten months, Kathy continues to improve and will probably be able to taper off both naturopathic and also medical treatment under supervision, providing that her doctor agrees. At present she is having only four attacks per month.

Fibroids

Fibroids are benign tumours which may occur in various parts of the body, but most commonly occur in the uterus. They vary greatly in size from that of an almond to several kilograms. Associated problems are heavy bleeding from the uterus, pressure symptoms and sterility. Occurrence of fibroids is more likely in women from thirty-five to fifty years old, although they can occur in younger women.

Causes

My understanding of this condition is quite different from standard medical theory. Fibroids are a toxic condition whereby the body attempts to wall off waste in a place which is not life threatening to the individual. Natural therapists recognise an inherited factor and this expresses through a sluggishness of the lymphatic system, allowing toxic material to accumulate.

When considering which energy centre is involved with a physical problem, it is usually that centre nearest to the physical organ, or that associated with the function of that organ. The sacral *chakra* is the one which will be associated with uterine problems and this centre may be sluggish, so that energy flowing through the centre is inhibited. Establishment of creative projects which are well-grounded or expressed at the physical level could be considered as a possible resolution here. Any sexual problems would also need attention for the sacral energies to be rebalanced.

Sometimes the physical aspect of fibroids may be the final working out of an inner problem which has already been resolved at the psychic level. A clue to this can be had from how quickly the client responds to physical treatment.

Treatment

Particular attention will be applied to cleansing the lymphatic system, and this may include exercise regimes and dietary changes. Specific remedies are:

1 Herbs: trifolium, violet leaves, burdock, dandelion, shepherd's purse.
2 Minerals: iron phosphate to reduce bleeding, potassium chloride for lymphatic glands.
3 Vitamin C for immunity and to assist absorption of iron.
4 Specific homoeopathic remedies for fibroids and to treat the inherited factor.
5 Constitutional homoeopathic treatment will be particularly important in a condition with tissue changes such as occurs in fibroids.[1]

Case History

Sometimes a patient will come to the clinic with a particular ailment which is closely related to another more obscure problem, the latter being the real focus for disease. Then when one ailment is resolved by natural therapies, the other problem either clears up automatically or comes to the surface where it can be treated more effectively. This phenomenon occurred in the following case.

Gillian had been treated for sinus over six months when it became apparent that she was suffering from fibroids. As she was receiving general lymphatic cleansing treatment for the sinus, the same remedies were useful for dealing with the fibroid condition. Her treatment included liver and lymphatic cleansing herbs, potassium chloride and iron phosphate mineral combination for both the sinus and fibroid. Calcium phosphate and vitamin E were given for chilblains.

After the fibroid was discovered, and in view of the fact that the sinus was not greatly improved, constitutional homoeopathic remedies were prescribed. These included high potencies of potassium chloride, and Thuja. Both of these have been found effective for sinus and fibroids. A homoeopathic tubercular nosode was also administered. A couple of months later her 'flooding' during menstruation ceased, and the doctor announced her free of fibroids.

The iris reveals that the patient's lymphatic system is still a weak point; and recently, after the sinus condition had been in total remission for many months, Gillian needed treatment again. Usually it is found that a second round of treatment allows the problem to clear up easily and quickly.

The relationship between respiratory lymphatic problems and uterine fibroids in this case can be explained as an inherited condition. Natural therapists find they are often able to help these conditions with the same remedies they would use for gonorrhoea. This is another way of saying that in most lymphatic problems, the gonorrhoeal taint would have manifested at some stage in the family tree, even if five or six generations ago. The continued effect of this problem manifests in pelvic problems of many kinds and lymphatic congestions affecting the respiratory area such as bronchitis and asthma. It does not manifest in the actual infection of gonorrhoea. This concept is also explored under the heading of vaginal discharges.

Fluid Retention

This problem does not always involve the kidneys, but frequently results from a sluggishness of the liver. By taking a careful case history and examining the patient for certain clinical signs via the iris, and hands and through bio-energetic or functional diagnosis, one is able to finely pin-point the cause of the problem.

Often, the fluid retention occurs just before the menstrual period in women. At this time each month, the ankles and feet swell, rings become tight indicating swelling of fingers, and breasts commonly become sore and enlarged.

Causes

The sluggishness of kidneys and liver may be an inherited tendency, or there can be mineral deficiencies due to poor diet and environmental factors. The medical profession does not have a great deal to say in cases of mild fluid retention apart from suggesting the use of diuretics. Serious forms of oedema relate to severe kidney disease and this is discussed under Nephritis.

Treatment

1 Herbs for kidneys and liver, for example, dandelion, burdock, parsley, pellitory, cornsilk, and centaury.
2 Sodium sulphate to regulate fluid balance in the body.[1]
3 Vitamin B-complex and C to promote a natural diuresis.
4 Selected homoeopathic remedies.

Case History

Shirley is a very vital business lady involved in the area of fashion. Her work schedule is demanding and she came to our clinic in the hope of improving her energy levels and of correcting the problem of fluid retention. Her periods were very heavy. Shirley's iris reveals her excellent constitution and it was not surprising that after two month's treatment, she was well in all respects. From time to time when her work becomes very pressurised, she needs to have a reappraisal of her health, and in between she takes maintenance doses of basic compounds for energy.

Her basic 'recipe' consisted of kidney and liver herbs for the fluid retention, potassium and magnesium phosphate, vitamin B-complex, and a homoeopathic nerve mixture for energy. Relaxing nerve herbs were used before bed for insomnia; these included valerian, skullcap, passaflora and mistletoe.

Food Allergies

see Allergies

Fractures

Fractured bones obviously need urgent orthodox medical attention. Natural therapies can be used as a very valuable adjunct to speed up the healing process.

Causes

Apart from the obvious precipitating cause of injury and trauma, deficiencies of calcium occur in post-menopausal women. Osteoporosis, and poor status of both calcium and magnesium through deficiencies in the diet contribute to the higher incidence of fractures. The average person thinks mainly of calcium in relation to bones which break easily, but the actual ratio of calcium and magnesium in the body is of importance.[1]

Ascorbate status, that is, vitamin C level in the body, is also important in bone healing as this vitamin is intimately concerned with collagen formation and forms the 'cement' of the bones.[2] Attention must also be centred on ligaments and tendons as weakness here will cause bones to move into more vulnerable positions during trauma. In this latter respect, calcium fluoride, another calcium salt already discussed in relation to elastic tissue, may be useful.

Treatment

The following supplements are of use:

1 Calcium salts of phosphate and fluoride.
2 Vitamins C and E.
3 Homoeopathic preparation of Comfrey and also Arnica — both useful after trauma and bruising, and homoeopathic Hypericum for pain associated with injured nerve endings.

G
Gallstones

In Western countries gallstones are found at autopsy in 20 per cent of women and 10 per cent of men over forty. There are not necessarily any symptoms from the presence of these stones. If they obstruct the common bile duct severe colic may occur with pain typically radiating under the right shoulder blade. Vomiting may accompany gallstone colic. Composition of the stones varies and is divided into three main types. The most common types contain 70 per cent cholesterol plus an admixture of calcium salts and bile ingredients. The less common pigment stones, which comprise 20 per cent of all gallstones, consist mainly of calcium bilirubinate.

The gall-bladder itself can become irritated and diseased from the presence of stones. Using natural remedies it is possible to gradually dissolve the stones but this is a very long procedure. Generally speaking, unless a stone is actually blocking the bile ducts, natural therapies can improve the health of the gall-bladder and prevent further crystallisation in the gall-bladder so that surgery is not necessary. In addition, the stones may gradually be dissolved if natural treatment is continued over a long period.

Causes

The gall-bladder has the role of concentrating the bile to four times its strength so that adequate fat metabolism is possible. The liver, which produces the bile, is a fundamental organ for attention by the naturopath. As the seat of all metabolic processes, sluggishness of the liver is found to underlie the many disorders related to poor digestive function. This is why so many treatments include liver herbs. Since using bio-functional diagnosis with the Vega instrument, the liver has been found to be the most stressed organ in the majority of cases.

Natural therapists consider that a sluggish flow of bile encourages the formation of gallstones. At the more subtle level, the liver is considered to closely reflect the emotional state of the patient.[1] Some therapists attribute particular emotions to specific problems in different parts of the body. For instance, haemorrhoids are associated with resentment and gallstones with hate. Like all the digestive organs, the liver expresses the amount and type of energy which flows through the solar plexus centre.

The diaphragm, lying directly above the liver, separates the energy centres below it from the heart, throat and head centres above. The base, sacral and solar plexus centres, situated below the diaphragm, express the personality life; the heart, throat and head centres express our spiritual development. Esoteric psychology holds that the liver expresses conflict arising between these two groups of centres in many people. Perhaps the close relationship between the liver and emotions accounts for why irritability has been often associated with an upset liver.

Treatment

Initially attention must be given to the diet and all fats removed so as not to stimulate the gall-bladder. Immediately after an attack of gallstones a diet of vegetable and fruit juices would be suggested. This has the effect of reducing inflammation in the gall-bladder and of resting all the digestive organs. It can also have a reflex action back on the astral body and induce a calm state.

Specific remedies for the gall-bladder and liver would be as follows:

1 Magnesium phosphate to reduce spasm.
2 Iron phosphate for inflammation of the gall-bladder.
3 Homoeopathic doses of herbs for liver and gall-bladder. (Herbs are too strong for the liver near the time of an attack and may provoke further discomfort.) Chelidonium, Chionanthus, Carduus mar, Hepatica and Berberis in low potency are a good selection of homoeopathic remedies which have worked well.[2] If the actual composition of stones is known, then the exact antidote in homoeopathic doses can be used.
4 Bach flower remedies, useful for the pain associated with gallstone colic.
5 Sodium sulphate over some months helps to tone the liver and to reduce the possibility of further stone formation.[3]

Case Histories

Ann, aged thirty-four, visited me in 1983. She had a history of small cholesterol stones in the gall-bladder and was suffering a lot of pain in the area of the gall-bladder and under the right scapula (shoulder blade). Other problems were headaches and haemorrhoids since the birth of the last baby. The iris revealed digestive problems and a nervous constitution.

Her first treatment included iron phosphate for inflammation of the gall-bladder, magnesium phosphate for spasm in the gall-bladder and associated ducts, and sodium sulphate to help dissolve the stones and to balance the acid/alkaline balance in the body. Vitamin B-complex was included as a general nerve tonic. The most specific part of the treatment involved a homoeopathic mixture specifically for the gall-bladder and to help dissolve the stones. This included Cholesterin 12×, Hepatica 2×, Berberis 12×, Chelidonium 6×, Carduus mar. 6×, Chionanthus, and Ipecachuana 6×.

It is of interest that Ann reacted violently to the drops. In her case this was classed as a healing crisis because the gall-bladder improved and elimination through the bowel was very violent. The drops were reduced in frequency of dose. There was no further problem with the gall-bladder. She needed only three months treatment, although for dissolving the stones a much longer period on the treatment would be necessary. It is difficult to convince clients to continue treatment once symptoms have gone completely.

Maureen visited me in 1983 for a pain in the chest which appeared to be associated with the gall-bladder. Over the years she had suffered headaches which we often find are associated with liver and gall-bladder problems. At the time of her visit she was in late middle-age and she and her husband were retiring out of Melbourne to buy a caravan park. A surgeon had been consulted but he did not wish to operate then.

At the time of her first visit she was taking vitamins A, B, C, and E. Her first prescription from me included the mineral salt sodium sulphate for its action on liver and gall, iron phosphate for any inflammation of the gall-bladder, magnesium phosphate for spasm of the area, and potassium phosphate for exhaustion and nerve tone. The most specific part of the prescription was a homoeopathic mixture for the gall-bladder. This included Hepatica, Hydrastis, Berberis, Chelidonium, Carduus mar, and Chionanthus.

On her return visit it was reported that headaches had gone, and pains in chest area were not so frequent, although still fairly severe. The magnesium compound was increased for the pain, and other supplements repeated. A herbal digestive tablet was added. At the third visit, Maureen reported easing of the pain, no headaches and she felt better in herself.

At the following visit both gall-bladder pains and headaches had recurred. This is obviously a critical situation to arise in the treatment progress; usually when a relapse like this occurs, an underlying psychological pain is found. In the case of Maureen, her son had left home and disappeared and all efforts to trace him over subsequent months and years have failed.

At this point, some of the treatment was changed to focus on the digestion from a different angle. Sodium phosphate replaced sodium sulphate and a herbal tablet containing slippery elm and liver herbs replaced the previous digestive tablet. A homoeo-pathic and herbal phosphate tonic was included for the nerve strain. Rheumatic herbs were included for a shoulder problem which was no doubt related to the underlying weakness of the digestion. This treatment was continued during the next few months.

There were no further problems with the gall-bladder and digestion from this time. The next phase appeared to be a retrac-ing phenomenon which involved a number of upper respiratory infections. From the naturopathic point of view, this is prefer-able to the more deep-seated problem with the gall-bladder and indicates that the body is healing itself from within to without. This latter phenomenon is taught as part of basic naturopathic principles. For this reason when any disease process moves towards the skin from more deep-seated structures, healing prin-ciples are at work.

Maureen visits for a check-up every few months or so and her basic improvement is maintained although the deep psychic wound caused by the disappearance of the son has not been fully resolved.

Gastritis

As the name suggests, this condition is inflammation of the stomach lining and is more commonly called indigestion. It manifests as discomfort in the area of the stomach, sometimes continual, sometimes just before or after meals. In severe cases, symptoms will be similar to that occurring in stomach ulcers. There may be gas, bloating, and burning.

Causes

Inflammation may be caused by chemicals, drugs, food allergies, and bacteria or viruses. More basic causes identified by natural therapies are vitamin and mineral deficiencies, and constitutional weaknesses of the stomach. In Chinese medical philosophy, there is great emphasis on studying the constitution of the client so that the correct types of food for that particular person can be suggested. Natural therapists regard the diet as needing detailed attention in all cases of digestive disturbance.

In the past few decades, we have seen a plethora of so called health diets; and the various proponents often forget that each person has their own particular needs, apart from general principles of healthy eating. The proportions of fat, carbohydrate and protein which are required by individuals vary considerably, although there are preferred sources of each type of food for each individual.[1]

Treatment

The most common mineral deficiency in gastritis is sodium, but large quantities of sodium chloride will not help here. It is the salt sodium phosphate which forms natural bicarbonates in body fluids and tissues.[2] Our clinical experience shows that foods rich in sodium such as celery and other alkaline vegetables are ideal for gastritis. In acute cases these may need to be prepared as juice or in strained soups.

The old medical approach of treating gastritis with an ulcer diet consisting mostly of milk products and eggs was only palliative. Specific medications of use for inflammation of the stomach lining are as follows:

1. Herbs such as melissa, angelica, centaury, dandelion, marshmallow, and slippery elm bark. These are soothing, healing and toning for the mucosa.
2. Vitamin A to promote healthy epithelial tissue, vitamin B-complex, and vitamin C in an alkaline form such as magnesium, sodium or calcium ascorbate.

3 Minerals such as sodium phosphate, zinc compounds if ulcer formation is likely. Iron phosphate is useful for acute inflammation.

4 Homoeopathic preparations to suit the individual case.

Case History

Susan, aged thirty, presented with a history of heartburn over a period of fourteen months. She suffered nausea after meals and this was worse with stress. The stomach had an 'acid' feeling. The condition was worse with dairy products. There was also a tendency towards constipation and headaches.

The iris revealed disturbances to the digestive function from the autonomic nervous system, a weakness in the liver and kidneys and general debility. The first month's treatment consisted of B-complex, and a combination of magnesium and potassium phosphate for the nervous system, iron phosphate for a tendency to blackout, and herbal tinctures for the digestion. Bach flowers were given for the more subtle constitution.

At her second visit, Susan reported more energy in the evenings. She still had a sensation of acid in the stomach especially in the morning before eating. Head symptoms were better and nausea was lessened. The treatment was continued over the next few months with minor changes such as a herbal tablet for insomnia. There were relapses with nausea at times of menstruation. At this time each month she experienced coldness, a sensation of a lump in the stomach, and a fuzzy head.

Magnesium orotate replaced magnesium phosphate when cramps developed in legs and feet after sport. Insomnia was worse at this time and the larger doses of magnesium helped this as well as the cramps. Vitamin E was added to improve circulation throughout the month. A month later the calcium and magnesium ratios were reversed and this finally eradicated the cramps for good.

It was nearly one year before the digestion was finally stabilised, and then the treatment was reduced to a maintenance dose of minerals and herbal treatment for the digestion. This may seem a long time of treatment for a gastric problem. The advantage over antacid powders is that the treatment is lasting once a balance is achieved. Fortunately, with the assistance of iris diagnosis, one can gauge from the basic constitutional tendencies how long the treatment is likely to take, and the patient can be advised accordingly.

In the case of Susan, her improvement from the first month gave encouragement to persevere throughout the short recurrent patches of nausea and discomfort which occurred during the first year's treatment. Her maintenance treatment amounts to one-third of the original treatment and she now only visits the clinic every few months.

Gastro-enteritis

See also Diarrhoea

Most of the treatment, including the food regime, will be similar to that for acute diarrhoea. The main difference will be the need for homoeopathic treatment for vomiting and nausea. Homoeopathic treatment is ideal for this condition because the remedy may be placed on the tongue. This is more tolerable to the nauseated patient than taking mixtures or tablets, which may be vomited immediately. The usual approach will be to give the homoeopathic remedies for a few hours until the vomiting has stopped and then the other more bulky medications can be introduced if necessary.

Causes

Perhaps a few comments could be made in addition to that which is stated in relation to diarrhoea. Gastro-enteritis is usually an acute problem and therefore the triggering factor is nearly always infection. It should be mentioned, however, that people who have good nutrition and who are in biochemical balance rarely have this problem. Such persons if infected will only be mildly affected.

From the point of view of naturopathic principles, consumption of large quantities of refined sugar and flour, and deficiencies of minerals and vitamins in the diet, are the main basic causes of vulnerability to gastro-enteritis.

Treatment

see Diarrhoea

German Measles

(Rubella)

This common childhood illness usually manifests in a mild fashion with the rash appearing on the first day, possibly accompanied by some enlargement of the lymph glands. It runs a short course and there are no complications except in the case of pregnant women. There is an incubation period of two to three weeks.

Causes

Apart from the immediate cause of the infecting virus, rubella, we find that persons who have poor immunity as a result of a congested lymphatic system are more prone. This applies in the case of all infectious fevers — it is noticed that severe bouts can be predicted in advance in most cases using the types of diagnosis used by natural therapists.

Treatment

It is useful in patients to speed up the process of eliminating toxins, and to improve the immunity with the following:

1 Liver homoeopathics to metabolise waste in the body more adequately.
2 Lymphatic herbs which may be given in homoeopathic form to babies and children.
3 Mineral salts to reduce inflammation of the skin and to tone the lymphatic system. These are iron phosphate, and potassium chloride.
4 Vitamin C to improve immunity and to assist detoxification.

Natural therapists are often asked about whether women of child-bearing age should have Rubella immunisation. Our approach to possible foetal malformation resulting from Rubella infection is to make women aware that any virus can affect pregnancy severely in the absence of good immunity. We are concerned that all women should protect themselves from viral attack by supplementing their diet during pregnancy and even before with adequate amounts of vitamin C.[1]

More specifically, natural therapists point to the findings of Dr Beverley Allen who carried out a research project involving immunisation of several hundred army recruits with Rubella. They were then tested for antibody levels, and exposed to Rubella. A significant proportion manifested the disease! She asked the question: What if these had been pregnant women?[2]

Glandular Fever

We have always found a degree of stress precedes this problem. Almost without fail, natural therapies can improve the immune system and greatly accelerate improvement. It has prevented the relapses so common in persons suffering from this condition. Due to the high incidence of glandular fever in the community, most people are aware of the symptoms of sore throat, headache, swollen glands and exhaustion which accompany the illness. The most distressing factor is that the symptoms can go on for months and can also recur for several years.

Treatment

I have noticed that almost without exception there are signs of both nervous exhaustion and of lymphatic congestion in the iris of persons with this problem. As the standard blood tests are notoriously vague for glandular fever it is valuable to have other means to gauge the problem. Treatment will be directed towards improving nerve tone and eliminating the congestion in the lymphatic system.

1   Vitamin C in large doses to improve immunity.[1]
2   Vitamin B-complex in large doses to improve energy.
3   Potassium phosphate to improve nerve tone.
4   Zinc salts to improve immunity if indicated.
5   Liver and lymphatic herbs, for example, violet leaves, red clover, burdock, dandelion and centaury. Tonic herbs such as hops, avena sativa and lime flowers.

Case Histories

Kylie attended me for treatment periodically over a period of several years together with her mother and two sisters. She had a history of asthma and hay fever and became tense easily with pressure of school work. Nerve tension was also observed in the iris. She developed glandular fever in her last school year at the age of seventeen.

Her treatment included the following over a period of three or four months. Liver toning and lymphatic cleansing herbs, a homoeopathic mixture to cleanse the lymphatic system, mineral combination of iron phosphate and potassium chloride to work on the lymphatic system, magnesium and potassium phosphate to give energy and rebalance the nervous system, two grams of vitamin C daily, and a high dose of vitamin B-complex twice daily. After the first two weeks treatment, Kylie felt much improved and there was no relapse with her condition. The treatment is always continued for a number of months to consolidate improvement and toning of the immune system and then the relapses which are so common with this disorder do not occur.

Neil, a records clerk aged twenty-two, attended me in 1979 with an acute attack of glandular fever. He had been off work for five weeks and had liver and spleen enlargement as associated problems. The first prescription included iron phosphate and potassium chloride, vitamin C and a lymphatic cleansing mixture containing phytolacca, burdock, dandelion, centaury, violet and trifolium. Magnesium phosphate and potassium phosphate was given as a general nerve tonic.

As this was an acute case, some of the remedies were given more than three times a day, and Neil was seen after two weeks instead of the usual four. By that time, he was generally better and the prescription was repeated with the addition of vitamin B-complex for giving more energy. Improvement continued but on the third visit stomach pain was still intermittent so homoeopathic liver drops were added. At the fourth visit, Neil reported all symptoms were improved.

Glaucoma

Glaucoma occurs in 2 per cent of all patients over the age of forty, although the person concerned may go without obvious symptoms for some years.[1] Symptoms include pain in the eye and halos around objects but it should be noted that these symptoms may result from other conditions also. In the case of glaucoma, these symptoms are often fairly late indications that the condition is well advanced.

Causes

The immediate cause is raised intra-ocular pressure so that the fluid for some reason is unable to escape into the anterior chamber of the eye. The consequent pressure gradually causes a deterioration in the optic nerve resulting finally in blindness.

From clinical experience, natural therapists have noted that in the majority of cases the client is accumulating too much waste in the body, especially in the lymphatic system. We have found that through using liver and blood cleansing herbs, the condition does not deteriorate, and may even reverse.

Treatment

1 Liver and/or lymphatic cleansing herbs.
2 Appropriate homoeopathic medication depending on the individual case and this will cover the inherited factor which is quite marked in the condition.
3 Magnesium compounds to reduce the pressure through relaxation of the eye structures thus allowing fluid to drain more adequately.
4 Vitamin C helps to lower the intra-ocular pressure.[2]

Glomerulonephritis

There are many forms of this disease both acute and chronic. The chronic cases can move in a few months towards chronic kidney or renal failure, whereas acute types may clear up without recurrence. Symptoms will vary according to the type, but the most characteristic finding is blood and protein (albumen) in the urine. General malaise may include vomiting, and headache.

The majority of nephritic problems are now understood to be

auto-immune disorders, meaning that a destructive process in the kidney is taking place due to circulating antigens and antibodies. These are thought to develop in response to an outer or inner factor affecting the body. It is the way in which the antibodies relate to the antigens and their effect on the kidney substance which causes the problem of tissue destruction. [1]

Final verification by renal biopsy confirms destruction to the tissue or tiny blood-filtering units of the kidneys known as nephrones. Whichever type of glomerulonephritis is discussed, from either orthodox or naturopathic viewpoints, a condition of inflammation and destruction of the kidney substance occurs. This will lead eventually to an inability of the kidney to filter the blood, and to chronic kidney failure with almost complete lack of urine flow in terminal cases. The usual treatment to prolong life in such cases is by dialysis — use of an artificial kidney — or by a kidney transplant.

Causes

Brief mention has been made of the immune problems and a full discussion of these is beyond the scope of this book. The question which interests natural therapists is why do antibodies and antigens behave destructively in some people and not in others? Do some people have healthier kidneys from the start? What is the trigger which causes the destructive process of the antibodies and antigens in the kidney? We have found that people with nephritis of most types always need large doses of the mineral salt calcium phosphate. [2] Does this point to an underlying mineral imbalance either from an inherited tendency or from a deficient diet?

As usual, natural therapists are thrown back on their clinical experience. It has been found from experience that, contrary to medical opinion, the destructive process may be stopped in some cases and in some cases reversed. If a seriously ill person returns to apparent good health and no longer has blood or albumen in the urine, after being told that only a transplant will save life, we can only conclude that natural therapies have helped.

As with all immune disorders of a destructive kind, the deeper causes of the problem may relate to self-destructive attitudes in the psyche. Whether cancer, multiple sclerosis, or nephritis, these problems are very deep-seated, and this is why negative energies from the psyche may perhaps manifest in the physical body as destructive antibodies if denied other outlets. Persons who respond to natural therapies for these disorders are people who are able to change deep-seated attitudes, whether consciously or unconsciously.

Perhaps it should be added that in cases of nephritis where the inherited factor is prominent, as in the case described below, the psychological factor may not be significant.

The *chakra* or energy centre associated with the kidneys is the base centre. The reader is reminded that this centre is fundamental to the will to live, and provides the basic energy for the whole system. An imbalance or distortion of the will aspect of our being can imbalance the energy flowing through the base centre, and this may in some cases stimulate a destructive process in the kidney.

Sometimes the shock of discovering a potentially fatal disease is enough to make people change their value systems. They may look for a creative change in their life. Others drop their bundle completely and rapidly move towards death This is an over-simplification of a very complex situation, but in these serious disorders it is my understanding that there may be a deep-seated problem in the psyche which needs resolving if the patient is to return to health.

Psychic disturbance is less likely to be the case in acute nephritis, as the majority of these patients make an uncomplicated full recovery. The treatment for both acute and chronic will not vary a great deal from our point of view, except that in chronic cases it covers a much longer time span.

Treatment

As nephritis rapidly moves towards a toxic state from the lack of blood filtration, diet is very important. Especially in acute cases, the patient will be put on a juice fast with fresh weak fruit juices alternating with fresh vegetable juices for a few days. Very often, the effect of this regime is to produce a diuretic effect which is soothing on the kidney substance at the same time promoting urine flow.

There will be an emphasis later on all raw and steamed vegetables, and a very strict control on refined foods. Chemical food additives will not be allowed due to the delicate state of the kidneys. Protein will be very restricted in acute cases, and in chronic cases only white meat in moderation will be allowed, with an emphasis on light protein such as bean curd, bean shoots, and light cheeses such as ricotta. Specific supplements would include the following:

1 Calcium phosphate, the tissue salt which has been found essential in all cases of kidney disease.
2 Iron phosphate, essential for the inflammatory process in the kidney as it reduces both bleeding and inflammation.
3 Zinc salts; these may be necessary to aid the immune system; zinc prevents scar tissue, accelerates healing and is responsible for many enzyme chains associated with the immune system.
4 Herbs, usually in homoeopathic form for chronic cases, and in fluid extracts for acute nephritis, may include cornsilk, parsley, pellitory, buchu, and berberis. Soothing or demulcent herbs such as marshmallow are also used.
5 Vitamin B6 is necessary, in addition the whole B-complex is usually advantageous.
6 Magnesium and potassium phosphate; used to improve the nervous system.
7 Vitamin C has such a close relation to the immune system and the healthy function of same; deficiency would be considered certain in nephritis. It is also concerned with collagen formation and is thus involved in any rebuilding process.
8 Bach flower remedies for negative and destructive emotions.
9 Constitutional homoeopathic prescribing, often essential for these deep seated disorders of the immune system.

Case History

The following case is from the files of my husband and involves Barbara, now aged forty-five. She was given a short time to live at the age of twenty-one when she first tried natural therapies for a severe bout of nephritis. There were other kidney problems in the family including that of a sister who lost one kidney at the age of eight. Their father had a history of tuberculosis and died from cardiac complications following this disease; this precursor to some familial problem is described under Tuberculosis.

In the case of Barbara kidney disease manifested early in her second pregnancy with symptoms of gross oedema of extremities, excessive vomiting, exhaustion and high blood pressure. Other health problems suffered by Barbara included a long history of migraines. In spite of her illness during the pregnancy, Barbara delivered a full-term baby girl of normal weight. She was only able to breast-feed for a very short period and her own health was fast deteriorating. The legs swelled to the knee each day and required almost daily injections from her doctor, blood pressure remained high, and she was given a short time only to live. Her disease manifested before renal dialysis or kidney transplants became relatively common procedures.

A relative suggested naturopathic treatment and Barbara commenced supplements which included calcium phosphate as the main tissue salt for the kidney, sodium phosphate to help absorption of the calcium, kidney toning herbs in liquid and tablet form, iron phosphate for inflammation of kidney substance, garlic and other herbs for blood pressure, and vitamin B-complex for general energy. Between one and five weeks on treatment, Barbara felt remarkably improved, and she was feeling really well with no oedema after four to six months. The blood pressure took about twelve months to decline and the albumen (protein) in the urine diminished and stopped at about this time. The migraines also disappeared.

Barbara has remained on natural therapies throughout her adult life, and regards it as health insurance. Emphasis has always been placed on keeping her calcium intake at optimal level, and she feels so well on a few supplements that she intends continuing this preventive measure for life. Barbara states that her diet was very good from early childhood. Very little junk food was consumed due to her tendency towards suffering migraine attacks. The strong inherited factor is therefore of interest in this case. Her positive approach to life, even when so sick at the age of twenty-one, must have helped her response to natural medication.

Glycosuria

see Diabetes

Goitre, Grave's Disease, Simple Goitre

To the average person this means a swelling in the thyroid gland which is situated in the front of the neck. The distinction needs to be made as to whether the lump comes from the gland being hyper- or hypo-active. In the former case, the term 'toxic goitre' is used and apart from the swelling, the whole metabolism is speeded up with palpitations, weight loss, sweating, nervousness, tremors, insomnia, and possibly high blood pressure.

A simple goitre or under-active thyroid is characterised by the opposite condition. All the metabolism slows down with possible weight gain, slow pulse, slightly subnormal temperature on first waking, hair loss, dry skin, poor circulation, and general sluggishness of the whole person.

Causes

All the endocrine glandular problems are most interesting if one is interested in the more subtle anatomy of the individual person. An imbalance of throat *chakra* is understood as the main cause of under- or over-activity of the thyroid. (The reader is referred to chapter 2 for a more complete explanation of the relationship between our creative energies and the healthy functioning of the thyroid.)

Over a period of years, the thyroid only needs to be slightly out of balance for changes in weight to take place as a result of metabolic shifts. Correspondingly, a change in energy flow through the throat *chakra* may be the basic cause of these metabolic changes. Generally speaking, we could say that we each have a tendency to move towards obesity or the opposite, and this would tend to be governed by the activity of the throat centre.

In the case of over-activity of the thyroid, I have noticed that women affected by this condition talk a great deal. One could conclude that the incessant use of the larynx could over-stimulate nearby structures like the thyroid gland. The esoteric view would be the reverse as explained below.

The throat centre relates to the lower mind and if this is over-active, there will be excess energy flowing through the throat centre, over-stimulating the thyroid and partly expressing as an excess of speech. This is a generalisation and there is always the exception which does not follow the rule. I have found, however, that in many cases, women with over-active thyroids are highly intelligent with an over-active mind. If they could learn mental relaxation through meditation, their thyroid function would possibly become normalised.

The other associated concern is that all women should develop creative outlets to channel their energy. By middle-age, the energies would then have somewhere to go apart from the demands of family life or routine office work. Without a suitable outlet, the energies may turn back on the physical area and thus over-stimulate the gland to produce an excess of thyroxine.

The chain of events may be sequenced as: an over-stimulated mind with no fulfilling outlet, stimulation of the emotions, imbalance in the etheric energies, imbalance of the autonomic nervous system, finally manifesting in over-stimulation of the thyroid.

Although medical opinion is that the cause of the disease is unknown, there is quite a body of research to indicate that Grave's disease or thyrotoxicosis is related to an auto-immune disorder, hence the logical possibility that, as previously suggested, it is basically a destructive process which is causing the thyroid gland to become disturbed.[1]

At the other end of the scale, an under-active thyroid has to be examined in the opposite sense of a sluggish, under-stimulated mind, resulting in insufficient energy flowing through the endocrine system, hence there is an under-production of thyroxine. A more exoteric cause relates to insufficient iodine in the diet. The usual example mentioned is the increased incidence of simple goitre in people who live in mountainous areas like Switzerland, away from the sea which is our main source of iodine. The more subtle physiological relationship between iodine, the thyroid and goitre has been well explored by medical homoeopaths.[2]

Treatment of Simple Goitre (Hypo-thyroidism)

From my point of view, for a lasting cure the quality and energy of the mental life would have to be improved, as well as physical measures taken. The person would have to understand the relationship between the energy centres and the endocrine glands. More mental stimulus and creativity are needed in the lives of those with an under-active thyroid.

General endocrine tonics in the way of herbs and homoeopathic remedies will be used, and either crude or homoeopathic kelp as a source of iodine. Other stimulating measures would be the use of vitamin B-complex and the mineral salt potassium phosphate. These could be listed as:

1 Kelp tablets, tincture of Fucus (seaweed), or homoeopathic kelp or iodine.
2 Vitamin B-complex and potassium phosphate for stimulation of the nervous system.
3 Herbal extracts traditionally used to stimulate the endocrine system.
4 Constitutional homoeopathic remedies, important for regulating the individual endocrine system.
5 Liver herbs to help eliminate toxins which often accumulate in a sluggish system.

Treatment for Toxic Goitre, Grave's Disease or Hyperthyroidism

In this case, the need for both mental relaxation and development of suitable creative outlets must be examined. This means a look at the total life-style. These can be tricky cases to regulate, and time is often against one if circulatory symptoms are pronounced. The following supplements have been found very useful:

1 Magnesium orotate which gives a large dose of that mineral which is most relaxing in its effect on nerves, heart and other vital tissues.
2 Sedating herbs such as valerian, vervain, motherwort, passaflora, and mistletoe, the latter being applicable for any circulatory stress.
3 Homoeopathic iodine — the crude kelp should be administered with great care in cases of overactive thyroid. Small amounts remove deficiencies which may result from the over-active gland.
4 Small doses of B-complex; large doses are too stimulating.
5 Homoeopathic constitutional remedies are very valuable as high potencies of the various iodine salts can reverse the effect of over-activity.

Case History

Pat is a talented weaver of rugs and tapestries, and it is of interest to consider her recurring thyroid problem in the light of comments about the thyroid *chakra*. She has that type of mental over-activity and creativity which can result in over-stimulation to the thyroid. Hence meditation and relaxation programmes featured as an important part of her life-style changes. Pat is a trained nurse and has worked in hospitals for many years, hence she understands the physical parameters of her condition.

There were other health problems for which Pat gained help from our therapies, in particular from her first visits which were for bad dermatitis. Later, menstrual problems were treated, and around that time it was noticed that the thyroid was slightly enlarged. It was not until a couple of years later as menopause approached that the thyroid became a real problem. Hot flushes also featured.

During the first month's treatment for the thyroid, large doses of magnesium orotate were given to stabilise the nervous system. Also administered were herbal sedatives, liver herbs for detoxification, homoeopathic drops for flushes, homoeopathic drops for regulating the glands, and homoeopathic Fucus (seaweed) as a mild tonic for the thyroid. In this case the latter medication was actually found to stimulate the thyroid and had therefore to be changed for a different homoeopathic medication. Bach flower remedies were also used, and a small B-complex supplement provided general nerve toning.

By the third month, Pat was considerably improved, and treatment was continued for another two months. Pat is typical of that large group of clients who keep in touch for general health checks and maintenance over many years, and who will have a course of treatment for six months or so, followed by a break of up to a year or so during which they manage their health well without any intervention. Pat has continued naturopathic treatment intermittently for ten years.

Gonorrhoea

This is one of the conditions which naturopaths are advised not to treat. Natural therapists are occasionally asked to improve the general health of a client after they have had the usual courses of antibiotics. More commonly of late, natural therapists have treated many persons with venereal herpes and this is discussed under Herpes.

In the section on Fibroids and also that on Vaginal Discharges, I have attempted to explain the deep-seated effect on the health of future generations from persons who have had gonorrhoea. It is paradoxical therefore that the left-over inherited taints of this type of venereal disease attract the attention of every skilled homoeopath, even though the average natural therapist cannot by law touch the actual disease in its infectious form.

The basic homoeopathic philosophy in relation to gonorrhoea explains that suppression of this problem with crude drugs causes a modified version to go deep into the lymphatic system. This will firstly manifest as pelvic problems of many kinds in future generations.[1] It may also affect the lymphatic system in relation to the respiratory organs.

It is not my suggestion that such a devastatingly infectious problem as gonorrhoea should be treated only with natural therapies. Rather, it is suggested that the problem may not end with antibiotics. Perhaps this is an area where a combination of different healing approaches is needed. It is possible that the long-term effects of venereal disease result from an imprint on the subtle part of the physical body known as the etheric vehicle. This section of our inner constitution appears to be intimately connected with immunity.

Because of their great power of penetration into the etheric body, homoeopathic remedies can remove inherited tendencies which result from illnesses from our forebears. This aspect of homoeopathy has been extensively explored and practised by the early homoeopathic pioneers, most of whom were first trained in the orthodox medical tradition.[2]

Gout

It may surprise the reader that this is one of the easiest of conditions to treat as it responds very quickly to natural supplements and to dietary changes. The condition usually presents with severe inflammation around the area of the big toes, but theoretically a gouty condition may occur in other joints. The condition often comes on suddenly with hot, red, glazed and excruciatingly painful joints.

Causes

This condition is a metabolic problem involving the formation of too much uric acid and it is accepted that there is an inherited factor. From the naturopathic viewpoint, the diet is important, even though dietary changes are no longer encouraged in the orthodox medical treatment. Stress may precipitate an attack and must be considered as part of the assessment of the total life-style.

Treatment

As far as possible, acid forming foods in the diet should be reduced, in particular, red meat, cheese and refined flour and sugar products. Alcohol should be kept to a minimum due to the stress it places on the liver. Treatment and toning of the liver is most important as it is faulty liver action which is the main cause of this metabolic error. This does not mean that the liver would be affected enough to show on a liver function test, but this is a very crude test from our point of view.

Treatment prevents uric acid formation by altering the metabolism, and also neutralises and eliminates the crystals which are already present. Remedies may include the following:

1 The mineral salt sodium phosphate which forms natural bicarbonates in the system and hence has an alkaline effect.[1]
2 Liver herbs such as dandelion, wahoo, centaury, and kidney herbs like burdock, parsley and pellitory. Rheumatic herbs will also be used for their anti-inflammatory effect.
3 Vitamin B6 is very important in gout but usually the B-complex is used.
4 Vitamin C is useful for general detoxification.
5 Mineral salt iron phosphate is given to relieve the acute inflammation.
6 Homoeopathic colchicum is often very useful.

Case History

Barry, aged forty-six, visited me in 1981 after passing four kidney stones. He had severe frequency of bladder function during the night. He was on medication for gout and had a life-long history of sinus problems. This is a good case to consider in a holistic fashion because natural therapists would see a causal chain involving all these conditions.

The biochemical imbalance which caused the kidney stones would be related to the build-up of uric acid crystals in the joint causing the gout. In both cases there is the need to work on the metabolism so that acid/alkaline balance in the tissues is restored. According to iris diagnosis Barry had problems in the right kidney, bladder and prostate. There were also imbalances in the autonomic nervous system and thyroid gland.

Treatment for the first month included magnesium orotate to rebalance the calcium levels in the tissues and to prevent spasm in the urinary structures, vitamin B-complex, and in particular vitamin B6 to prevent further formation of kidney stones. A herbal mixture was an important part of the treatment and included kidney, liver, bladder and antacid herbs. Homoeopathic drops and a mineral combination were given for the prostate.

On his second visit, Barry reported less bladder frequency at night, and lessening pain in the kidney region, but his sinus condition had flared. This was understandable given the usual retracing effect whereby the body heals itself from within outwards. A temporary exacerbation of the sinus would indicate elimination of toxic waste through the normal channels.

The treatment was repeated with the addition of a zinc compound for the prostate gland and vitamin E. During the second month, Barry experienced a bad bout of gout and this was also consistent with the retracing phenomena. The body was re-experiencing previous problems on its way back to health. The ache in the kidney area was back again during this month.

Treatment was continued over the next three months and there was no further problem from the gout. The sinus also became much better. No further problems of pain in the kidney occurred and the bladder only required emptying once per night.

Growing Pains

I remember well as a young child, waking in the middle of the night with an ache like toothache in the tibia bone of the leg, and the family talking about a strange malady known as 'growing pains'. Natural therapists, or more particularly homoeopaths, understand that these pains manifest as a result of the child inheriting a particular constitutional problem from the parents. It is actually a miasmatic taint and is widely spread, hence many young children present with this problem. In the forties, whenever it occurred we were given two aspirins crushed up in jam for the problem!

Treatment

Due to the inherited tendency of this problem, deep-seated homoeopathic treatment is often needed, and the condition in children then clears up very quickly. Specific remedies may be:

1 Calcium phosphate or magnesium phosphate depending on the constitution.
2 Rheumatic herbs.
3 Vitamin B-complex.
4 Specific homoeopathic remedies to counteract the inherited problems which may manifest following suppression of syphilis earlier in the family tree, see Syphilis. [1]

Case History

Anna, aged three years, woke at night with pains in the legs, and at times hands and joints were involved. She had a good diet, being fond of raw fruit and vegetables, and this ruled out the more common rheumatic ailments which go with a poor diet lacking in alkaline foods. She also suffered recurrent colds, a lot of mucus, and eye infections.

By taking a careful case history it was found that her normal milestones of teething, crawling and walking were out of the usual sequence and this gave a clue to a particular range of homoeopathic remedies based on barium salts. The basic remedies given were vitamin C to improve immunity to colds and mineral salts, iron phosphate and potassium chloride to reduce inflammation of respiratory passages and eyes and to reduce mucus. Calcium phosphate was used to help with the bone pains, and homoeopathic doses of lymphatic cleansers and liver herbs reduced production of excess mucus.

The most specific part of the medication was the homoeopathic preparation of the selected barium salt. This was needed for one month only. The other basic treatment was given for a total of four months. There were still occasional problems with respiratory infections, but by the second month no further problems were experienced with the legs.

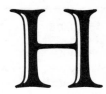

Haematuria

Haematuria simply means blood in the urine. There are a number of different causes. These include cystitis, pyelonephritis, glomerulonephritis, kidney stones, papilloma and cancer. The causes are many, and skilled differential diagnosis is needed to decipher the causal chain. Pathology may need to be undertaken if the cause is not easily recognised. Treatment will depend on the diagnosis and is discussed separately under the relevant section named above.

Haemophilia

This condition is entirely due to a genetic problem and natural therapists can do no more than improve the general health of the person concerned. It is due to a deficiency of anti-haemophilic globulin in the plasma, which results in uncontrollable bleeding from even minor cuts and abrasions.[1] The condition is transmitted by females but only manifests in the male.

Haemorrhoids

This painful ailment is another name for varicose veins around the anus. As with all varicosities and weakness of elastic tissue, natural therapists find it to be a biochemical problem. Apart from the pain of the protruding haemorrhoids, they can bleed, and at times itch. Unless the biochemical problem is corrected, surgery may not end the problem.

Causes

In most cases of varicose veins there appears to be a familial weakness in absorption of particular calcium salts, namely calcium fluoride, no matter which part of the body is affected.[1] The most characteristic place to find this weakness illustrated is on the tongue. Cracks on the tongue indicate a deficiency of calcium fluoride in some part of the body. According to the life-style, this weakness will manifest mildly or profoundly. For instance, food allergy can be a precipitating cause for haemorrhoids.

In linking any possible subjective causes to haemorrhoids, it has been noted that the emotion of resentment features strongly in sufferers. When this has been tactfully discussed there has been acknowledgment of the problem in a number of cases. In those cases which have remained defiant to the most carefully selected supplements, I have had the impression that deep-seated resentments have not been resolved. Resentment is an expression of suppressed anger. In 'holding' this emotion, congestion at the final part of the bowel is an appropriate but unfortunate physical reaction.

Treatment

Treatment needs to be continued over a long period of time, especially for varicose veins of the legs. For some reason not fully understood, the assimilation of calcium fluoride is slow. This may be in direct consequence of the inherited disposition. In varicosities, we are looking at a change of structure, that is, pathology. It is not surprising that response is slow.

Specific treatment for haemorrhoids may include:
1 Calcium fluoride in some form.
2 Astringent herbs as fluid extracts or homoeopathic potencies, for example, hammamelis and horse chestnut.
3 Liver herbs: dandelion, centaury, burdock.
4 Vitamin C in combination with the bioflavanoids.
5 Vitamin E to improve circulation and prevent thrombosis; especially important for varicose veins of the leg.
6 Constitutional homoeopathic remedies.

Case History

David, an accountant aged fifty, visited for treatment after suffering haemorrhoids intermittently for twenty years. Other problems included dyspepsia from the age of twenty-four and a history of high blood pressure and gout. The haemorrhoids bled at times. His general life-style was poor with constant drinking of coffee plus the smoking of twenty cigarettes per day.

Considering his previous life habits, progress was quick and lasting. Improvement took place in digestion and haemorrhoids from the first month and continued throughout treatment and after it was discontinued. David brought a number of other patients to the clinic after his treatment was completed and we therefore knew that his improvement continued.

The main constituents of his treatment over the nine months were as follows; calcium fluoride and sodium phosphate in combination for elastic tissue and dyspepsia respectively, herbal liver tablet, herbal tincture of horse chestnut and other astringent herbs, iron phosphate for the bleeding tendency, and bromelain, an enzyme from the pineapple, for digestion. He was already taking B-complex himself.

Hallucinations

see also Schizophrenia

The conditions chosen for description in this book are not only those most commonly suffered, but also those more peculiar and less common conditions which respond dramatically to natural therapies. Hallucinations are often a symptom of schizophrenia and other psychiatric disorders.

Causes and Treatment

A group of Canadian psychiatrists spearheaded by Abram Hoffer discovered the chemical chains in the body which result in hallucination as it occurs in schizophrenia.[1] They have found that the use of large doses of niacin or B3, and in some cases B6, have removed hallucinations and restored health.

I have found this to be true. Several young people have been treated and returned to completely normal life-styles as a result of the B3 plus a few other natural remedies. While it is a fact that hallucinations may occur in conditions other than schizophrenia, from a biochemical viewpoint the same parameters may prevail. The reader is referred to the section on Schizophrenia for further details and a case history.

Hay Fever

This is a common condition which natural therapists encounter in their clientele every spring. Fortunately we can offer more than the antihistamines which are commonly available and prescribed. There is no need to describe the streaming, itching eyes, or the blocked or running nose of the average sufferer.

Causes

Here natural therapists have something controversial to offer — hay fever is not caused basically by pollen, dust, feathers and allergies or numerous other foreign proteins, but rather by the biochemical imbalance of the body as a result of a sluggish liver and inability to digest the chosen diet adequately. Often, the bowel is found to be in a toxic state, and the mucus membranes have begun to function as eliminative organs.

This does not mean that the pollens or dust or allergies are not triggering factors in the attack, but they should be seen as such rather than as the cause. The chain of events is therefore as follows: an unsuitable diet which overloads the system with waste, or poor digestive functions which cannot even metabolise a good diet, followed by inadequate elimination of the waste thus formed. The result is a toxic build-up of waste, resulting finally in the incapacity of the body to deal with any further foreign protein such as pollen.

Further, more basic causes must be described as they indicate why hay fever is a difficult condition for even a skilled natural therapist to treat. These are inherited tendencies which lie behind the eczema, hay fever and asthma manifesting in families, and which indicate that correct homoeopathic prescribing is necessary to eradicate the hay fever, in addition to the prescribing of vitamins, minerals and herbs.

Treatment

1 At least 2g of vitamin C daily to boost the immune system and to reduce toxins in the system. [1]
2 Vitamin A to improve the epithelial tissue of nose, eyes and throat. [2]
3 Liver and lymphatic herbs to improve metabolism and to clear out the burdened lymphatics. A typical mixture may include dandelion, centaury, burdock, red clover, elder-blossom and violet leaves.
4 Homoeopathic remedies traditionally used for problems with the mucus membrane such as Alium cepa, Natrum muriaticum, Nux vomica, Sabadilla and Euphrasia.
5 Constitutional homoeopathic prescribing for the individual case.
6 Mineral compound of iron phosphate, and potassium chloride to reduce inflammation and mucus.

Case Histories

Bill, aged fifty-five, was a public servant who attended with hay fever and a history of bronchitis. A number of patients with respiratory problems tend to have symptoms alternating between the nose and chest. For his first month's treatment he was given the following: liver herbs for improving metabolism, herbs for the mucus membrane of the nasal passage, the mineral combination of iron phosphate and potassium chloride to reduce inflammation and mucus in the nasal passages respectively, vitamin C for the same reason, vitamin A to improve health of epithelial tissue lining the nose, and specific homoeopathic drops for nasal catarrh.

On the second visit, Bill reported less sneezing but chest congestion had developed. This was not surprising, given the common retracing phenomena which cause a manifestation of old ailments after natural medication begins. The same treatment was continued plus a herbal chest mixture containing liquorice, trifolium, lobelia, coltsfoot and marshmallow.

On each of the next four visits, Bill reported continuing improvement and the only further addition to the treatment consisted of codliver oil capsules as winter approached. This is often included to aid calcium absorption in the case of respiratory weakness.

May, a fifty-eight-year-old librarian, attended our clinic in 1980 for help with conditions of weight gain, exhaustion, and pain in one hand. She had a history of hay fever. Her first treatment included iron phosphate and potassium chloride and herbs for the nasal mucus and congestion. Liver herbs were included to reach the more basic metabolic problems which give rise to hay fever, and rheumatic herbs covered the problem in the hand. For the extreme tiredness, a high dosage vitamin B and a mineral combination of potassium phosphate and magnesium phosphate were given.

On her second visit, May reported marked improvement in all respects and this continued through the third month except for a bad bout of hay fever at the beginning of November. As the hay fever season was in full swing, this was expected. May had not yet had sufficient treatment to get to the cause of the problem. The prescription was repeated with the addition of specific homoeopathic hay fever drops, and May continued through the next three months completely free of all problems before the treatment was discontinued.

As with many causal chains, the metabolism was the main problem which gave rise first to the nasal problem, and more recently to the rheumatic problem of the hand. The body heals itself by retracing back in order of last symptoms to appear. Therefore in May's case the hand cleared up first, vitality improved and then the hay fever really came to the surface in season, and probably in part, as a result of the treatment. With hay fever, the cause often needs to be treated for about two years.

Headache

Tension headaches will be dealt with here, and migraines under the appropriate section later. It may be of interest to the reader to know that the natural therapist asks a lot of questions about headache so as to give the appropriate remedies. Frequency, area of head affected, position on head, type of pain, time of day, and other factors are taken into account.

Causes

Causes of headaches are multiple, but the most common types of headache are usually brought on by stress and tension. More basic causes are related to deficiencies of mineral salts of magnesium and potassium. These salts keep the nervous system in balance.[1] In addition, vitamin B-complex is related closely to many aspects of healthy nerve function.

Another fairly common cause relates to toxic waste burdening the cerebral areas and this can be seen at a glance with iris diagnosis. This form of analysis also reveals lack of adequate blood circulation to the head, which may give the experience of a 'fuzzy' head rather than actual pain.

Treatment

The general life-style of the patient including nutrition is investigated so that any deficiencies of mineral salts and vitamins may be corrected after supplements are reduced. Some people need a few supplements on a continuing basis and choose this approach as health insurance. This continuing need results from stress in the modern world, from inadequate farming methods which denude the soil of nutrients, and from pollution. People with high pressure jobs in cities are often in the category where supplements are used as an insurance policy. Specific supplements for tension headaches include:

1 Potassium phosphate and magnesium phosphate to balance the nervous system.
2 Vitamin B-complex.
3 Liver herbs to tone liver so that metabolism of waste is improved.
4 Antispasmodic herbs to reduce nervous tension, for example, scullcap, vervain, passaflora, valerian and mistletoe.
5 Individually prescribed homoeopathic and Bach flower remedies.

Case Histories

Lorraine is aged fifty-six and is director of nursing at a large medical complex just out of the city. She has sought intermittent naturopathic treatment over a number of years. Her professional position is stressful and she regards naturopathic treatment as good health insurance. Following a total hysterectomy, she attended me during 1986 with problems of headaches, poor sleep and constipation. There was a history of skin allergies.

The first prescription included B-complex and a mineral combination of potassium and magnesium phosphate to both relax and tone nerves. She was also given calcium phosphate to prevent the possibility of osteoporosis. A herbal mixture included herbs with oestrogen content — liquorice, sarsaparilla, and angelica. These herbs were to replace the need for pharmaceutical oestrogenic products following removal of the ovaries. Liver stimulating herbs were prescribed for reducing the constipation. Linseeds were advised to stimulate the bowel to secrete more mucus. Homoeopathic drops were included to balance the endocrine glands following the hysterectomy.

On her first return visit, Lorraine reported that the bowels were quite regular again, and the headaches were less often. Sleep had also improved. Tiredness was still profound, but she felt this was due to the professional stresses at the moment. At this visit the basic prescription was repeated plus some homoeopathic drops which included Carbo vegetabalis for flatulence.

Improvement continued, with constipation and headaches entirely diminished by the third visit. As the tiredness persisted, further reflection on this problem took place. Using the Vega instrument for bio-functional diagnosis, it was discovered that the thyroid was sluggish. Kelp tablets were added to stimulate the thyroid gland through their iodine content. The B-complex was increased in potency and a homoeopathic phosphate tonic included for more energy.

At the next visit, Lorraine reported all problems to have been resolved, and improvement has been maintained since. At the six-month mark, remedies will be tapered off.

This is a good case to illustrate the synergistic approach which may be needed for a common problem. The constipation was probably contributing to the headaches. The sluggish thyroid may in turn have contributed to the constipation. The constipation was treated in a number of ways: improving nerve tone to the bowel, stimulating the thyroid, toning the liver, and working on the mucosa of the bowel.

This case also indicates the difficulty of undertaking clinical trials as they are conducted in orthodox medicine. In the natural therapy approach to diagnosis, we are looking at the causal chain and the relationship between a multiplicity of factors. This is the meaning of approaching the client in an holistic manner. Likewise with natural therapy treatment, it is impossible to itemise a particular remedy as being the sole factor producing improvement in a particular condition.

Angela first visited me at the age of twenty-nine, about six years ago, suffering from headaches. On occasions they were bad enough to need medical attention in the form of injections. She also suffered from hay fever in the usual season and some dermatitis. Recurrent thrush was another problem.

Her treatment included a mineral compound and cleansing herbs for the thrush, and potassium phosphate and magnesium phosphate and vitamin B-complex for the headaches. Liver herbs were also included because of the relationship between the liver and headaches found in clinical practice. After the first two months of treatment, the severe headaches had ceased, but a lot of tension headaches were still present. Antispasmodic and nerve toning herbs were added.

Headaches cleared after six months or so but have returned in less severe form from time to time. Angela has been treated for general health during two pregnancies, and has remained free from headaches in the main over the six years I have known her. In a case like this, she may have a few months' treatment every two years or so, remaining well and free from headaches and other problems in between visits.

Heartburn

see Gastritis

Heart Disease

see Atherosclerosis including Angina

As the most common form of heart disease is blocked coronary arteries, the only other pathological problem not covered under atherosclerosis would be valvular problems, and less commonly inflammations as in pericarditis, and endocarditis. These latter conditions would need skilled orthodox medical help apart from any natural therapies.

Causes of Valvular Problems

Valvular problems are often related to heart murmurs and these can be congenital or resulting from rheumatic fever. The valves may have lost their elasticity or have become misshapen in some way.

Treatment

Obviously results will not be spectacular, but with the use of calcium salts and selected constitutional homoeopathic remedies, improvement can take place. Remedies will include:

1 Vitamin E.
2 Calcium fluoride in suitable preparations.[1]
3 Vitamin C.
4 Constitutional homoeopathic prescribing. I have used high potencies of barium salts with good results on babies who matched this particular remedy.
5 Magnesium compounds are needed for most heart problems.[2]

Hepatitis

As the most common form encountered in the general public is acute viral hepatitis, this infectious form will be discussed. The viruses are mainly in two groups known as A and B, of which hepatitis A is the most common, being spread through poor sanitation and hygiene. Type B is known as more serious in its long-term effects on the patient.

Symptoms are variable but may include nausea, vomiting, fatigue, headache, and influenza-like symptoms and these can precede the onset of jaundice by one to two weeks. A low grade fever may also be present. After the jaundice commences, the liver becomes large and tender indicating the inflammation. If the condition is not adequately resolved in any form of hepatitis, then long-term serious effects are fibrosis and possible cirrhosis.

Causes

Natural therapists would not argue with the immediate cause being infective, but through various methods of diagnosis, we are convinced that many people have a sub-clinical liver problem which renders them more prone to hepatitis. These sub-clinical problems which we identify in various organs of the body do not show up on standard pathology tests, as the organ weakness is not yet pathological.

This attitude illustrates the basic difference between the two professions. Natural therapists are concerned with preventive medicine and their forms of diagnosis are used in this context. Orthodox pathology and diagnosis is concerned to measure the disordered biochemistry and tissue changes which have formed the sphere of orthodox medicine.

It is significant that natural therapists often treat patients for various toxic lymphatic conditions and general malaise, and on questioning find a history of hepatitis, sometimes for as long ago as ten years. This reinforces our understanding that the liver really is central to all the metabolic processes of the body, and is often the first cause in a chain of problems.

As with other digestive disturbances, it is relevant to note the relationship between the liver and that more subtle part of the anatomy, the etheric body, and in particular to the solar plexus *chakra*. The liver is intimately connected to our emotional life through the solar plexus *chakra*, and as such can become weakened and disturbed by fears, suppressions and emotional conflict. This in turn makes one vulnerable to infection. [1]

More rarely, hepatitis may occur as a result of drugs, chemicals and from other diseases. In these cases the naturopathic treatment will not basically vary as it is still directed towards healing of the liver tissue and improving immunity.

Treatment

This is one area of treatment where the natural therapist could be of great assistance to the orthodox profession. There is very little in the way of orthodox drug treatment which is safe in the case of an inflamed liver. This is because the liver has to detoxify all drugs entering the body, and it cannot be further embarrassed with drugs in its diseased state.

People suffering from hepatitis and its after effects are frequently not given any dietary advice. This is an area of treatment emphasised by the natural therapist. The client is advised to have a diet including a lot of fresh vegetable and fruit juices as these have been found to detoxify and cleanse the liver. Pineapple, grapefruit, lemon, and grape juice are particularly suitable fruits, and celery, carrot and beetroot are some of the more useful vegetables.

For the first few days of treatment, juices alone can be used, and this can be followed by a diet of steamed vegetables, raw salads and fruit, lean meat and fat-free curd cheeses such as ricotta or cottage cheese. Fats and oils are totally restricted for some weeks, and are only very gradually resumed. Complex whole grain carbohydrates are encouraged.

Specific supplements may include the following:

1 Mineral salt sodium sulphate which has a direct tonic action on the liver and helps reduce swelling.[2] Iron phosphate is used to reduce inflammation.
2 Liver herbs are initially used in homoeopathic form so as to start the toning effect gently. These may include chelidonium, carduus mar, chionanthus, and berberis. Other digestive herbs will be added later as needed.[3]
3 For the exhaustion, mineral salts magnesium phosphate and potassium phosphate are used, plus vitamin B-complex.
4 Vitamin C is very important to aid the immune system, and to help both the detoxification of the liver, and the repair work.[4]

Case History

Usually natural therapists find themselves treating post-hepatitis cases but in this instance, Ron, aged twenty-eight, had been under medical supervision for five months with a continuing positive blood test for hepatitis B. He was very tired and was suffering still from headaches and nausea. Diet was good in Ron's case and he was keeping off all fat and endeavouring to have plenty of fruit and vegetables.

Clinical findings included tenderness in the liver area, heavily coated tongue, and a moderate degree of toxins showing in the iris in association with the bowel area. A disturbance in the dermatoglyphics or finger pattern on the hands indicated acid waste as the result of faulty metabolic processes.

The prescription for the first month included potassium and magnesium phosphate combined with a strong potency B-complex for improving nerve tone and energy, a mixture of liver and cleansing herbs, sodium sulphate as a mineral liver tonic, iron phosphate for inflammation of the liver, and vitamin C to boost immunity and to help the detoxification process. After this month of treatment, headaches and nausea had gone, and energy was improving. The blood test was negative for hepatitis after two months of treatment.

The treatment was continued for three more months with minor alterations and improvement continued after it finished. There was a further bout of digestive problems six months after leaving off treatment, and this again responded well with appropriate medication. After many months off treatment, Ron has had no further relapse with his liver.

An important point is illustrated here. Natural therapists find that at least six months is needed to consolidate the treatment following a serious acute or chronic illness. In this case the client chose to discontinue after four months and this was apparently not quite long enough to restore the lasting function of the digestive system. Although the hepatitis did not return, other digestive problems cropped up as a result of digestive weakness not being fully corrected.

Hernia

Under this heading it is logical for the naturopath to consider all types of hernias as we are mainly concerned with the biochemical reasons for the weakness of tissue which results in a hernia. The most common type of hernia which natural therapists treat is the hiatus or diaphragmatic hernia. This is found to be present to a greater or lesser extent in 60 per cent of persons over sixty.[1] Less commonly, natural therapists treat abdominal, umbilical and inguinal hernias. The latter group are more amenable to surgery, and as they often involve the bowel, there is the possibility of bowel strangulation unless corrective measures are taken.

The main symptoms of the diaphragmatic hernias near the junction of the stomach and oesophagus occur from stomach acid regurgitating into the oesophagus and throat. This is aggravated by lying down after a large meal and by exercise which involves bending forward. There can also be a feeling like a stone sitting under the sternum. Particular foods will aggravate the condition, especially acid foods.

Causes

The problem with elastic and fibrous tissue which forms the gastro-oesophageal junction as it passes through the diaphragm is a deficiency in the tissue salt, calcium fluoride. This calcium salt has been found essential for healthy tissue and its deficiency or lack of assimilation results in a number of diverse problems.[2] These include all those structures which contain elastic tissue such as ligaments, tendons, veins and will therefore manifest in varying problems at many different sites in the body.

In treating hiatus hernia, natural therapists also find an associated digestive weakness which appears to contribute markedly to the problem. We often find in clinical practice that symptoms of discomfort entirely disappear long before the hernia could have healed with the use of calcium fluoride; a slow acting remedy at best. It is logical that congestion in the liver, and any excessive turbulence of the stomach will cause more pressure on the weakness in the diaphgram.

Treatment

1 Digestive herbs for both stomach and liver as, for instance, dandelion, centaury, wahoo, melissa, angelica, and marshmallow.
2 Sodium phosphate to alkalinise the overacidity of the digestive process.
3 Calcium fluoride as the tissue salt or in homoeopathic potency. This will be needed for up to two years.
4 Magnesium phosphate to correct spasm in the upper digestive tract.

Case History

Russell, aged fifty-seven, is a retired scrap merchant and a typical case of hiatus hernia. He was sent by his wife who was previously treated by me. His main symptoms were acid regurgitation of food, and he described a diet high in sweets and junk food. After explaining the relationship between the diet and indigestion, Russell was motivated to considerably change his diet. On the second visit he reported cutting down on sweets and refined food.

The therapy for the first month included a herbal mixture for the digestion as described earlier, liver herbs in tablet form, fluoride in a base of astringent herbs and vitamins C and B-complex in the form of yeast tablets. He was slightly better after one month and the same prescription was continued for a further two months. He reported feeling well at the third visit and there were no relapses. The treatment was continued for eight months altogether to consolidate progress. During the last two months, the remedies were reduced and tapered off.

Herpes

Clients with herpes simplex virus 1 and 2 are very common and it has been estimated that between 20 and 40 per cent of persons in the USA have been infected by the virus.[1] The type which manifests on the face is usually virus 1 and that which is commonly called venereal or genital herpes is type 2.

The usual symptoms, apart from a feeling of general malaise, fever, and enlargement of lymph nodes, are actual skin lesions on the face, oral mucosa, or genitals. These lesions, usually in the form of vesicles, develop in groups on lips, around the nose, or on the genitals. In type 2, which features on the genitals, the vesicles become ulcers in several days. The cervix in the female may also be involved, and the genital area around the lesions is often swollen.

Causes

As usual, the natural therapist is looking for the first cause beyond the immediate infective virus. We do, however, recognise the very infectious nature of the condition and would not be so naive as to say that even a healthy person could withstand continual sexual contact with a person infected with type 2. Nevertheless, as it is expected that two out of three women with the infection will have relapses, natural therapists can report that those treated with natural therapies appear to become immune for long periods.

Natural therapists would also comment that certain types of constitutions are more prone to the problem, and that in homoeopathic language, particular inherited miasms make one more likely to manifest herpes. It has been found that the great majority of persons tested are positive for antibodies, with greatest incidence amongst lower socio-economic groups, and with prostitutes having the highest incidence.[2]

Perhaps therefore, one could dare to suggest that one subjective cause may be an imbalance of the sacral centre, resulting in promiscuity. This is a generalisation and obviously does not cover those cases who unfortunately contact genital herpes with their first sexual partner, nor does it necessarily relate to infection with virus 1 in the face area. These latter cases would express an inherited disposition, and unless we apply some of the concepts of reincarnation, the relationship of promiscuity to the sacral centre will not be placed in correct perspective.

It is worth mentioning that the energies which substand the physical body, and which are likened to an electromagnetic field, appear to be intimately related to immunity in the following manner. If a chaotic pattern is set up in our electrical field by interaction with electrical fields from motors, high tension wires, radiation, or by intimate interaction with a number of other human fields as occurs in promiscuous behaviour, immunity to infection appears to be lost. Poor diet is also understood to affect our electrical field.

Medical orthodoxy already accepts that disorders like hepatitis, glandular fever, and herpes manifest when people have reduced their immunity through stress of various types. The more technical explanation for lowered immunity may be demonstrated in the future as an electrical imbalance which precedes any biochemical disturbance and specific pathology. It is not a very big jump from recognition of the effect of man-made electrical fields on immunity to the effect of another person's electrical field on our own, once validity of the human electrical field has been established. Acquired Immune Deficiency Syndrome (AIDS) should perhaps also be evaluated in this manner.

Treatment

Treatment may need to be over a couple of years, given the recurrent and virulent nature of herpes. Specific supplements will include the following:

1   Vitamin C in large doses — for acute attacks, intravenous vitamin C will cut short an attack due to its inhibiting effect on the virus.[3]

2 Vitamin B in doses of at least 50mg of each component daily.

3 Zinc salts to promote immunity and healing.[4]

4 Iron phosphate and potassium chloride to reduce inflammation and to dry the vesicles.

5 Lymphatic cleansing herbs such as violet leaves, trifolium, burdock, sarsaparilla, and liver herbs for metabolising toxins.

6 Potassium phosphate and magnesium phosphate for improving the health of the nerves.

7 Homoeopathic Natrum muriaticum is almost specific for herpes, but the potency and frequency must be selected carefully.

8 The amino acid lysine has been found valuable in therapeutic doses.[5]

9 Vitamin A in large doses is usually given in a water soluble form and strengthens the immunity of epithelial tissue to the infection.

Case Histories

Mary, aged thirty, attended the clinic for facial and genital herpes in the winter of 1984. As her work involved public relations, it was important for her health to be restored as soon as possible. Her history included severe asthma from the age of three to fifteen; also a paternal aunt had died of asthma. Her mother had a history of facial herpes.

This was a case where there was co-operation between the medical and naturopathic professions. After we resolved the first very bad attack of herpes, Mary was advised that future attacks could be shortened by the use of intravenous vitamin C. During the first six months' treatment she had a minor attack following influenza; its strength may well have been lessened by the use of intravenous vitamin C which was administered by a registered medical doctor at the first sign of the attack.

Her naturopathic treatment included liver and lymphatic herbs, vitamin A in large doses, the amino acid lysine, vitamins B and C, zinc, and the mineral combination which we use for so many skin inflammations and vesicles — iron phosphate and potassium chloride. During the first month, homoeopathic sulphur was used in high potency, an interesting deviation from the usual Natrum muriaticum which is almost specific for herpes.

Two months later in the treatment, vitamin E was introduced to resolve scarring tendencies on the face.

As Mary has a very high pressure job, and as she is very pleased to use the treatment for health insurance, most of the basics mentioned have been continued for eighteen months, although she does not attend the clinic often. When seen several months ago, her progress had been maintained.

Felicity, an accountant aged thirty-six, suffered recurrent bouts of genital herpes. Other problems included poor sleep, and constipation. Felicity admitted to a poor diet and the herpes appeared to manifest whenever she was under extra stress at work. Her treatment included lymphatic cleansing herbs, vitamin B-complex and vitamin C, magnesium and potassium phosphate, liver herbs for the constipation and homoeopathic Natrum muriaticum as specific for the herpes virus.

This treatment was continued for nine months and although she had three bouts of herpes during the first half of this time, the attacks cleared very quickly. The bowel became regular and energy improved.

Hiccoughs

This phenomenon is included because it can occasionally affect a person so dramatically that treatment is needed to balance the nervous system, and to prevent the acute embarrassment resulting from the disturbance.

Causes

From the medical point of view it is classed as a nerve irritation involving the diaphragm. From the naturopathic viewpoint we find that repeated hiccoughs occur in people who are particularly deficient in magnesium. Magnesium is needed for all conditions where nerves and muscles need sedating or relaxing. [1]

Case History

In my fifteen years of practice I have only had to attend two very severe cases of this problem. In each case there was hiccoughing followed by burping every 15–20 seconds. In the case of Karen, aged twelve, the problem had been manifesting for four weeks and she had to have special seating arrangements outside her classroom. Indeed the continuous sounds were so extraordinary that it was difficult to know if one felt like laughing or crying at her predicament!

For her first week's treatment, Karen was given magnesium phosphate, B-complex, and two homoeopathic mixtures in different potencies. The first included homoeopathics for the liver as it was obvious from the iris that a toxic element involving the liver was in part irritating the diaphragm. Bach flower remedies were also included in this first mixture. The other homoeopathic remedies were magnesium phosphate and Dioscoria, both in high potency.

One week later, it was obvious from Karen's intermittent silence that improvement was taking place. The treatment was continued with the addition of a herbal sedative. Her mother reported that the problem disappeared while Karen was asleep even though severe during the day. This illustrates the obvious nerve factor and, in Karen's case, her mother felt there was a psychosomatic factor also. The Bach flower remedies covered this aspect.

After three weeks the burping and hiccoughing disappeared and improvement continued while we tapered off treatment during the fourth month. During the third month's treatment, as happens with so many cases, there was a healing crisis involving a respiratory infection. Appropriate treatment was added at this stage with an emphasis on cleansing the lymphatic system.

Hodgkin's Disease

Hodgkin's disease is not one which the natural therapist will be called upon to treat often. It is a fairly rare malignant process involving the lymph glands. In my years of practice, I have had the opportunity of using natural therapies to help the general health of only two cases, and both persons responded well and enjoyed long remissions. Chemotherapy was also used in these cases.

Causes

The reader is referred to the section entitled Cancer. One specific point in relation to this type of cancer is of interest. One would imagine that the lymphatic system as depicted in the iris would indicate great congestion prior or during the process of Hodgkin's disease. In discussion with colleagues, it appears that this finding is variable, indicating the many complex causes of the cancer process. The two cases mentioned by me were not good examples of lymphatic congestion as depicted by iris diagnosis. However, in a further case, who unfortunately died within a couple of years after having the disease diagnosed, an extraordinarily prominent lymphatic rosary was noted in the iris.

Treatment

This tends to be directed towards the improvement of general health; in addition most clients would be having standard medical treatment such as chemotherapy. The main thrust of natural therapy treatment would be to tone the vital organs such as liver and kidneys, and to promote the immune system by the use of herbs and vitamin C.

Hypertension

see Atherosclerosis and Blood Pressure

Hyperthyroidism

see Goitre

Hypoglycaemia

Perhaps this condition is the most popular malady of the 1980s, for many patients present at our clinic with the information that they are sufferers. Although it is used almost as an excuse for a group of symptoms which seem to accompany an erratic blood sugar curve, there is no doubt that modern society inclines us in the direction of energy imbalance.[1]

Common problems associated with the condition include depression, craving for sugar, tiredness, insomnia, nervousness, anxiety, headache, and lack of concentration. As this list is rather common to many conditions and to modern society in general, the only specific diagnosis can be through the challenge of a large dose of glucose, followed by blood tests to trace how the body is handling sugar — the traditional glucose tolerance test.

Causes

The immediate observable cause is low blood sugar which is greatly aggravated by the regular eating of refined sugar foods.[2] This gives a temporary rise but is then followed by a large drop in the blood sugar. Coffee provides a similar experience to some extent.

More basic and interesting causes relate to the general life-style of the patient. How do they come to have irregular meals of refined carbohydrate, stressful jobs, lack of regular sleep, and to be lacking in those elements in the diet needed to give a normal blood sugar?

Treatment

Obviously the life-style is of considerable importance to the natural therapist, and time is spent exploring the diet, work life, home life and any other stresses. In relation to the diet, regular meals featuring slow release carbohydrates like millet, oats, whole wheat, almonds and sunflower seeds are promoted. In addition, a diet with an abundance of vegetables, both steamed and raw, and moderate amounts of protein is encouraged. Coffee, soft drinks, and even excess fruit either juiced, whole, or dried is discouraged. Honey is reduced to a couple of teaspoons daily.

Specific supplements may include the following:

1 The vitamin B group has a stabilising effect on the nerves and blood sugar.
2 Vitamin C is used as an anti-stress vitamin.
3 Zinc and magnesium have been found necessary as they are minerals involved with many enzymes in the process of sugar metabolism.[3] Chromium is often deficient in problems with the pancreas.[4] The reader is referred also to the section on Diabetes which may have some connection with hypoglycaemia.

4 Potassium phosphate is often combined by the natural therapist with magnesium phosphate for balancing the autonomic nervous system, and thus improving the digestive processes. [5]

5 Liver herbs are always given to tone that organ and this has considerable effect on sugar metabolism.

6 Constitutional homoeopathic prescribing is invaluable for these type of cases.

Case History

Mark, aged twenty-four, was a fairly simple case to treat although he had suffered with his digestion for a period of eight years. He was lethargic after meals, and had lack of concentration and faintness. He was worse in the morning and worse after taking sugar. Most of his symptoms indicated hypoglycaemia or low blood sugar. As he has a high pressure job in advertising, it is important for him to feel consistently energetic throughout the day.

Improvement was immediate and lasting after taking a few months' supplements including liver herbs, zinc compound, magnesium and potassium phosphate compound, kelp and calcium phosphate. Mark had probably been deficient in these basic minerals for many years. He had already been using vitamin C and B-complex supplements and these were continued during treatment with the minerals.

As the minerals are the basic building blocks of so many tissues and biochemical processes in the body, natural therapists find repeatedly that vitamin supplements alone do nothing for a condition like hypoglycaemia. Once the mineral deficiency has been made good, stability can be maintained with a good diet.

Hypotension

see Blood Pressure

Hysteria

see Anxiety

Immune Deficiency Disorders

see Auto-immune Disorders

Immunity and the promotion of a healthy immune system are both central to all naturopathic treatment. In terms of the common infectious disorders like the common cold and influenza, the childhood infectious fevers, glandular fever, hepatitis, and the more chronic disorders of rheumatoid arthritis, multiple sclerosis, and other auto-immune disorders, natural therapists understand the treatment of the whole person to be essential.

Causes

The psychology of the person, general life-style including nutrition, the environment and work factors are all considered to have a role in maintaining an efficient immune system.

Specific causes of poor immunity may be deficiencies of zinc, vitamin C, and vitamin A, chemical pollution, electronic pollution, lack of rest and suppressed emotions, and in the more esoteric sense, a lack of alignment between the various levels of our inner constitution. Lack of thymus secretion which is directly related to an under-active etheric heart *chakra* is another more subjective cause. Thus one could say that imbalance at both the subjective and physical level is the general problem to be addressed although this is a very broad topic and therefore encompasses many aspects of treatment.

Treatment

This is covered under the heading Auto-immune Disorders and to some extent under each of the diseases listed in the first paragraph of this section. At the subjective level, counselling and a suitably selected meditation programme can achieve a great deal, and at the objective level, cleansing herbs and vitamin C are nearly always included, but there are many other variables applicable to each condition.

Impetigo

Impetigo is a common infectious skin condition usually manifesting in children. It manifests as a pink flat spot which rapidly becomes a vesicle, then a pustule which later develops into a scab. The face is the usual site and the condition rapidly spreads.

Cause and Treatment

The cause from the point of view of naturopathic philosophy is a deficiency of calcium salts on the basis of a tubercular heredity. Deficiencies of basic vitamins also plays a part. Specific treatment includes:

1 Calcium phosphate, iron phosphate for the inflammation, and potassium chloride for the serous discharge of the vesicles. [1]
2 Vitamins A and C to improve immunity.
3 Liver and lymphatic herbs or homoeopathics.
4 Specific anti-tubercular homoeopathics.

Case History

This condition is usually encountered in young children but Stephen presented with a king-size bout at eighteen years. It was of interest that he had previously suffered asthma, as natural therapists often find that when chest conditions are working out of the system the area involving the nose or face becomes affected. In this case the whole of the lower part of the face was affected and had become pustular and scabby.

Stephen responded well in a few weeks with large doses of vitamin C, calcium phosphate, 3g of vitamin C daily and large doses of blood cleansing or lymphatic herbs. He was given papaw ointment to apply locally as this is both antiseptic and soothing.

Influenza

see Colds

Iron Deficiency

see Anaemia

Insomnia

This problem is not given much space in standard medical texts and yet it affects about 30 per cent of the population during the course of one year.[1] Insomnia is a very common condition treated by natural therapists as many people object to taking drugs for sleeplessness and they prefer to look for a more lasting and curative solution.

Causes

Natural therapists find there are two basic causes. About 50 per cent of people respond to a selection of natural remedies to balance the nervous system. This group would be classed as suffering from deficiencies or biochemical imbalances. The remainder have more subtle problems of psychological and psychic origin. These persons may have problems with their life-style and various unresolved conflicts and will respond to counselling, relaxation and meditation techniques and to homoeopathic or Bach flower remedies.

Treatment

To discover the right approach to any particular individual with insomnia, a detailed case history will be necessary. The following information may be necessary especially for homoeopathic pre-scribing: whether there is trouble getting off to sleep or in staying asleep, times and positions for sleep, type of dreams, and disturbing thoughts which occur during wakefulness. Specific remedies may include:

1 B-complex in small doses in the morning. Large doses at night can be over-stimulating.
2 Magnesium compounds for relaxing nerves and muscles. [2]
3 Herbal sedatives; valerian, passaflora, vervain, mistletoe, scullcap are all popular and useful. [3]
4 Tryptophan, an amino acid, has been found useful in selected cases.
5 Constitutional homoeopathic remedies.

Case Histories

Usually, natural therapists find that people do not come just for insomnia, but it is included amongst a number of other problems. The following three cases are typical of this experience.

Susan, a student teacher aged twenty-two, required treatment for ailments including nervous irritability, poor sleep, scanty and irregular periods, and numbness in one foot. She also complained of catarrhal problems. It actually took five months to sort out all these problems including the sleep.

The particular part of her treatment for the balancing of the nervous system and improving of sleep included calcium, magnesium and potassium phosphates, and a herbal tablet composed of valerian, scullcap, hops, and passaflora. B-complex also contributed to her improvement.

Neil, a records clerk aged twenty-two, came for treatment following an acute attack of glandular fever. His stomach and spleen were still enlarged and he was suffering from headaches as well as insomnia. His sleep improved after the first month, and the main ingredients for the nervous system were potassium and magnesium phosphate in combination with vitamin B-complex. There is no doubt that in his case the abdominal congestion was contributing to the sleep problem and this was resolved with a herbal mixture for the liver, spleen and lymphatic system.

Fiona, aged twelve, was treated for insomnia, irritability, headache and hypoglycaemia and difficult behaviour. In a number of cases, the same biochemical imbalances which give headache will also produce insomnia. As with most children, Fiona was considerably improved after the first month. Her remedies included magnesium and calcium phosphate in the ratio of 2:1, vitamin B-complex plus extra B3 and B6 for the behaviour problems described by her mother, and the nerve herbs listed in the first case. Fiona had three months' treatment and she had no relapses during this time.

Ischaemic Heart Disease

see Arterial Disease

J

Jaundice

see also Hepatitis

There are many forms and causes for jaundice, but in each case it is characterised by a yellowish tinge to the skin and sclera or white of the eye, and the urine is usually dark as a result of the extra bile pigment present.

Causes

The immediate cause is a back flow of bile into the blood as a result of pressure on the bile ducts which lead into the duodenum. This pressure may be due to swelling and inflammation as with infective hepatitis, pressure from a tumour, or a blocking off through the presence of stones.

Causes which interest the naturopath are more fundamental, such as the disturbance in biochemistry which leads to the formation of stones in the liver or gall-bladder, and perhaps the disturbance in psychology which underlies the change in biochemistry. Haemolytic anaemia is a more rare cause of jaundice, involving the premature breakdown of red blood cells within the blood stream.

Treatment

see Hepatitis and Gallstones.

There will be individual differences because of the different causes, but in the main, most of the principles covered under the section on hepatitis will prevail except for the more mechanical problem of gallstones.

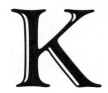

Kidney Stones

Calcium stone formation takes place more frequently in men from the third decade onwards.[1] The problem is strongly familial. Uric acid stones are also mainly formed by men. Struvite stones are mainly found in women and usually follow bacterial infection. Oxalate stones have been ascribed to fat malabsorption. Stones are not necessarily painful, although the most common symptoms of their presence is pain and haematuria (blood in the urine). Renal colic is associated with a stone which is lodged in the ureter.

Causes

Causes include both primary and secondary metabolic diseases such as hyperparathyroidism, excess vitamin D supplements, destructive bone disease, Cushings' syndrome and sarcoidosis. More immediate causes for stone formation involve insufficient fluid consumption, and biochemical imbalances which promote increased excretion of stone constituents.

From the naturopathic viewpoint, an imbalanced diet will foster formation of stones, especially if lacking in fresh fruit and vegetables.[2] An excess of proteins and carbohydrates, foods high in calcium such as dairy products, low fibre and high alcohol intake have all been cited as causes.[3] A deficiency in magnesium and vitamin B6 is considered to predispose towards stone formation.[4] More deep-seated causes involve the sclerosing tendency examined in anthroposophical medical literature, and problems involving the base *chakra*.[5]

Treatment

Dietary considerations will be very important. For the most common problem involving calcium stones, the client will increase fibre, complex carbohydrates, leafy green vegetables and foods rich in magnesium such as brown rice, oats, soybeans, avocado, bananas and rye bread. Foods rich in purine such as yeast, poultry, fish and meat will be reduced, as will dairy produce. For oxalate stones, spinach, strawberries and rhubarb will be deleted from the diet. Unfortunately, not many clients have a biochemical analysis of their stones, making dietary choices more difficult. A healthy and interesting diet, however, can be arranged by taking all these factors into account.

Supplements will include:

1 Magnesium orotate or phosphate for preventing further stones and for reducing spasm in the ureter.
2 Vitamin B6 which has been found to prevent further stones.
3 Iron phosphate for reducing bleeding and inflammation of kidney and/or ureter.
4 Parsley piert, pellitory, and other herbs traditionally used for kidney stones.
5 Sodium sulphate which has also been found valuable to prevent further stone formation and to act as a kidney tonic. This tissue salt balances body fluids.[6]
6 Homoeopathic berberis in varying potencies has been found to be specific for dissolving stones and curing renal colic. The famous English homoeopath who treated the royal family, Dr Margery Blackie, commonly used a high potency of berberis to stop renal colic and to promote the passing of stones.[7] This homoeopathic remedy would also act as a biochemical regulator.

Case Histories

Frank, aged seventy-one, had attended the clinic intermittently over several years for a variety of ailments. He had a history of high blood pressure and this was diagnosed at the beginning of 1986 as associated with kidney problems. An X-ray of the kidney revealed three stones. Other problems included frequency associated with a slightly enlarged prostate gland, and rheumatism which gave him pain in the legs.

His treatment consisted of liver and rheumatic herbs, sodium phosphate, magnesium and potassium phosphate, B-complex and a separate supplement of B6. This prescription was repeated for another two months, and he felt well during this time. Homoeopathic kidney remedies were also used and several kidney stones were painlessly passed over a period of six months. The blood pressure reduced to within normal limits for his age and the leg pains disappeared.

It was interesting that kidney lesions did show in Frank's left iris, indicating a tendency to kidney problems. Vega diagnosis indicated weakness of the kidney and also of the pancreas. On enquiry it was found that several elderly relatives developed diabetes in old age, indicating a familial pancreatic weakness. A couple of months later, during a health crisis, mild diabetes manifested. Frank had already been on homoeopathic drops for the pancreas following the Vega diagnosis, and this may have minimised the diabetes. There have been no further kidney stones.

Maurice, aged forty-eight, visited the clinic after a diagnosis of calcium oxalate kidney stones. Five years prior to this time, he had calcium carbonate stones. The iris indicated a lesion in the left kidney, and a degree of acid waste showed in the iris, indicating a biochemical imbalance of the tissues.

He was given magnesium phosphate for spasm, vitamin B6 to prevent further stone formation, sodium phosphate for acidity, liver herbs for cleansing, iron phosphate for inflammation and a high potency of Berberis as a specific homoeopathic remedy. On his return visit, health was found to be good with no renal colic. The prescription was repeated. At the next visit, he was in the middle of an attack of renal colic. The magnesium phosphate was then given hourly with a homoeopathic mixture of hepatica which is used for blockage of small tubes in the body. A herbal mixture containing marshmallow, burdock, pellitory and trifolium was taken six times daily.

An X-ray later in the month revealed that the stone had moved down to the end of the ureter and it was later passed without too much trouble. In this case, treatment should have been continued as there was obviously a metabolic problem which needed at least six months' treatment.

Laryngitis

Laryngitis is something we have nearly all experienced as part of a respiratory infection; it literally means inflammation of the larynx. It is characterised by a sore throat and husky voice. In severe cases the voice disappears completely for several days or more.

Causes

The obvious immediate cause is a respiratory virus but the underlying cause is lack of immunity which may in turn result from a poor life-style. Immediate considerations are vitamin C status, congestion of the lymphatic system, stress and other environmental factors such as pollution.

The more interesting cause relates to the state of the throat *chakra* which has an intimate connection to the throat, thyroid and respiratory system in general. The throat *chakra* literally sounds forth the creative note of our being, and if we are unable to make any vocal sound except a hoarse squeak, there is a temporary disturbance or imbalance involving the energy which should be flowing through the throat *chakra*.

In this connection, we could consider a school teacher daily facing a group of thirty or more hyperactive students. Does she repeatedly succumb to respiratory infections which start as a sore throat because of so many children coughing or blowing over her, or is there a more subtle contributing factor? Representing as it does the creative activity in humanity, the throat centre can easily become irregular in its action through frustration and inability to express ourselves fully.

The typical modern classroom produces difficulty in the teaching situation as a result of many children suffering from hyper-activity caused by poor nutrition. Many teachers attending the clinic have reported on the growing problem of unmanageable children — especially teachers who have been in the profession for twenty years or more. The frustration of this situation would be sufficient to cause a disturbance in the throat *chakra*, which in turn would make the area more vulnerable to infection.

This is just one example of many which could be suggested in relation to the throat area and the underlying effect from the throat *chakra*. In any situation where the voice has to be con-stantly raised and strained such as when trying to enforce disci-pline, one can imagine the two-way effect on the physical and psychic constitution.

Another point of interest could be added about creativity as an expression of a developed throat *chakra*. Perhaps those teachers and lecturers who are most truly creative are those who have no trouble in attaining discipline. This would be a positive example of the right kind of energy flowing through the throat centre. One wonders if these people would also have greater immunity to infection.

Treatment

Basic aids to immunity are provided, and in the case of engorged lymphatic glands in the neck area, the treatment for cleansing the lymphatic system would need to be continued for several months to prevent recurrence. Sometimes it is necessary to strengthen the thyroid gland by the use of kelp which contains iodine. Attention to life-style is important in terms of work-style, relaxation and rest patterns. The need for suitable creative expression is emphasised.

Specific aids may include:

1 Vitamin C and the bio-flavanoids to improve immunity and to assist detoxification of the lymph glands.[1]
2 Iron phosphate for the inflammation and potassium chlo-ride for mucus.
3 Vitamin A to increase resistance of epithelial tissue.
4 Lymphatic herbs and homoeopathic preparations of same to cleanse the lymphatic system, for example, violet leaves, trifolium, burdock, echinacea, phytolacca.

5 Specific homoeopathics for the larynx and for the individual constitution.

Case History

Mrs M.G., aged fifty-four, came to visit the clinic following an
attack of laryngitis which had lasted for one week. She had been
feeling unwell generally with an arthritic tendency, an inclina-
tion to accumulate fluid, hot flushes, and loose bowels. Her
menstrual periods appeared to be phasing out.

After one month's treatment she had more energy, excess fluid
was not noticed, and she reported that the laryngitis had cleared
quickly. Treatment was continued for the hot flushes for another
two months. Her prescription included Causticum in homoeopathic potency for the laryngitis, another group of homoeopathic
remedies for the hot flushes, kidney herbs and sodium sulphate
for the excess fluid, rheumatic herbs, vitamin B and C, and liver
herbs.

Particular improvement was noted after she took sodium sulphate in a high potency, and this indicates the benefit of using
the mineral salts in both small physical and in homoeopathic
doses if indicated by the constitution of the client.

Leukaemia

see also Cancer

As with other forms of cancer, the natural therapist treats this
problem in conjunction with a registered practitioner. Leukaemia is of several kinds, and the usual medical treatment is
chemotherapy. Some of the main problems associated with this
cancer of the blood cells relates to the disappearance of other
types of cells which are necessary to protect against infection.
Platelets, which supply the normal clotting factor of the blood,
may also be reduced. Thus some of the problems in advanced
stages of the disease are lack of immunity to infection and haemorrhage. The bone marrow is usually severely affected and is
unable to produce normal white blood cells.

Causes

As with all cancer, these are multiple. The naturopath accepts the rapidly growing medical opinion that cancer is basically a problem of the immune system, and especially in the case of lymphatic leukaemias, this is evident from iris diagnosis.

The far-reaching psychic causes are of interest because one type of leukaemia has a peak incidence in children between the age of two and four years. If we reflect on the more subtle influences and causes, the implication of karma from previous lives would need to be considered. These more distant causes would be locked into the karmic relationships between parents and child. In many cases, the suffering of the parents of children with malignancies appears greater than that of the children concerned.

Treatment

Naturopathic treatment is directed to being supportive of the general health and to improving immunity. We have also found that natural therapies mitigate the side effects of chemotherapy to a considerable degree. Basic minerals, vitamins and cleansing herbs are administered with nutritional guidance, and where indicated, specific homoeopathic remedies could be useful. Megadoses of vitamin C may be of particular importance in controlling leukaemias.[1]

Lymphomas

see Cancer

M

Measles

This childhood disorder usually begins with symptoms like a heavy cold accompanied by fever. The rash appears on the fourth day and manifests as pink macules (raised spots) behind ears and on face, and rapidly spreads to the trunk and limbs. Complications such as broncho-pneumonia, infected ears, and gastro-enteritis are not uncommon in untreated children and are caused by secondary infection.

Causes

The obvious cause is a virus called morbilli, but natural therapists are concerned with the reasons for susceptibility to the virus. The naturopathic concern is with the lack of immunity which children suffer as a result of poor diet, although inherited factors play a part. Lack of immunity relates to poor vitamin C status in many cases, and to a congested lymphatic system.[1] Natural therapists can often predict through iris diagnosis the likely severity of measles.

Treatment

I have never known complications occur in a case of measles where a few natural remedies were given from the beginning of the appearance of the rash. Natural therapists are opposed to vaccination for measles because of the research which has been undertaken by medical scientists which indicates the possible harm and general lack of usefulness of vaccination.[2]

The parents are advised to give the child a very simple diet of raw juices, steamed vegetables and fruits. Specific treatment is as follows:

1 Vitamin C — at least 2g daily.
2 Iron phosphate for the fever and inflammation of skin, and potassium chloride for the lymphatic system.
3 Lymphatic cleansing herbs or homoeopathics — the latter are easier to take.
4 Liver homoeopathics to tone that organ as an aid to detoxification.
5 Pectoral herbs for the lungs may be needed if a cough is present.
6 Homoeopathic antidote to the measles virus.

Melanoma

see Cancer

It may be useful to make the comment that in a recent medical survey reported by *The Age* newspaper, Australians were informed that the incidence of melanoma was highest in the state of Victoria — the coldest Australian state except for Tasmania. Yet Australians have the highest incidence in the world because of their addiction to sunbathing! It is more logical to conclude that the Australian life-style or diet is more conducive to the disease. The deficiency of selenium in Victorian soils may be responsible for the higher incidence: it has been shown that selenium levels are related to cancer incidence.[1]

Meniere's Disease

This syndrome of vertigo or recurrent dizzy spells usually commences in about the fifth decade of life, although it can occur earlier. It may be accompanied by nausea and vomiting and progresses towards tinnitus (ringing in the ears) and deafness. In some milder cases, the patient may complain only of head discomfort and lack of concentration.

Causes

These are not altogether clear-cut according to medical authorities. It is understood that the pathological changes involve
dilation of the endolymphatic system, followed by degeneration
of the vestibular and cochlear hair cells. The actual vertigo
relates to a disorder of the labyrinth or semi-circular canals
within the ear structure, but it is not known how the former
problem of the hair cells is related to the labyrinth disturbance.[1]

From the point of view of natural therapy and diagnosis, it is
interesting that the first disturbance is now believed to involve
part of the lymphatic system. Natural therapists have often found
various kinds of ear disturbances involving vertigo to have a
catarrhal basis involving a congested lymphatic system. The final
deafness which accompanies the nerve destruction is understood
therefore, to originate from a lymphatic disturbance.

The more esoteric cause may be a disturbance involving the
energy centre called the Ajna *chakra*, situated between the two
eyes. As this centre unfolds and develops, temporary problems
with eyes, ears and nose can occur. As with most disorders, there
is probably an inner and outer factor with Meniere's syndrome.
The Ajna *chakra* is related to a stage in our development during
which we integrate all the personality forces in our being, and it
is easy to imagine the temporary energy disturbances which could
occur during this process.

Case Histories

Jean, aged sixty-four, visited the clinic in the hope of gaining
relief for her condition of Meniere's disease which had been
diagnosed more than ten years before. She was continually giddy
in spite of medical treatment, and had pain across the top of her
eyes. Iris diagnosis showed plaque formation in her arterial system. This congestion of the arteries could have been a definite
contributing factor to her ear problem.

During the first month's treatment, she had only one attack of
dizziness, and this was less severe than usual. General energy was
much improved. The first month's treatment included calcium
fluoride and silica to start clearing the arterial condition, potassium phosphate as the main mineral salt for vertigo, vitamin
B-complex to augment the general nerve toning, liver herbs for

cleansing, and specific homoeopathic remedies for Meniere's disease which included Cocculus indicus. Later, garlic was added to help clear the arteries and the lymphatic system.

This basic treatment was continued for a number of months, and other ingredients were added during temporary health crises caused by influenza, her mother's death, and an operation for bunions. There was only one short relapse of vertigo at one of these critical points, probably brought on by the need to make important decisions.

Recently, Jean returned for further therapy. Her return followed removal of benign tumours in the neck region. There had been no relapse of the Meniere's disease and she continues to maintain basic preventive treatment for this syndrome. In the older age group and with this type of condition, clients are very glad to stay on maintenance doses for a long time, as their relief from the problem is so greatly valued.

Elois visited me at the age of fifty for vertigo of three months' duration. Her giddiness came in waves. She had been using the standard medical medication. A history of osteoarthritis in the neck may have been a contributing factor to the vertigo, and she had a history of migraine.

Her first prescription included the specific homoeopathic remedy for vertigo — Cocculus indicus in the 30th potency, liver and rheumatic herbs, magnesium and potassium phosphate to stabilise the nervous system, and the mineral combination potassium chloride and iron phosphate to deal with any catarrh affecting the ear and also for the inflammation of the cervical spine caused by the arthritis.

On her second visit she reported that the dizziness had gone but an acute situation with the gall-bladder appeared to have developed. The first prescription was repeated with the addition of a homoeopathic mixture for the gall-bladder. Improvement was then maintained with the Meniere's problem for several months until a slight relapse occurred with the death of her mother. Adjustments were made to the remedies at this time, but the basic treatment for vertigo was continued.

Elois then went on holiday and I did not see her for a few months. After this break she returned; her arm and wrist were very painful with rheumatism for the next two months. Vertigo had also returned. Post-menopausal flushes made their appearance and were improved with the addition of vitamin E.

It was at this stage that it was suggested she might be helped by learning the Vivaxis techniques as I had found them very valuable for vertigo. Using a particular form of 'scanning' it was found that Elois had a severe oxygen deficiency in the skull area. Vivaxis techniques are based on developing radiaesthesia and visualisation skills. Interested persons may wish to study my manual on this subject.[2] In the case of Elois, the oxygen disturbance was found to be caused by using a brand of hair spray. As soon as the spray was discontinued there was permanent relief from the dizziness.

Elois continued treatment for her Meniere's syndrome and arthritis for another five months. There was no relapse with the dizziness except for a few minor disturbances. The treatment was changed in minor respects in relation to the arthritis and various challenges to her health, such as a bout of insomnia during the sale of the family home, and recurrence of hot flushes.

Meningitis

This condition is a notifiable infectious disease and as such does not feature often in the practice of the natural therapist. I have never seen a case during my time of consulting practice. If presented, however, with a child suffering high temperature, headache, and neck rigidity or stiffness, one would certainly not waste time and the patient would be referred immediately for orthodox medical investigation and treatment. Meningitis is caused by acute inflammation of the meninges or covering of the brain, and it is this serious development close to the cerebral tissue which makes the disease so dangerous to life. The severe irritation to the brain causes the headache, fever, possible delirium and neck stiffness which characterise the illness.

Causes

The cause of meningitis is always of infective origin in the first analysis, and may be either the meningoccocal bacteria or a secondary infection of the meninges from a virus from which the person is already suffering, such as measles. Diagnosis can only be certain by obtaining a specimen of cerebro-spinal fluid through lumbar puncture, and its microscopic examination and culture.

While not ignoring the immediate infective cause, naturo-pathic principles teach that the deep structures of the body only become infected in a very toxic organism. In other words, natu-ral therapists see infectious disease moving into the vital organs such as lungs, liver, kidneys and brain in direct proportion to the health and immunity of the individual.

Given a reasonable life-style, and correct treatment of any disease processes which manifest as the child grows and develops, it is unlikely that a serious infective disorder such as meningitis will occur. A similar principle could be stated in cases of pneu-monia. It is extremely unusual for people to develop pneumonia following a respiratory infection provided they have a good life-style, and well chosen natural remedies for any chest problem as soon as it manifests.

Treatment

This will have to be instituted following the orthodox medical treatment and will be geared to cleansing the lymphatic system and thus improving immunity, plus strengthening the cerebral area with appropriate mineral salts in both physical and homoeopathic doses.

Menopause

This should not be a difficult change which takes place in a woman's life when the ovaries slow down around the age of forty-five to fifty. The common symptoms of hot flushes, insomnia, anxiety, depression and general nervousness are attributed to hormonal changes and this is obviously true. Why, however, should a natural process be full of such disturbances?

The anthroposophical approach to menopause is very appeal-ing and concurs well with the basic esoteric understanding.

Anthroposophical medicine says that at this time in her life, a woman has etheric energies which are freed from their connection with the ovaries and which can be used to acquire and develop wisdom as an aid to creative service.[1]

The transfer of energy from the sacral *chakra* to that of the throat has been discussed in chapter 2. At menopause this is a naturally occurring activity and provided the woman has developed creative activities earlier in life, the energies from the sacral centre will flow naturally through the throat centre into the environment. Without any creative outlet, the throat centre will not be correctly stimulated and the energies may flow back into the body over-stimulating the thyroid, causing hot flushes, and over-stimulating tissues in various parts of the body. This may be a logical explanation for breast and other cancers which occur between the ages of thirty-five and fifty.

In the presence of environmental pollution, toxins, and accumulated waste in areas of the body, unused energies can be a problem and may stimulate disease.[2] The transfer of energies from the sacral to throat centre does not mean that a woman should lose all interest in sex, but rather that life attitudes and emphasis will be different and values may change. Menopause is therefore an opportunity to use additional energies which have been freed for creative use. It is the responsibility of the woman to decide in what way they shall be used.

Treatment

Treatment will be combined with suitable counselling programmes if necessary, and it may be a good time to introduce meditation into the life. Basic nutrition will be discussed and natural remedies are very useful for a number of conditions and may include:

1 Iron phosphate for heavy periods.
2 Lymphatic cleansing herbs if there is a fibroid tendency.
3 Homoeopathic drops for hot flushes.
4 Vitamin B-complex for energy.
5 Magnesium phosphate for palpitations.
6 Potassium phosphate if energy is low.
7 Calcium phosphate for any tendency towards osteoporosis.
8 Constitutional homoeopathic prescribing.
9 Bach flower remedies to balance the *chakras*.

Menstrual Cramps

Dysmenorrhoea is the medical term for this common and painful condition which afflicts many women, particularly in the younger age group. The uterine cramps usually manifest on the first day of menstruation, but some women have pains both before and during the first three days. In severe cases, there can be vomiting and diarrhoea associated with uterine cramps.

Causes

It is considered that an imbalance in production of the hormone prostaglandins may be responsible for the condition.[1] In clinical practice, natural therapists find that the cause is also due to deficiencies of calcium and magnesium, particularly the former in the case of young girls.[2] It is possible that the imbalance at the hormonal level is basically a biochemical problem. Natural therapists often find an associated lymphatic congestion involving the pelvic area.

Whenever the hormones are implicated, we can usefully give some thought to the more subtle constitution. The *chakras* are understood to govern the glands and are therefore conditioning the hormone balance throughout the body. The sacral *chakra* is the centre which governs the reproductive organs and its associated problems in consciousness involve the successful balancing and expression of our basic appetites for food and sex. In the teenage girl and young woman, these areas often involve conflict and are still in process of resolution. These conflicts result in physical congestions and imbalance of energy with cramps as one indication of an astral or feeling problem.

Treatment

1 Calcium and magnesium phosphate in the correct ratio for the person concerned.
2 Anti-spasmodic herbs as for instance valerian, skullcap, passaflora, motherwort, and verbena which is specific for pains down the thighs.

3 Lymphatic cleansing herbs if necessary.
4 Primrose oil capsules to balance prostaglandin secretion.
5 Vitamin E to improve circulation in the pelvic area.
6 Selected homoeopathic remedies for the individual.

Case History

Jeanette, aged fourteen, visited me in 1978 with painful menstruation on the first day. The pain was accompanied by colic. It was noted that a thyroid weakness showed in the iris. Another problem involved catarrh of the nose. Remedies for the first month included calcium phosphate, antispasmodic herbs, kelp for the thyroid and for general nerve toning; potassium and magnesium phosphate plus B-complex. Vitamin E was given also from the first month.

Improvement took place with the next menstrual period and continued throughout treatment during the next eight months. Remedies were then tapered off. Jeanette returned for spinal manipulation two years later following a fall and there was no mention of menstrual cramps.

Migraine

Migraine is a term used very loosely by many practitioners and patients. It should be confined to those periodic headaches which are hemicranial (one-sided). The problem can begin in childhood, adolescence or early adulthood. Headaches in this category often begin with visual disturbances or other neurological disturbances such as tingling or numbness on one side of the body. The neurological symptoms can be dramatic enough to mimic a stroke in some cases. Neurological symptoms may last from fifteen to thirty minutes and will be followed by a unilateral or generalised throbbing headache which can continue from several hours to two days. Nausea and vomiting may accompany the headache.

There is a familial incidence in 60–80 per cent of patients involving near relatives.[1] Women are slightly more susceptible than men and their migraines occur commonly in relation to the menstrual cycle. Generally speaking, the migraine attacks diminish after middle-age.

Causes

Clinicians do not consider they have the whole story of causes, although all agree that the migraine attack consists of a neuro-vascular disorder involving the intra- and extra-cranial vascular supply. There is an initial restriction of vascular flow followed by an excess of flow.[2] Triggering factors to the attack can be sunlight, stress, particular foods such as chocolate, exercise or alcohol.[3]

The naturopathic viewpoint results from the clinical success of treating migraine sufferers with liver herbs, magnesium compounds, potassium phosphate, vitamin B-complex and selected homoeopathic remedies. Antispasmodic herbs have also been found very useful.

The way we differentiate migraine from tension headaches stems from our knowledge of the digestive processes and their dysfunction in migraine. Rudolf Steiner, the pioneer of anthroposophical medicine, considered migraine to result from disordered digestive processes of which we become conscious in the cerebral area. While the average natural therapist may see this as a slightly extreme viewpoint, it is generally agreed that the liver in particular is often congested in people suffering migraines, and attention to this organ is always stressed.

Nausea is always associated with liver disturbance in naturopathic medicine, and the food allergies which often feature in association with migraine are further evidence of lack of strength in the digestive organs. In contrast to this emphasis on the digestion, natural therapists find that tension headaches are more specifically related to that nerve tension which results from mineral deficiencies alone.

Although poor function of the digestive processes is understood as the main factor in producing migraine, mineral imbalances causing nerve spasm are also contributing factors as in tension headaches.

It is interesting to consider the more subjective causes of migraine. The energy centre known as the Ajna *chakra* is probably imbalanced in most types of headaches. The Ajna *chakra* expresses the synthesis of all energies in the personality life. In keeping with this philosophy, natural therapists find that migraine sufferers are usually highly intelligent people, often displaying an ambitious nature. The Ajna *chakra* connects to the eyes and this may indicate another cause behind the common visual disturbances.

The inner problem may therefore be associated with an imbalance of energies in the head area, due to a temporary imbalance from a rapidly integrating personality. Further to this connection with the Ajna centre, migraine is considered to express a disturbance in the magnetic field between the pineal and pituitary glands. These two glands are connected with the Crown and Ajna *chakra* respectively. The strength of the magnetic field between these two energy centres and their respective glands develops as we begin to align the integrated forces of the personality with our inner essence or soul.

Treatment

1 Vitamin B-complex for a pronounced tonic effect on the central nervous system. In cases of migraine, only small doses are given as large amounts are found to be overstimulating and may worsen the condition.
2 Magnesium phosphate for its antispasmodic effect on nerves and vascular structures.
3 Potassium phosphate in small doses for its tonic effect on the nervous system.
4 Antispasmodic herbs such as passaflora, vervain, skullcap, and valerian.
5 Liver herbs and homoeopathic remedies.
6 Selected constitutional homoeopathy.

Case Histories

Leanne was twenty-seven when she visited the clinic in 1980 with headaches which had lasted two weeks. She had a history of migraines. Her symptoms at the time of visiting included buzzing across the forehead and a light-headed sensation. She had a history of hepatitis in childhood and glandular fever in her teens.

It is important to mention hepatitis in keeping with my previous reference to liver disturbance in connection with migraines. Natural therapists find that although the liver has great powers of regeneration, it rarely resumes full vigour of function after hepatitis without natural medicine.

Leanne was a teacher, and the nervous strain of this profession perhaps contributed to the nerve exhaustion which is part of the basis for migraines. In classic style, her migraines were one-sided, more on the left than right. Her first prescription included B-complex, potassium phosphate and magnesium phosphate to balance the nervous system, antispasmodic herbs, a herbal liver tonic and vitamin C for detoxification. Following this first month of treatment, Leanne reported less headaches and absence of buzzing sensation. The prescription was repeated, and improvement continued with the exception of one bad headache when the new term of teaching began.

Two months of further treatment were undertaken; the treatment was fairly similar except for the addition of kidney herbs to aid further elimination of waste. Improvement was maintained but at the end of term, as stress levels increased, a relapse occurred. Treatment was maintained and during the fifth and sixth month health was good. When the daily work is constantly providing stress as it does in teaching, it is likely that a maintenance dose of treatment will be needed until the job can be modified or changed.

Michael, aged sixteen, had suffered migraines for one year. Vomiting and visual disturbances accompanied the headaches, otherwise his health was good. The following treatment was given over a period of one year with a break of a couple of months at one stage: vitamin B-complex, liver herbs, antispasmodic herbs, and magnesium and potassium phosphate. Only one headache was reported during this period of treatment.

Monilia

see Thrush

Morbilli

see Measles

Motion Sickness

This is one area where natural medicine is very useful through application of simple remedies. The condition may manifest as car, train, plane, or sea sickness and can turn family trips into nightmares. Symptoms vary from nausea to excessive vomiting.

Cause

The exact mechanism is not entirely understood, but the vestibular apparatus of the ear is involved, and the natural therapist would add that the liver usually needs attention as it does with any problem involving nausea.[1] While not wishing to elaborate on esoteric causes for such a simple sounding problem, the solar plexus *chakra* will probably be in a state of imbalance, and the Ajna *chakra* will no doubt be related to the ear disturbance.

Treatment

1 Homoeopathic doses of the Indian cockle shell — Cocculus indicus is an almost specific remedy and can be given to young and old.[2] The shell is shaped in a labyrinth design, and gives the homoeopathic effect of curing problems with similar shaped structures in the body such as the inner ear.
2 Liver homoeopathic remedies.
3 General nerve treatment with B-complex and phosphate salts may be needed.

Mouth Ulcers

This is a common condition; the underlying cause will usually be found in the lymphatic system. There is also an inherited factor and in these cases treatment can be quite long and difficult. Environmental triggers can include imbibing of certain chemicals such as fluoride in toothpaste, or dietary excesses involving the use of refined sugar. In ulcers of any kinds, there may be a zinc deficiency.[1] Adequate vitamin A levels are also essential for healthy and resistant epithelial tissue, whether of external skin or mucus membrane.[2]

Case History

Mouth ulcers can be easy or difficult to treat, depending on the underlying cause. In the case of Elizabeth, aged twenty-one, treatment was speedily effective. Elizabeth, a trained nurse, had tried the usual medication applied locally. By the time she visited me, she also had a sore tongue and inner lip. Accompanying tiredness was another problem.

She had ten months' treatment not for the ulcers alone, but to totally balance the biochemistry, and build up her general health. Treatment included liver and lymphatic herbs for cleansing, calcium phosphate for a deficiency noted by iris diagnosis, a high potency B-complex and potassium and magnesium phosphate for toning the nervous system, and a zinc compound specifically for the ulcers. The ulcers cleared in a few weeks.

Homoeopathics are often needed for mouth ulcer cases and in these cases treatment may be more difficult as there are inherited factors present. In this case, note that the quick response took place after only basic cleansing and toning, and there were no deep-seated factors needing treatment.

Multiple Sclerosis

This is known as a demyelinating disease which means patchy

destruction of the myelin sheaths in the central nervous system, accompanied by an inflammatory response. In multiple sclerosis, the problem usually involves the spinal cord, optic nerves and brain. Attacks may be spaced far apart with intervals or remissions of up to twenty years. MS is inclined to be a progressive disease, especially if occurring after forty. [1]

Symptoms depend on which part of the nervous system is involved but commonly include impaired vision, decreased perception of vibration, bladder weakness, tremor, and weakness with gradual paralysis of one or more limbs.

Causes

The medical profession admits to no known cause of MS. An infectious factor with auto-immune problems has been postulated but not proven. Natural therapists have quite strong thoughts about the cause in relation to mineral deficiencies of the main two tissue salts which we find necessary for healthy nerve function. These salts are magnesium phosphate which is essential for the health of the myelin covering of nerves and which is attacked in MS, resulting in greyish patches or plaques, and potassium phosphate, essential for transmission of nerve impulses. [2]

Natural therapists have also found there is a toxic factor involved with MS and this expresses itself as profound congestion of the lymphatic system in these people. Quite likely it is this factor which causes the inflammation found in the disease and the consequent invasion of the myelin matter by inflammatory cells.

It is interesting to speculate on the more subtle causes of the disease. The relationship between the etheric body and the gross part of the physical body takes place through etheric channels called *nadis* which underlie the physical nerves. The energy carried by the *nadis* to the physical nerves is conditioned by our emotional and mental states. Any psychological problems will directly affect the nerves, and in those cases of MS which do not repond to natural therapies, negative emotional states, sometimes very subtle but potent, have been observed. The question to ask is which comes first, the psychological or the physical condition?

Treatment

This will have to be carried out over a number of years and many patients are not prepared to persevere. Improvement will be slow in well-established cases, but not always so in new cases. The following supplements are of use:

1 Magnesium phosphate for myelin sheaths and potassium phosphate for nerve transmission.
2 Vitamin B-complex in high doses for nerve stimulation.
3 Liver and lymphatic herbs for cleansing as, for instance, burdock, dandelion, trifolium, clivers, violet leaves.
4 Vitamin C for immunity and detoxification.
5 Zinc salts to boost immunity and improve nerve tone.
6 Homoeopathic constitutional prescribing.

Case History

The following case appeared to go into a long remission and it is hard to know with a young person whether this will last. Vonnie first visited me at the age of twenty during her first pregnancy. She had been diagnosed as MS one year earlier. Headaches were constant and worsened by light. Her legs were weak and sight badly affected. She was on fifteen analgesic tablets daily for the headaches.

The first prescription included magnesium phosphate, iron phosphate, sodium sulphate, B-complex, vitamin C, liver and lymphatic herbs. On her return visit after one month, Vonnie reported a lessening in the head pain, and she had improved her diet. She was now four months pregnant. Calcium phosphate was added for the developing baby and antispasmodic herbs were included to further improve the headaches. Improvement continued and by the end of the third month of treatment, analgesic tablets had been reduced from fifteen to four daily. She was feeling very well and continued working until seven months pregnant. At this stage, her specialist told her she was cured and did not require further visits.

The baby was born apparently healthy and Vonnie had a good labour. Vonnie continued treatment for another eighteen months during which she became pregnant again. She went through the pregnancy in good health and had a second healthy baby. We lost touch with her when she moved into a country area, but she did return after a bit of a relapse for a few more months' treatment. When last seen a few months after the birth of the second baby, Vonnie was still in good health.

Mumps

This common childhood infection has an incubation period of about twenty-one days. It usually runs a mild course unless occurring after puberty in which cases complications involving the ovaries or testes can occur. The infection often begins with general malaise and fever and swelling of the salivary glands on first one side and then the other. This swelling can be minimal or very pronounced, giving the typical moon face. Fever and swelling usually subside in a few days.

Causes

The immediate cause is infection with the virus called epidemic parotitis. As with other infectious disorders such as measles and chicken-pox, it is worth noting that the natural therapist finds those most severely affected to have a congested lymphatic system. Thus, their immunity and resistance is weak. The use of natural remedies at the first onset of infective fevers almost always prevents any complications.

Treatment

1 Potassium chloride and iron phosphate to reduce fever, inflammation and glandular swelling.
2 Vitamin C as in all infective disorders to boost immunity.[1]
3 Lymphatic cleansing herbs or homoeopathic remedies.
4 Liver herbs to help metabolise viral toxins in the body.
5 The homoeopathic nosode Parotidinum in the 30th potency is very useful to prevent complications and to protect other members of the family.

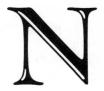

Nephritis

see Glomerulonephritis

This condition literally means inflammation of the basic structural unit of the kidney — the nephrone. If the disease is progressive, extensive destruction of the kidney may take place; this is known as the nephrotic syndrome and is characterised by loss of plasma protein into the urine — albuminuria. The final result can be renal failure.

The subject is treated more extensively in the section on Glomerulonephritis.

Neuralgia

Explained simply, this condition is characterised by acute pain often occurring in the facial area; it usually involves the trigeminal nerve, although the term is often loosely used for nerve pains in other parts of the body.

Cause

Natural therapists find this problem results from a combination of mineral and vitamin deficiencies plus an accumulation of rheumatic toxins. Reasons for mineral deficiencies include poor diet and constitutional factors. An excess of refined food also gives rise to toxins and this is a cause for accumulation of acid waste in the tissues. The acid waste inflames the facial nerves. Sluggish activity of the liver and kidneys may be a contributing factor as in the case of all rheumatic problems.

Treatment

1 Vitamin B complex is very specific for problems with nerves.
2 Vitamin C for its properties of detoxification.
3 Sodium phosphate to balance acid waste in tissues.
4 Magnesium and potassium phosphate for nerve tone. [1]
5 Rheumatic herbs.
6 Specific homoeopathic remedies which usually have a brilliant effect in a very short time. [2]

Neuritis

This is the term usually applied to a disorder of a peripheral nerve. The term neuritis means literally inflammation of the nerve; however, the main cause for the problem is found to be trauma. The radial, medial (carpal tunnel syndrome) and ulna nerves are three of the nerves most commonly affected. Numbness, tingling, loss of power and wasting of associated muscles, and pain are common symptoms.

Causes

Although trauma is said to be the main cause, the natural therapist finds in clinical practice that there is a definite biochemical basis for these nerve problems. Mineral deficiencies of the phosphate salts of potassium, magnesium, calcium and iron are all found to predispose persons to this type of nerve problem. Deficiencies of these mineral nutrients are gauged by a number of clinical signs and symptoms.

It is probable that the compression which the medical specialists have found to be the traumatic cause takes place partly because of swelling and thickening in the surrounding tissues. This fits in with natural therapists' finding that clients often have an associated rheumatic condition of surrounding tissues which may cause fibrosis and thickenings.

Treatment

1 Iron phosphate for inflammation of the nerve.
2 Potassium and magnesium phosphate for improving the actual tone of the nerve.
3 Vitamin B-complex as a general nerve tonic. As mentioned under carpal tunnel syndrome, vitamin B6 appears to have helped reduce the swelling in many cases. [1]
4 Rheumatic herbs to remove any toxic waste from the area around the disturbed nerve. This will help to reduce any swelling and thickening in surrounding tissue.
5 Selected homoeopathic remedies.

Neuroses

There are many neuroses and in the main, true neuroses fall within the province of the registered psychologist or psychiatrist. It should be mentioned, however, that many clients who have been diagnosed as neurotic by the medical profession improve with life-style changes involving nutrition, work, relaxation and through the learning of skills to develop creative expression.

Causes

In some cases, apparent neuroses are found to be caused by mineral deficiencies or lack of vitamin B-complex in the diet. We have discovered in clinical practice that a deficiency of potassium phosphate causes worry and insomnia plus nervous exhaustion, while deficiencies of magnesium salts cause tension and stress in nerves and muscles.

Lack of thiamine or vitamin B1 can cause depression and

other psychological problems.[1] The need for B3 can cause insomnia and in extreme cases hallucinations, while B6 has been found very helpful in cases of premenstrual tension.[2] Exhaustion caused by stress is helped by B5 which tones the adrenal glands. The causes involving deficiencies of the B vitamins can be genetic.[3]

Treatment

This is an area where, due to the enormous range of psychological and psychic differences between clients, one can make only very broad suggestions as to the supplements which can help the physical side of the neurosis. Natural therapists find that if we improve general energy, sleeping, and assist physical relaxation, clients are in a much better state to work on the psychological situation which may predispose them towards neuroses.

From the esoteric point of view, the balance of the *chakras* will be considerably disturbed in any neuroses, and the etheric body is often severely lacking in energy, which in turn affects the physical energy. The most positive way of dealing with neuroses from the esoteric viewpoint, is to encourage the client to develop creative outlets and therefore to take their eyes off the point of friction within the personality. Furthermore, if through suitable forms of meditation, they can touch their own inner essence or soul, healing energies will sweep through their personality and they can often become detached from previous worry and the habit of focusing on problems.

Specific remedies may include the following:

1 Potassium phosphate and magnesium phosphate or orotate.
2 Vitamin B-complex sometimes in doses up to 500mg of a particular component of the B group.
3 Herbal nervines such as passaflora, vervain, motherwort, valerian, scullcap.
4 Bach flower remedies selected for the particular emotional state of client. It should be mentioned that the flower essences are the most specific natural medication for the many negative emotions which we can suffer.[4]
5 Constitutional homoeopathic remedies can have a very dramatic effect provided the client is also making a psychological effort to resolve their problem.[5]

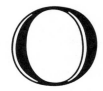

Obesity

Problems with obesity often respond only minimally to natural therapies. Although one can often improve associated problems such as fluid retention, joint pains, and tiredness, I cannot honestly say successes with weight loss feature strongly in my cases. Hence it is with unexpected delight that the case of Lorelle, aged twenty, will be described.

Causes

These are so complicated that one can hardly dare to begin in a short manual of this nature. Orthodox medicine does not currently consider an imbalance of the endocrine glands as a major cause of obesity. However, naturopaths do consider that subtle endocrine changes are a contributing cause, especially in cases of familial obesity. There is, however, no doubt that many cases of obesity are due to a lifetime of poor eating habits and also that various kinds of stress will cause people to overeat.[1]

Nevertheless, sufficient cases have been observed in connection with their eating habits to conclude that nutrition is not the only factor involved. In severe cases, particularly of women, it appears that the tissues are composed of 'water-logged' cells, and hence even if there is no actual oedema from extra-cellular fluid, the intra-cellular fluid may be imbalanced. This would account for those women who really do not eat much, and yet because of an unusual amount of fluid within the cells, weight gain is significant and permanent.

In other cases, the problem appears to relate to a sluggish thyroid gland and this may have a familial basis. The sluggish metabolism results in weight gain plus a slowing down of all bodily processes.

The hidden esoteric factors of obesity are based on an imbalance in the energy centres, especially on that involving the sacral *chakra* and the throat centre. The problem may involve a congestion in the sacral *chakra*, and this may include disturbance in appetites for food and sex, plus a sluggish throat *chakra* in relation to creative outlets. Development of creative activities may help the throat problem, provided the problem with the sacral *chakra* can be first resolved.

The base *chakra* can be affected as it connects to the adrenal glands, and the pituitary gland which controls the thyroid, adrenals and gonads to some extent may also be involved. As weight gain may be caused by a very slight deviation from normal in the thyroid, and as blood tests to investigate thyroid imbalance are a fairly crude analysis, one cannot rely completely on standard pathology tests to evaluate the balance of the endocrine glands in relation to obesity.

Case Histories

Lorelle has always suffered from a weight problem and other family members have the same problem. She has a history of severe depression and had been hospitalised intermittently for three years from the age of fourteen to seventeen. From this history, it is likely that her thyroid hormonal output has always been below par. When she came to the clinic, she had just finished a gardening course. The main accompanying problem was tiredness. Her whole condition pointed to sub-normal thyroid activity.

The supplements included kelp for the thyroid, calcium, potassium and magnesium phosphate for the nervous system, liver herbs to increase the metabolic processes, and a selection of Bach flower remedies. After one month, energy was much improved, and after two months she had lost twenty-four kilograms. Improvement continued over the next six months and she has now achieved the loss of over fifty kilograms.

On searching through my files, I found a few other cases of obesity where there had been a reasonable loss of weight in a short time. Sylvia, aged thirty-two, had gained twelve kilograms in two years and had already attended Weight Watchers plus having a course of acupuncture, without results. Other problems included poor circulation which manifested as numb toes and chilblains, and backache.

Once again, the main thrust of treatment was towards toning the thyroid and Sylvia was given large doses of kelp, a general mineral tonic, calcium phosphate and vitamin E for poor circulation, liver herbs for general cleansing, and vitamin B-complex for nerve toning. Vitamin C was also included. On her first return visit after one month she reported a loss of eight kilograms and was feeling much better. All signs of backache had gone.

The treatment was repeated for several more months and then Sylvia discontinued attending so we are unable to say whether her improvement was continued or maintained.

Osteoarthritis

see Arthritis

Osteoporosis

In osteoporosis, the bone mass is decreased, indicating that the rate of bone resorption is exceeding that of bone formation. This causes likelihood of easy fractures, and is a major problem particularly in post-menopausal women. Over the final three decades of life, it has been found that there can be a loss of bone mass in the order of 30–40 per cent of that present at age thirty or forty.[1]

Causes

Although calcium deficiency is found to be the main factor in some cases of osteoporosis, there are other causes in idiopathic, senile or post-menopausal osteoporosis. In the latter cases oestrogen is usually found to be deficient but this may not be the only cause of osteoporosis in post-menopausal sufferers. The condition also occurs in prolonged cases of obstructive jaundice, in patients following gastrectomy, and in cases of lactose intolerance.

There are suggestions that subtle alterations in pituitary, adrenal and gonadal levels of the associated hormones may be related to osteoporosis. This prompts natural therapists to suggest again the subtle relationship which exists between the *chakras* or energy centres and the endocrine glands. In the future, medical science may discover that after middle-age changes take place in the psyche as it withdraws from active life either intentionally or unintentionally; changes which correspond to fluctuations in the energy centres governing the glands. The bones are our most material part, and if inner factors disturb our incarnation at the material level, the final result may be a lack of density of the bone. Anthroposophical medicine is deeply concerned with these subtle processes, and is one example of therapy which takes such esoteric factors into account.[2]

Treatment

1 Herbal and homoeopathic endocrine tonics to balance the glands.
2 Calcium phosphate in combination with sodium phosphate as a homoeopathic preparation which is easily assimilated. The latter salt provides an alkaline medium so that the calcium is deposited in the right places.
3 Homoeopathic remedies of a more constitutional nature.
4 Nutritional advice so that the diet is biochemically balanced particularly in relation to calcium, magnesium and phosphorous.

Ovarian Cysts

Ovarian cysts are a very common problem presenting to our clinic. In some cases the diagnosis has already been made by a medical practitioner and in others we know by the clinical signs and symptoms that there is the likelihood of a cyst.

Vega diagnosis is very valuable to discriminate in a situation where any one of a number of pelvic problems could be present. Through the use of the test ampoules which are introduced into the testing circuit as a 'challenge' to various parts of the pelvic organs, poor function and pathology can be pin-pointed. Differentiation can then take place between, for instance, blocked fallopian tubes, ectopic pregnancy, appendicitis, and ovarian cysts. This is a much cheaper and more convenient diagnosis than a laparoscopy.

All the above conditions can have overlapping symptoms, the main ones being pain in the right or left iliac fossa (above each groin). Inflammation, congestion or swelling in these areas can also interfere with normal bowel functioning, making differential diagnosis more difficult. With ovarian cysts, the menstrual cycle can also be affected.

Causes

Apart from hormonal causes, the orthodox profession does not have much to say in the way of etiology which throws light on the situation. From the naturopathic point of view, we usually discern a basic mineral imbalance with a more deep-seated cause related to an inherited tendency. The subjective or inner causes will be related to the energies flowing through the sacral *chakra*. When considering subjective causes, if one accepts the concept of reincarnation, the present problem may have very ancient causes. It is here that the right counselling approach could be of extraordinary value, combined with constitutional homoeopathy to deal with the inherited factor.

Treatment

1 Calcium phosphate is found to be the most commonly needed mineral salt.
2 Sodium sulphate may be needed for rebalancing fluids in the body.
3 Specific homoeopathic remedies for cysts.
4 Homoeopathic remedies to counteract inherited miasms or taints.
5 Constitutional homoeopathic prescribing.

Case History

Pat was diagnosed as having an ovarian cyst in 1983. Her main symptoms from this problem were niggly pains in the ovarian area and very heavy periods as a result of hormonal imbalance. She was very exhausted.

Treatment for the first month included iron phosphate both as replacement therapy for iron loss with the heavy periods, and because of its therapeutic mode of constricting blood vessels.[1] Vitamin P, a common term for the bioflavonoids, was also given as this complex resolves a bleeding tendency in many cases. Due to the signs noted in the iris including a familial tubercular taint, the mineral salt calcium phosphate was given.[2] A herbal mixture included female tonics, astringent herbs, and blood cleansing and liver herbs. Vitamin B-complex was added in large doses for energy.

Pat reported on her first return visit that energy was improved, pains reduced and period was less heavy. The same prescription was repeated and on the next visit pain was missing but her period lasted for eleven days. At this stage, more specific treatment for the bleeding was introduced with iron phosphate administered in the 12th dilution for homoeopathic effect, and a tubercular homoeopathic nosode in high potency was added. These additions marked the real turning point, and Pat progressed well over the next few months with no relapses.

It is worth pointing out the extraordinary effect of the minute homoeopathic dose in this case as a means of fine-tuning the treatment. Even though Pat faced the sudden unexpected death of her husband a few months later, her condition remained stable.

Paget's Disease

This problem with resorption of bone occurs in about 3 per cent of persons over forty.[1] Cases occasionally present to the natural therapist. The loss of calcium and subsequent skeletal deformity is not uniformly spread throughout the skeleton as in osteoporosis. The earliest symptom is often lower back pain which can worsen at night. In advanced cases the skull is enlarged, and perhaps the most commonly noticed symptom which lay people recognise in elderly relatives is bowing of the legs. Another common skeletal change is kyphosis (hunchback) There can be circulatory disturbances with tachycardia (fast pulse). Deafness is common from compression of the auditory nerve.

Causes

From an orthodox medical point of view, the causes and etiology of the disorder have not been clearly established. The calcium imbalance which causes losses of bone in parts of the skeleton and thickening in other parts is easily observed, but the reasons for this imbalance are not fully known.

From our naturopathic understanding, improvement and remission from this problem can be established by working on the biochemistry of the individual using herbs, minerals and vitamins. We find in clinical practice that calcium balance can be restored using natural remedies. I have not treated many cases of this disorder. Proof of reversal in the disease can of course only be truly demonstrated through radiography before and after treatment.

Case History

Molly visited me at the age of seventy with a diagnosis of Paget's disease, and with a further calcium imbalance manifesting as arthritis in the spine. She had pain right down to her feet. Other problems involved eczema on her arms and bronchial asthma. There was a greenish bronchial and nasal mucus associated with her respiratory condition.

Her treatment included a combination of calcium phosphate and sodium phosphate to balance the calcium in the skeleton, and liver and rheumatic herbs. For the respiratory problem, she received potassium sulphate for the green phlegm in the form of both the mineral salt and homoeopathic remedy, vitamin C, and iron phosphate and potassium chloride for the general inflammatory state of her nasal passages and bronchial tubes. Lymphatic cleansing herbs were also included. In spite of her age, she responded quickly and after the first month phlegm and leg pains were both reduced. Eczema was also clearing.

Pancreatitis

The literal meaning of this disorder is inflammation of the pancreas. The problem may be acute or chronic. This is not a common condition and is mainly seen in alcoholics. Abdominal pain is the major symptom of acute pancreatitis. This pain, steady and boring in character, is felt around the umbilical region and often radiates into the back. Nausea, vomiting, and abdominal distension can also accompany the disorder in its acute form.

The natural therapist is more likely to encounter and treat chronic rather than acute pancreatitis. In these cases, gallstones are frequently an associated cause and factor. In chronic cases, the pain may be intermittent or absent. There are usually abnormal fatty stools and there can be other signs of malabsorption syndromes.

Causes

These are not fully established but the main associated physical disorders are alcoholism and gallstones. The necrosis or destruction of the pancreas which can take place in chronic cases appears to be sometimes related to the autodigestion by pancreatic enzymes which for a variety of reasons are activated within the pancreas, rather than in the digestive canal. Obstruction in the ducts of the pancreas, and hypersecretion of pancreatic juice are two other theories for pancreatitis. [1]

From the more esoteric viewpoint, the relationship between the solar plexus energy centre and the pancreas must be mentioned once again. Any disease or imbalance in pancreatic secretion, either exocrine, or endocrine, has a subjective cause in an imbalance of energy flow through this *chakra* or energy centre. As the outlet for the emotional life, the solar plexus centre is disturbed by negative or suppressed emotions, and also by an excess of emotions. The emotional problem will need to resolved if any physical therapies are to be successful.

The natural therapist is likely to be approached by chronic cases of only moderate severity, which may or may not have been diagnosed as a pancreatic problem. As the pre-clinical phase is the sphere of preventive medicine, only a careful case history and skilled observation and interpretation can identify this problem. Iris diagnosis is of particular assistance in any digestive problem as the pre-clinical signs of most digestive problems are clearly shown. Bioenergetic diagnosis using the Vega or Theratest instruments can also be of great assistance in the pre-clinical phase where pathology is not clearly indicated.

Treatment

This will vary considerably depending on whether the condition is acute or chronic. As the latter is the most likely situation for the natural therapist, treatment for chronic pancreatitis will be described.

1 A nutritional regime which will rest the pancreas will be advocated. This will include an initial two to three days on fresh vegetable juices only. A diet emphasising whole grain cereals (with the exception of wheat), salads, vegetables, light protein, and restricted in all refined carbohydrates, excess fats and protein, would be gradually introduced.

2 A selection of digestive herbs according to the individual parameters.

3 Enzyme tablets carefully selected for the case.

4 Homoeopathic and Bach flower remedies for the particular constitution.
5 Vitamin B-complex as a general nerve tonic.
6 Sodium sulphate in a specially prepared form as a tonic to the pancreas and liver.
7 Iron phosphate to reduce inflammation.

Case History

Val is a retired businessman who has been receiving naturopathic treatment for a number of ailments, most of which involve the digestive system to some extent. He first presented for treatment in 1978, and his problems included sciatica, nocturnal epilepsy, Meniere's disease, and digestive disturbances. Pancreatitis had been diagnosed some years earlier, and his iris contained a typical pattern for weakness of the pancreas.

Over the next few years, Val had treatment for all these ailments, and especially for the digestive system. During the first year's treatment, there were times when he had quite severe pain in the region of the pancreas. Whenever there was an acute flare-up, he was advised to have a juice fast for forty-eight hours and this proved to be useful and ameliorating on several occasions.

Important supplements for Val's health included papaya enzyme tablets and homoeopathic digestive drops for the pancreas, magnesium and potassium phosphate to stabilise the central nervous system, Bach flowers which worked on the solar plexus *chakra*, and homoeopathic drops containing Cocculus indicus for the vertigo which comes from Meniere's syndrome. He also benefited from rheumatic herbs which helped his sciatica and later trouble with the cervical vertebrae.

As Val has been attending me now for eight years, it has been of great value to see the pronounced changes which have taken place in his iris. The 'autonomic wreath' which was quite square when he first commenced treatment is now moderately regular. The square shape indicates digestive weakness. Val was fifty-eight when starting treatment, and reflecting on his several chronic conditions, his health is now very stable. He rarely has digestive disturbances now, but still suffers pain in the rectal area for which no definite cause can be found. Medical examinations have found nothing, and from the naturopathic viewpoint the problem is intermittent spasm of the rectum. His arthritic tendency is in remission, and the Meniere's syndrome under control.

Papillomas

A very common request to natural therapists from people of all ages is a cure for recurring papillomas. In many cases these have been burnt off with liquid nitrogen only to return shortly later. Although most papilloma cases involve the sole of the foot, a number of clients have been treated successfully for papilloma of the bladder. The naturopathic understanding of a papilloma on any part of the body is closely related to the development and treatment of warts, so the reader is referred to that section.

Parkinson's Disease

(Paralysis Agitans)

A number of elderly persons with this ailment have been treated at the clinic, but it should be explained that once the disease is established, natural therapies can only retard to some extent further degeneration and cannot reverse the process.

The characteristic picture and experience of this condition is a rigidity which affects the facial expression, and tremor which often starts in one hand and is given the very descriptive tag of 'pill rolling'. Due to the developing rigidity, the patient becomes stooped and their posture is affected. The tremor may gradually spread from the hands to the lower limbs and to the face. A shuffling gait develops. Those affected are usually in middle or late life.

Causes and Treatment

The cause of the degeneration of certain areas of the brain in this condition is not fully understood. The natural therapist is more interested in prevention in connection with this problem. We can contribute our own theory for Parkinson's disease. If the brain is liberally supplied with the particular mineral salts necessary for health and with sufficient quantities of the B-complex group of vitamins, natural therapists do not believe a person would develop this disease.[1]

The mineral salts which natural therapists understand to be essential to keep the white and grey matter of the brain in health are magnesium phosphate and potassium phosphate. These mineral salts are given to clients suffering from the disorder in the hope that further degeneration may be retarded.

I have treated only two patients with this condition over any length of time. Their general health was improved in various ways, but the tremors gradually worsened over a couple of years. Hence the natural therapist's main contribution is probably in the preventive sphere and in improving the general health of the sufferer.

Peptic Ulcer

see Stomach Ulcer

Pertussis

see Whooping Cough

Pleurisy

The literal meaning of this problem is inflammation of the

pleura, which is the covering of the lungs. The inflammation can be dry or associated with fluid (effusion). In the first case the main symptom is pain when breathing. The diagnosis is confirmed by the 'pleural rub', a superficial grating or crunching sound which is heard through the stethoscope during examination of the chest. In the case of pleurisy with effusion, apart from pain there may be fever, sweating, and general malaise.

This is not a condition often treated by natural therapists due to the fact that it usually follows other conditions which normally require medical intervention. On occasions, however, pleurisy arises spontaneously from direct infection of the pleura, or following bronchitis. In these uncomplicated cases, intervention with natural therapies may quickly resolve the problem.

Causes

There are a variety of causes; the most common are pneumonia, injury, tuberculosis, lung abscess, and malignancy in the lung or chest area. As with other respiratory disorders the natural therapist will be mainly concerned with prevention. Natural medicine can also assist, however, in cases where the antibiotics are not having the required effect, or especially in mild cases where there is no exudate.

Treatment and Prevention

1 Vitamin C for immunity. [1]
2 Iron phosphate for reducing inflammation.
3 Potassium chloride and sodium sulphate to reduce any exudate.
4 Herbs such as marshmallow, angelica, pleurisy root, elder and yarrow. [2]
5 Specific homoeopathic remedies such as Bryonia which is a classic remedy for pleurisy associated with pain which is worse on movement. The choice of an individual homoeopathic remedy will have to match the situation, however, and factors taken into account will be the type of pain, the side of the chest involved, and other clinical signs and symptoms.

Pneumonia

This is another chest condition which the natural therapist prefers to prevent rather than to treat. It is our clinical experience that if a chest infection is handled appropriately with natural remedies at the onset of infection, pneumonia is very rare, except in cases with other complicating factors such as malignancy.

Nevertheless, natural therapists are trained to recognise the clinical signs of pneumonia. On finding a patient with fever, rapid breathing, sweating, and perhaps bluish discolouration of parts of the face, and absence of breathing sounds in parts of the lung, the patient will be referred for immediate medical attention. By the time the patient has got to this stage of infection it is best for them to have antibiotics so as to resolve the consolidation of the lung as soon as possible.

Natural therapies can often enhance the action of antibiotics in pneumonia, and can certainly aid in the elimination of toxic waste so that the patient returns to health more quickly. This type of treatment, if continued after the cessation of antibiotics, can also improve immunity and strengthen the health of the lungs so as to prevent a recurrence.

Causes

Natural therapists would not argue with the concept of an infecting organism, either bacteria or virus, but are concerned also with the more basic causes of lowered immunity such as congestion of the lymphatic system, and the environmental stresses, for example, pollution, which may all be conditioning factors. We are also concerned with breathing, posture, and with treating any other associated bronchial conditions, for example, asthma.

Treatment

1 Vitamin C to improve immunity and for its anti-bacterial and anti-viral effect. [1]
2 The mineral combination iron phosphate and potassium chloride to reduce inflammation and reduce congestion.

3 Herbs; for instance, marshmallow, garlic, horehound, colts-foot, trifolium, and in the case of staphylococcal infection — the herb echinacea.[2] Sage and wild cherry are also useful in this type of chest condition.

4 Well-selected homoeopathic remedies can have a spectacular effect in pneumonia, lowering temperature and resolving the consolidation of the lung.

5 Vitamin A will be used more as a preventive measure by increasing the resistance of the epithelial tissue lining the lung.[3]

Pregnancy

It gives natural therapists joy and a creative feeling to treat women during pregnancy. We know that the baby will have the best start possible from a biochemical point of view. Over the years, we have made links with doctors who are pleased to have women taking natural supplements and some of them welcome the use of particular items during labour. Natural therapists are able to help with common ailments like morning sickness, vari-cose veins and haemorrhoids, backache, dyspepsia and thrush. More serious problems of pregnancy like high blood pressure and toxaemia also respond to natural therapies.

Nutrition is one of the main areas which expectant mothers enquire about from natural therapists. It is almost a platitude to say that we encourage women to have a diet as natural as possible and which includes a quantity of raw salads, fruit, whole grain cereals and unprocessed foods. Increasing consciousness about the effects of smoking and chemicals on the unborn child makes this part of the natural therapist's job quite easy now.

Pregnancy is an especially good time for treating constitu-tional problems in a woman as at this time they often come to the surface. Homoeopathy will be used for these factors. Specific supplements for more general aspects of pregnancy include the following:

1 Iron phosphate for the first few months to prevent anaemia.

2 Calcium phosphate to promote a healthy structure in the growing foetus.

3 Liver herbs to tone metabolic processes in the mother.
4 Vitamin C to protect against the effect of all viruses.
5 Vitamin B-complex to give energy and especially the B6 component in large doses for morning sickness,
6 Selected homoeopathic remedies for morning sickness may include Pulsatilla, Sepia or Chelidonium according to constitution.
7 Vitamin E after four months or so to maintain the health of the foetal circulation, particularly that involving the placenta.
8 Raspberry leaves in tea or tablets to strengthen the uterine wall and to ensure a quick labour.
9 Caulophyllum in the 30th potency is given by a number of therapists after the sixth month to ensure that the baby takes the right position for birth. This remedy is found to have promoted the complete turning of a baby.
10 Homoeopathic Arnica and other remedies as needed can be very valuable during labour.

Premenstrual Tension

(PMT)
The media has given wide publicity to this problem suffered by many women from one to two weeks before each period. Symptoms include profound irritability, insomnia, sugar cravings, depression, fluid retention and headaches.

Causes

These are considered by natural therapists to be primarily biochemical, which in turn affects hormonal balance. An excellent review by John Piesse, an Australian doctor, explores the nutritional factors which may affect biochemistry in women. In this article the relationship between levels of magnesium, vitamin A, B6, and E, and essential fatty acids are examined in relation to PMT.[1]

In many women, the problem is caused by an excess of oestrogen in the second half of the cycle. This would correspond to the type where fluid retention and associated problems manifest. Other cases appear to be associated with general nerve depletion. It has also been suggested that in some women PMT can be induced by tubal ligation and through interference with female hormones following the use of the contraceptive pill.

Subtle factors will involve the regulation of energy flowing through the energy centres, in particular the balance of the sacral centre. Meditation is one positive approach to balancing the energy flows, but more importantly the whole rhythm of the life-style may be a fundamental problem and may need regulation.[2]

Treatment

1 Magnesium and potassium phosphate to balance the nervous system.[3]
2 Evening primrose oil, kelp and vitamin E to help normalise hormone levels.
3 Vitamin B6 in moderately large doses is given especially during the two weeks before the period.[4]
4 Useful herbs include agnus castus, cramp bark, black haw, and wild yam, as these herbs stimulate production of progesterone.
5 Homoeopathic Folliculinum in the 30th potency is fairly specific in many cases of PMT.

Case Histories

Lorraine, a twenty-two-year-old secretary, was in good health except for premenstrual tension. She felt she gave everyone a very bad time with her moods each month. Her only other problem was constipation.

In this particular case, I decided that the main problem was an imbalance and deficiency of magnesium and calcium salts in the body. The treatment was directed accordingly with supplementation of magnesium and calcium phosphate. A herbal tablet with antispasmodic and nerve toning herbs was given, plus liver herbs for general cleansing. The final item was a homoeopathic mixture to regulate the endocrine glands.

In the case of Lorraine, there was improvement in the first

month and this continued throughout the treatment. The bowel also became regular. Lorraine took nearly a year of treatment and there were no relapses after it ceased.

Mary, aged thirty-two, had depression and irritability for about a week before her period. Otherwise she was well. She responded very quickly to the treatment which included calcium and potassium phosphate, high potency B-complex, kelp, herbal nerve tonics and liver herbs. The main specific ingredients for the PMT were sodium sulphate compound and kidney herbs to regulate fluid balance, a homoeopathic mixture of Pulsatilla and Cimicifuga and the Bach flower mustard. This last mentioned mixture is particularly suitable when depression like a black cloud settles over the woman for some days before the period. The potassium phosphate was also used for this reason.

Prolapse

The most common ailment which natural therapists treat in the area of prolapsed organs is prolapse of the uterus. Provided the condition has not been allowed to develop too long, natural therapies have completely reversed the condition. Apart from the local symptom of the uterus dropping down into the vagina, causing pressure symptoms on bowel and bladder, backache can be an accompanying problem. Natural therapies can also help prolapse of the bladder.

Causes

The basic cause is weakness of the elastic tissue due to a malabsorption of calcium salts, in particular, calcium fluoride.[1] This weakness of the tissues is often familial. These clients may have indications of other similar weaknesses such as occur in hernias, varicose veins and haemorrhoids. The biochemical imbalance caused by this deficiency is slow to correct due to its inherited basis.

Treatment

When considering the whole life-style, women with a familial incidence of varicose veins or prolapse should certainly be quite regular about doing pre- and post-natal exercises. Strengthening of the muscles and ligaments through exercise is obviously a preventive measure. One of the best dietary measures for including liberal supplies of calcium fluoride is to take plenty of rice bran and celery. Specific supplements for prolapse of uterus or bladder include:

1 Calcium fluoride as the tissue salt or homoeopathic preparation.
2 Astringent herbs such as hammamelis.
3 Specific homoeopathic remedies such as Sepia and Helonias are spectacular if they fit the case.[2]
4 Vitamin E and vitamin C both have positive effects on tissue weakness.

Case History

Gwen, a housewife aged forty-one, attended me in 1972 during my first year in practice. She had suffered a slight prolapse for some time, recurrent cystitis, and bachache. Diarrhoea and vomiting accompanied her cystitis. A haemorrhoid tendency and a history of intermittent migraine were also present.

Her first month of treatment included iron phosphate, potassium chloride, bladder herbs and vitamin C for the cystitis. Calcium fluoride was given in a base of astringent herbs for the prolapse, and it was found that Sepia was her constitutional homoeopathic remedy. Sepia has many prolapse symptoms and was very useful for this case. Liver herbs and magnesium phosphate were given for the migraine tendency over a period of months.

The prolapse made steady progress and after about seven months there was no further trouble with bladder or prolapse. Eighteen months later, headaches began to develop again especially on Saturdays. These are the sort of gems looked for in homoeopathic prescribing and Silica in the 200th potency proved to be useful for these headaches. This remedy is well known for its usefulness in headaches which appear as soon as the individual relaxes after the working week finishes. A selection of antispasmodic herbs were used; these included valerian, mistletoe, vervain, and avena sativa.

Gwen had a course of treatment over a period of eighteen months at this stage as there were menstrual problems with the start of menopause. When everything was stabilised, treatment was tapered off. There was no further trouble with the bladder or prolapse during this time or afterwards.

Prostatitis and Enlarged Prostate

Due to the natural therapist's particular approach to homoeostatis or the biochemical balance of the body, it is appropriate to consider inflammation of the prostate (prostatitis) and enlarged prostate together. Inflammation may affect the prostate gland in men of all ages, but generally speaking, enlargement of the gland affects men who are usually over fifty years of age.

Symptoms in both these conditions may include frequency and discomfort passing urine, lower back pain, and in the case of acute inflammation, blood can be present in the urine. When the prostate is enlarged, there can be interruption to the flow of urine and difficulty in emptying the bladder in addition to frequency.

Causes

When considering the biochemistry of the body, the diet appears to have a very significant effect as a precipitating cause in cases of prostatitis, just as it does in cystitis. This is logical if it is remembered that the acid/alkaline balance is often a critical factor in the growth of organisms which are found in or near the excretory organs.

It is true that in the case of prostatic inflammation, an infecting organism is not always found. This still reinforces the naturopathic understanding that the biochemistry is disturbed, for we find that by placing the client on an alkaline diet with lots of vegetables, salad, and vegetable juices, inflammation is reduced.

The enlargement of the prostate is also found to be partially due to a zinc deficiency.[1] Soil used for farming is often deficient in zinc, and unless we eat husks of cereals or brewers yeast, it is difficult to get much zinc in the diet.[2]

An inner or subjective cause may relate to the sacral *chakra* and will be connected with a disturbance in the energy flow through the area. It would be interesting to know whether those men who have a continuing and satisfactory sex life into old age have less trouble with their prostate. The inference here is that the damming up of forces connected with the sex life may congest structures in the vicinity of the sacral *chakra*. Only recently has there been any consideration of sexual needs in people of late middle-age or older.

The orthodox medical reasons for trouble with the prostate are not very specific beyond the finding sometimes of infective organisms in prostatic fluid. In the case of enlargement, hormonal changes are cited as the main associated feature in ageing men with prostatic hyperplasia.[3] The finding that the problem is almost universal in men after fifty may perhaps relate to a universal zinc deficiency in this age group.

Treatment

1 Iron phosphate to reduce acute inflammation.
2 Sodium phosphate to increase alkalinity of the urine.
3 Zinc compounds.
4 Urinary tract herbs and herbs to promote lymphatic drainage, plus specific herbs for the area; sabal serrulata and damiana.
5 Homoeopathic potencies of Silica or Conium for enlarged and hardened prostate, Pulsatilla which may be specific, and constitutional remedies for the individual.
6 Vitamin E, useful for increasing vascularisation of the hardened prostate.

Case History

Bernard, aged thirty, had been diagnosed as suffering from an enlarged prostate and his main symptom was a burning sensation on urinating. It was significant in terms of my previous comments about the diet that he had eight cups of tea per day with three spoons of sugar in each!

His first month's treatment included sodium phosphate to alkalinise the urine, zinc compound as specific for enlarged prostate, iron phosphate for the inflammation and burning, vitamin C in a buffered form to reduce any infection, and specific homoeopathic drops for the gland. He reported back in one month with less burning but had suffered a bout of pharyngitis for which he took antibiotics. He had made an effort to reduce his sugary tea.

Similar treatment was continued for three months with the addition of lymphatic cleansing herbs. The pain and burning of his prostate disappeared and after four months' treatment he was left with just a slight disturbance of the urinary stream. No doubt this final problem would have responded had treatment been continued.

Psoriasis

This is one of the most difficult conditions to treat either from orthodox or naturopathic viewpoints. It is characterised by red oval scaling patches which can cover nearly the whole skin area. They are not usually of the itching kind like eczema, although a common site where itching does occur is the scalp. Other common sites for psoriasis are on the knees and elbows, and the nails may be affected.

Causes

There is a definite familial incidence and from the naturopathic viewpoint, a tubercular taint would be present in the family heredity. This may go back many generations and not be known by any living family member. An interesting cause is discussed by the Edgar Cayce medical group. They are of the opinion that people suffering from psoriasis have a thinning of bowel walls. Toxins are absorbed too readily through the bowel wall. The skin as an excretory organ is then called into activity in an attempt to eliminate the toxins. The Cayce group do have some good results with the condition, but the treatment is so involved that the average patient would not be interested.[1]

Treatment

The naturopathic approach to all rashes on the skin involves toning of all the excretory organs, cleansing of the lymphatics, and toning of the liver. In the case of psoriasis, specific minerals and vitamins are needed, and the particular homoeopathic remedies required for elimination of inherited tubercular tendencies. Specific remedies may include:

1 Iron phosphate for reducing inflammation of the skin.
2 Potassium sulphate for the scaling tendency of the skin.
3 Vitamin A to reduce thickening to the epithelial layer of skin.
4 Vitamin B-complex and C for general toning and cleansing respectively.
5 Liver and blood cleansing herbs.
6 Specific homoeopathic remedies for heredity, constitution and skin condition.
7 Zinc compounds. [2]

Case Histories

Colleen, aged forty-two, is a school principal. Her condition of psoriasis involved mainly the skin on the elbows and scalp. She also had sinus problems. The iris indicated a considerable build-up of acid waste in the tissues, and the nervous system was severely depleted of essential minerals.

Treatment included liver and blood cleansing herbs, vitamin B-complex and vitamin C, a zinc compound, potassium chloride and iron phosphate, potassium sulphate in a high homoeopathic potency as well as the physical salt, and linseed oil. After one month on this regime, a number of improvements had taken place. She stayed on the treatment for four months by which time both skin and sinus had improved.

A recent phone call found that she had relapsed when off the treatment. Being out of town and a busy professional person, she had been unable to get back for a visit. We do find that psoriasis is one of those conditions where treatment must be persisted with over a very long period of time.

Alexander came for treatment with psoriasis at the age of seventy-one. He had suffered the condition on his legs for two years and he had a bad patch of raw skin on his left ankle. His skin condition tended to alternate with attacks of hay fever. The hay fever commmenced immediately on his return from the Second World War. He also had a history of recurrent bronchitis and pleurisy. The alternation of the skin problem with respiratory symptoms is typical with clients as they shift from the acute stage of skin manifestations to the more deep-seated sub-acute manifestations of the respiratory system.

The first month of treatment consisted mainly of a blood cleansing herbal mixture which included phytolacca, burdock, yellowdock, marshmallow and centaury. A mineral combination to reduce inflammation and thickening of the skin contained iron phosphate and potassium chloride, and another supplement provided for general nerve toning with a combination of calcium, potassium, and magnesium phosphates plus vitamin B-complex.

After a month on this combination, Alexander manifested considerable improvement in the skin condition; this improvement continued during the next three months of similar treatment. A person in this age group with a pronounced skin condition should continue treatment for many months but Alexander gave up treatment after two months. It was not surprising that he returned two years later with a further acute manifestation on the skin requiring a further course of treatment. On this occasion the condition was not as deep-seated as psoriasis and manifested more as a severe bout of eczema.

Kenneth, aged forty-nine, had psoriasis on his trunk and on the hair line of the scalp. His case is included because he responded so quickly to treatment, which is unusual for psoriasis. The iris indicated the typical acidity which is commonly found in this condition, and there was imbalance indicated in the autonomic part of the nervous system.

His brief two-month period of treatment included vitamin B-complex, liver herbs, a homoeopathic mixture for the lymphatic glands, potassium sulphate for the dry flaking skin, and potassium chloride and iron phosphate for the inflammatory process of the skin. Treatment in this client was most probably accelerated by response to a high potency homoeopathic by the name of Mezereum.[3] As with all homoeopathic remedies, it is only administered when specifically indicated for the person concerned, but I have found it almost in the class of a specific for many cases of psoriasis.

Raynaud's Syndrome

This problem is caused by spasm to the digital arteries and may result from a variety of causes. The hands are hypersensitive to the cold and beginning at the fingertips become white, cold and numb when subject to cold weather or on touching cold objects.

Cause

This is a vasospastic disorder and is therefore connected with an imbalance in the autonomic branch of the nervous system. From the naturopathic viewpoint, a mineral imbalance involving calcium or magnesium is often suspected. Inability of the body to absorb or use magnesium causes spasm in different parts of the body, while deficiencies of calcium are often found in relation to hypersensitivity to cold and to numbness and tingling.

Biofeedback where individuals learn to control the temperature of their hands and feet can be a valuable aid.[1] Improvements using these techniques indicate the involvement of the psyche in this type of nerve imbalance.

Treatment

Clients have been helped while on the minerals calcium and magnesium depending on consitutional type, but tend to relapse when off supplementation, indicating the value of pursuing more deep-acting approaches using meditation or biofeedback. Vitamin E can be of assistance in improving the general circulation, and the use of nicotinic acid (B3) gives a temporary flush to the circulation.

Renal Calculi

see Kidney Stones

Repetitive Strain Injury

(RSI)

This common malady amongst typists, key punch operators and other workers who engage in repetitive arm movements appears to be widely spread in Australia. It has been reported that workers in USA and UK who perform the same tasks do not develop this problem. As this is a new development in industry over the last five years, it is difficult to find an authoritative medical text dealing with the aetiology or development of the problem.

Common symptoms include various degrees of pain on moving the affected arm, and there is sometimes associated swelling and tenderness to touch. The problem can go on for months and years after the person has ceased their usual work routine. The condition has also affected professional musicians.

Causes

This is a very controversial area and medical specialists do not agree on the causes of RSI. A number of commentators have pointed to the likelihood of a strong psychological factor, given that workers on exactly the same tasks in other countries do not have this problem to the extent of Australian workers. There does not even seem to be agreement as to what particular structures in the arm and hand are affected. Muscles, ligaments and nerves have all been implicated.

Natural therapists find that there is usually a rheumatic factor involved, plus in many cases, an imbalance of calcium which has weakened muscles and ligaments. The diet of the Australian worker is possibly worse than workers in other countries although it seems unlikely that American office workers would differ markedly in this respect. It is hard to ignore the psychological factor which has developed in Australia in terms of fear about developing the condition known as RSI.

From the subjective point of view we have a rich field for speculation connected with RSI. We understand that energy follows thought, and it is very possible that a type of mass hysteria underlies the complaint. This does not mean that the person concerned does not have pain and discomfort, but from an esoteric point of view, the psyche can produce profound physical changes in the body. Perhaps this only happens when there are also certain outer factors such as mineral deficiencies and rheumatic tendencies.

Treatment

1 Balancing of mineral status, particularly that of calcium phosphate.
2 General nerve relaxing and toning treatment with minerals, herbs, homoeopathic and Bach flower remedies.
3 Liver and rheumatic herbs to metabolise waste round the affected area.
4 Counselling as to aims and life plan of the individual.

Case History

Denise is a key punch operator aged thirty. She had undergone chiropractic treatment for fourteen months following a diagnosis of repetitive strain injury (RSI). Both arms were affected and she still had pain even after not typing for many months. Denise was on a good diet and already taking vitamin A, B-complex and E. Her iris revealed a poor constitution with marked mineral deficiencies. Lymphatic congestion was also prominent. In her case, the physical basis for the complaint appeared obvious.

The first month of treatment consisted of calcium phosphate, calcium fluoride, sodium phosphate, liver and rheumatic herbs, lymphatic herbs, iron phosphate, and magnesium phosphate. The pain rapidly disappeared with this prescription which has now been repeated five times. Recently, Denise resumed typing when an important job had to be finished by her firm. As she typed for several hours without a break it is not surprising that pain recurred. The pain, however, was not as severe as that before treatment and it is expected that as treatment progresses she will be able to resume typing without distress.

Rheumatic Fever

This fever is not as common now due partly to the widespread use of antibiotics to control streptococcal bacterial infections. It is still, however, a major cause of death and disability amongst children and adolescents in socio-economically depressed areas of the world. Most cases occur in children between the ages of eight and fifteen. The attack of rheumatic fever nearly always follows seven to twenty days after a streptococcal throat infection.

The illness commences with fever, pain, stiffness and sometimes swelling in one or more of the larger joints. The pain and swelling travel from one joint to another. The small joints are rarely affected. There may be an accompanying skin rash. The most serious problem following this type of infection involves the heart. The valves of the heart may become diseased giving heart murmurs and inflammation of the heart muscle may occur accompanied by enlargement.

Causes

The immediate cause is infection with group A streptococcal bacteria. The natural therapist is concerned with the basic immunity of the person and therefore considers that if the person is in biochemical balance, the bacteria cannot affect deep structures of the body such as joints and heart. Only a small percentage of people who are infected with streptococcal bacteria develop rheumatic fever.

Treatment

It is only in areas with a high incidence of the disease through environmental factors such as weather and poor socio-economic conditions that this disorder will be encountered by the natural therapist. As there is very little government support for the mainstream of natural therapies in countries with these predisposing conditions, rheumatic fever is rarely encountered by graduates of natural therapies.

It is unfortunate that natural therapies cannot be applied, because large doses of intravenous ascorbate (vitamin C) would be a very quick and simple way of annihilating streptococcal bacteria. This procedure must only be carried out by a registered person and will therefore need the support of the established medical profession. As rheumatic fever commonly recurs, natural medicine could be used to great advantage in persons recovering from the initial attack. Some specific aids would be:

1. Vitamin C in doses of several grams daily. Deficiency in this vitamin was linked to carditis as early as 1937.[1]
2. Lymphatic herbs to improve immunity.
3. Herbs to improve strength and function of the heart.
4. Herbs for any joint problems.
5. Magnesium phosphate and potassium phosphate for improving the tone of the heart muscle. Iron phosphate for any residual inflammation of heart or joints.
6. Calcium fluoride or other selected homoeopathic remedies for valvular problems of the heart.
7. Vitamin B-complex as a general nerve tonic, and vitamin E as a cardiac tonic.

Rheumatoid Arthritis

See Arthritis

Rickets

As a recognised deficiency syndrome, rickets was perhaps one of the first biochemical problems recognised by the orthodox medical profession as a deficiency disease. Even school children are taught that sunshine is needed for the production of vitamin D in our skin. This in turn allows for adequate use of calcium in relation to the bones.

If vitamin D is lacking, the classic deformity of the bones results in bowing of the femur and tibia, that is, thigh and shin bones. Fractures may occur more easily as a result of calcium deficiency in bones, and dentition may be delayed and accompanied by problems with teeth enamel.

Causes

Deficiencies of vitamin D and calcium may arise from lack of sunlight, lack of dietary sources, and malabsorption syndromes involving the digestive functions.[1] Some kidney disorders may also cause the problem although these are rare.

Treatment

Treatment is fairly clear-cut, involving supplementation of vitamin D and calcium in a suitable preparation. Natural therapists would be inclined not to give synthetic vitamin D, but would emphasise the use of natural sunlight and edible fish oils. A calcium phosphate preparation is given in combination with sodium phosphate to counteract any acidity in the tissues which would inhibit calcium absorption.

Rubella

see Chicken-pox

S

Scabies

Infection with the scabies mite is still quite prevalent. The mite burrows into the skin and the lesion appears as a fine hair-like line on the skin which ends in a tiny vesicle, barely visible to the naked eye. The burrows occur mainly in the folds of the skin. The mite causes intense itching which is worse at night in the warmth of the bed. The infection is spread mainly by sleeping with an infected person.

Cause and Treatment

The obvious immediate cause is infection with the scabies mite. It is of interest to note that the founder of homoeopathy, Samuel Hahnemann, placed great emphasis on what he saw as the inherited cause of the scabies itch and he called this disease factor the Psoric Miasm. Psora was considered to be the father of all disease. Dire consequences to the family tree in terms of inherited disease was understood to eventuate if the itch was suppressed by lotions and ointments.[1]

If Hahnemann had lived today and had access to modern medical diagnostic technology, he may perhaps have expressed his understanding of scabies in a different way. His basic concept is that itching rashes should be treated internally rather than by suppressing the skin manifestation. In relation to eczema and dermatitis, this philosophy is still accepted by homoeopaths and natural therapists, and clinical experience underlines the value of this approach.

Nevertheless, in relation to the actual scabies infection, I have not met any natural therapists who have eradicated a well-established scabies infection through the use of natural therapies alone. It is true that natural therapists would see some people as more constitutionally prone to infection. These individuals would gain from the application of natural remedies in addition to medical lotions. Supplements would include calcium salts, vitamin C and liver herbs to help detoxify the body from the rather potent chemical lotions which are used, and treatment for the nervous system.

Scarlet Fever

This disease is not so dreaded as it was in the early part of the century. Quite apart from the advent of penicillin, like many other diseases which manifest in cycles, scarlet fever just does not seem to be prevalent over the last few decades. Very few natural therapists have experience handling the problem; orthodox medical treatment will be given promptly in the form of antibiotics.

Nevertheless, it is worth discussing the problem because an increasing number of people are seeking natural medicine for every manifestation of ill health; therefore when registration comes about for natural therapists they must be able to deal with or refer every manifestation of disease.

Scarlet fever begins after a short incubation period of less than a week with an abrupt onset of fever, shivering, sore throat and, often, vomiting. The tonsils and surrounding area are red and swollen. The rash appears on the second day and is formed from minute red spots which give a bright scarlet colour. The rash appears first behind the ears and side of the neck and spreads rapidly over the whole body, except for a characteristic pallor around the mouth. Complications can include pneumonia and nephritis.

Cause and Treatment

The immediate cause is a streptococcal infection of a particular strain. It is probably worth repeating that natural therapists do not consider that children or adults with an adequate diet and life-style are prone to this manifestation of streptococcal infection. If treated promptly with the correct natural medication, complications would not be expected, and natural therapists consider the disease could be managed without the use of antibiotics.

Treatment will be similar to that for measles (morbilli), so the reader is referred to that section. In the case of each infectious fever, there is an appropriate homoeopathic nosode, specific for each disease. This adds a specific supplement to the general toning and eliminative therapies. It is also worth repeating that the homoeopathic treatment of individuals suffering from any particular infection will vary according to their individual constitution. As with all infectious fevers, vitamin C is of great assistance.[1]

Schizophrenia

This is the only mental disorder which will be mentioned in this book, and it is covered because of the spectacular results which can be obtained using vitamins and minerals. Important pioneering work in this area has been accomplished not by natural therapists in the first instance, but by a group of registered medical doctors in Canada who call themselves orthomolecular physicians.

The main pioneer in this area is Abram Hoffer, M.D., Ph.D. Following his training and preliminary work as a psychiatrist, Hoffer and colleagues researched the biochemical basis for schizophrenia, and have now established a growing medical association whose members successfully treat the problem with vitamins and minerals.[1] The *Journal of Orthomolecular Psychiatry* documents the history, scientific research, clinical trials and longitudinal studies which have been accomplished over several decades in this area of medicine.

Causes

The research mentioned previously indicates that some individuals have a genetic need for very large quantities of certain vitamins due to a metabolic problem, and a consequent inability to use adequately particular substances available in the average diet. In the absence of these nutrients, hallucinatory chemicals are produced in the brain and this disordered biochemistry gives the signs and symptoms of several types of schizophrenia.[2] Clinical signs and biochemical tests are able to distinguish between different well-documented biochemical problems, and the treatment with vitamins and minerals is administered accordingly.

In the light of previous discussions on the esoteric causes of disease, one cannot pass over lightly such a serious psychic disorder without attempting to put the problem into a larger perspective than that of a biochemical abnormality. The question arises as to why we are born into a particular family who may transmit abnormal biochemistry to their descendants. There is also the question as to why some schizophrenics are prepared to persevere with the necessary supplements over many months; perhaps for the rest of their lives, while others do not seem to have any underlying motivation towards health.

Some of these basic differences in the psychology of schizophrenics cannot be completely attributed to biochemistry, but to our inner nature which natural therapists call the soul of the individual. This expresses itself through a particular psychology and biochemical arrangement, perhaps determined by the previous life cycle or karma. The underlying motive towards health can be fostered by physicians of many kinds, but the ultimate choice must always remain with the patient.

Many schizophrenics are highly intelligent in spite of varieties of aberrant behaviour, and there is usually some appropriate time when the mineral and vitamin therapy can be explained. Provided there is some kind of family or community support for the regime, and provided the patient can co-operate to some extent, excellent results can be achieved.

The main vitamin to reduce the hallucinatory experience is vitamin B3 which can be administered as nicotinic acid or niacinamide. Up to 8g daily may be needed initially, with maintenance doses of 1g possibly for the rest of the life. Vitamin B6, zinc, vitamin C and other members of the B group are selected according to the particular biochemistry concerned.[3] Homoeopathic literature also indicates the usefulness of a number of potent remedies for the schizophrenic problem.[4]

Case History

The following case concerns a teenager who was brought to my practice with a diagnosis of schizophrenia, and who returned to a completely normal life in the community. It is one of a number of cases that have been helped using natural medicine.

Rosemary, aged sixteen, attended the clinic in 1980 with a history of hallucinations over a one-year period. Other problems included absence of menstrual periods for three months and eczema in the ears. She was on orthodox medication for the hallucinations. Her first prescription included 3g of niacinamide per day, magnesium orotate 400mg daily, 1g daily of vitamin C, yeast tablets for the B-complex content, liver herbs, and homoeopathic drops for the eczema.

After one month, there were no further hallucinations and Rosemary reported having a menstrual period. Improvement continued over the next year and the basic prescription was continued. The menstrual cycle took many months to stabilise; periods were every two weeks and sometimes were accompanied by painful cramps. Calcium phosphate, and vitamin E were added for the menstrual cramps and homoeopathic drops were added to regulate the cycle. Antispasmodic herbs such as passaflora and valerian were used to help sleep.

After a year on treatment, the niacinamide was reduced to 50mg and administered in a B-complex tablet, and the magnesium was also reduced and given as a potassium, calcium and magnesium phosphate compound. Acne and rashes continued for a further few months and were treated with a zinc compound and lymphatic cleansing herbs, plus the mineral combination of iron phosphate and potassium chloride.

Rosemary gained employment after a few months' treatment, moved interstate and married after about three years. We have kept in touch with her movements through other family members and recently she returned for a visit and was found to be in excellent general health.

Scleroderma

The disease is also known as Progressive Systemic Sclerosis. This is an appropriate label as patients gradually develop fibrosis of the skin and epithelium of some internal organs, notably gastrointestinal tract, lungs, kidney and heart. The first symptom is often Raynauds' phenomena whereby the hands go numb and white and this may include symmetrical swelling or stiffness of fingers. The skin develops pigmentation as it becomes firm, thickened and leathery. Occasionally, the internal organs are affected before the skin. The digestive problems usually start with fibrosis of the oesophagus and this causes difficulty in swallowing.

The firm tight skin may precede internal manifestations by several years Death from renal failure occurs in almost 50 per cent of patients and the onset of renal involvement is frequently within three years of the initial diagnosis.[1]

Causes

From an orthodox medical point of view, the causes are not known. The clinical experience of natural therapists has shown that some patients with scleroderma have worked with lead during some period of their life. The question could well be asked whether lead poisoning may be a significant factor in the etiology of this disease.

The anthroposophical medical groups in Germany and Switzerland have commented extensively on sclerotic diseases. They see patients as tending to move towards sclerosing or inflammatory conditions according to their psychic and physical constitutions. The sclerosing diseases include all fibroses, hardenings, and problems involving stones or crystals, plus the cancer process.[2] Scleroderma in this context would be understood as an excessive move towards the normal sclerosing factor which occurs in many people during old age.

Anthroposophical medical doctors consider that our modern environment encourages sclerosing in the population through the emphasis placed too early in educational institutions on accumulation of knowledge and facts. They also cite the emphasis on technology and the neglect of more artistic and rhythmic activities between the ages of seven and fourteen as a major conditioning cause of imbalances which may later lead to scleroses of various kinds.

Treatment

Some therapists have had experience in treating this disease with vitamins, minerals and herbs and this therapy has retarded the sclerosing process for some years. Treatment is directed towards helping the digestive processes, and to supplying the optimal levels of nutrients so that the skin elasticity is preserved sufficiently to prevent ulceration. Natural therapies can help any ulceration which does occur.

One case in our practice was given considerable help through the taking of homoeopathic lead. She had worked extensively with lead during the course of her teaching work in the art department of a tertiary institute. Natural therapies helped her to gain weight, healed a number of large ulcers on the legs, and improved her general health for many years. The following remedies are often of assistance:

1 Vitamin C to boost immunity.
2 Vitamin E to assist healing and retard fibrosis. Zinc compounds will be used for a similar purpose and to prevent scarring.
3 Digestive herbs to help the fibrosing of the digestive tract.
4 Lymphatic cleansing herbs.
5 Homoeopathics to reverse the sclerosing process when possible.

Case History

Greg, a clerk aged twenty-four, was diagnosed as having scleroderma six months before visiting me for treatment. The problem commenced with tight cold hands. He also developed epileptic fits. Large meals caused vomiting and this indicated that the disease was affecting the lining of the digestive tract. His diet was good but sleep was poor. The iris revealed gross deficiencies of calcium and other minerals, an accumulation of acid in the tissues and moderate lymph congestion.

The first month of treatment included calcium, magnesium and potassium phosphate to stabilise and balance the nervous system, iron phosphate and potassium phosphate for the lymph congestion, a lymphatic cleansing mixture, and vitamin A to work on the hardened epithelial tissue throughout the body. Vitamin C was included for immunity and its effect on the collagen of body tissues.

This selection was continued for nine months with the addition of vitamin E for circulation and zinc to work on healing and to prevent adhesions in the gastrointestinal tract. The treatment kept Greg in reasonable health, although he had an amputation of one finger which was badly infected as a result of poor circulation. The fits were kept under control and he was able to keep working during this period. Sleep also improved.

With this condition, treatment would be needed continuously. Unfortunately, Greg is one of the few cases which was unable to be followed up while preparing this book.

Scurvy

Scurvy is generally considered to be a serious vitamin C deficiency. This condition is thought by many medical authorities to be a thing of the past, but natural therapists are often confronted with cases of sub-clinical scurvy. These clients have a variety of symptoms including bleeding gums, lack of resistance to infection, a tendency to bruise very easily, and a number of ailments where mucus production features.[1]

The most simple way of diagnosing a vitamin C deficiency is to test the urine with a dip stick designed for vitamin C evaluation or to use a sublingual test with the appropriate reagent on several consecutive days. This evaluation soon demonstrates the fallacy of recommending a uniform dietary intake of vitamin C for everyone. It will be found that the body's needs vary enormously from day to day.

Senile Dementia

The incidence of severe dementia in the population over the age of sixty-five is estimated to be about 5 per cent, with moderate dementia in about 10 per cent of aged persons.[1] Over 50 per cent of these cases are considered to have Alzheimer's disease. This disease is characterised by pathological changes in the cerebral cortex including plaque formation and 'tangles' involving the nerve fibres. There is a disturbance in neurotransmittors within the brain involving enzymes and the neuronal transfer of choline. Senility and dementia in the elderly needs to be distinguished from depression and withdrawal which is common in people over sixty.

Causes

Aluminium has been cited as a main predisposing factor in the development of Alzheimer's disease.[2] Many old people in nursing homes and retirement homes of various types are fed meals which are cooked in aluminium utensils. It is not surprising that the incidence of this problem increases after the elderly are put into such homes. A valuable synthesis of all the nutritional factors involved with senility is available from a book by Abram Hoffer M.D., Ph.D. and Morton Walker D.P.M. Their research and clinical practice indicates the need for studying closely the disordered biochemistry leading to senility.[3]

From the naturopathic viewpoint, natural therapists would also see deficiencies particularly of magnesium and potassium phosphate as causing poor memory, lack of concentration, depression, insomnia and lack of energy. Many old people who eat poorly are deficient in the water soluble vitamins of B-complex and C. The other main consideration is lack of blood to the brain from hardening of the cerebral arteries. Evidence of this can be obtained easily by iris diagnosis.

The more subjective causes should be mentioned as many people find it very difficult to accept the personality changes which take place in relatives as a result of senility. Without a larger perspective of humanity than that involving the physical body through which the personality expression manifests, one is at a loss to explain where the real individuality has gone in cases of senility. I have found when lecturing on esoteric subjects that group members are particularly interested in discussing and exploring this subject.

If we accept that the esoteric constitution includes activity and expression at the astral, mental and soul levels of being, we can more readily understand that a slow withdrawal can take place many years before death.[4] The apparent regression which takes place in senility can be seen as the viewing of a tired old shell which no longer houses the real self which has now begun to go about its business on other planes or levels of being. Ideally, as we approach death we should retain all our faculties until the last. With natural medicine and a good life-style this is possible in many cases.

In cases of senility, we have a blurred transition whereby the soul is still connected to the diminishing life form, but the channel of communication between the indwelling consciousness and the central nervous system is so feeble that only the instinctual life remains at the physical level. It may be postulated therefore that senility has both an inner and outer cause. If the indwelling soul loses interest in outer life well before death it is far more likely that the outer factors for senility will develop.

Obviously, prevention is the best approach to this problem. If any one factor could be isolated to prove the difference between soul development, it would seem to be attitudes to life and death as people approach old age. Those who are concerned to be useful and creative into old age start taking sensible measures in middle-age including responsibility for their own health. I have noticed repeatedly during the years of clinical practice how extraordinarily people vary in this respect. Admittedly there are cases of hardship and personal circumstances where a person appears fated to have a difficult old age, but even in these cases, attitudes vary a great deal.

Treatment

Treatment will differ considerably according to what factors appear to be causing the problem. The following supplements are very useful:

1. Kyolic garlic in cases where cerebral arteries are clogged. Other dietary measures can also be taken such as the Pritikin diet.
2. Magnesium and potassium phosphate for insomnia, lack of concentration, exhaustion and poor memory.
3. Vitamin B-complex is useful for all the previous conditions.
4. Vitamin B12 is very helpful in particular kinds of dementia.
5. Vitamin C for reducing cholesterol deposits.
6. Homoeopathic aluminium in selected potencies to antidote bad effects of aluminium.

Shingles

This distressing ailment presents as severe nerve pain over the area involving the distribution of a nerve root or roots. There is often an accompanying swelling of associated lymph nodes, and a few days later a vesicular rash appears over the affected area.

The pain can continue for months and years in some cases after the rash disappears, especially in elderly patients.

Cause

The immediate cause is a virus identical or very similar to the herpes virus which causes chicken-pox. The naturopath is interested to apply the basic philosophy so the deeper structures of the body are not affected by infection in a healthy person. As we become older and vitality diminishes, toxins accumulate more easily in the various structures including nerves.

In the younger person who contracts herpes, the main expression will be confined to the skin and the disease is then called chicken-pox. If the deeper structures have become toxic through accumulation of waste, the virus will find soil for growth in these areas.

This philosophy will be further explored in the condition known as venereal herpes. In the case of shingles, natural remedies can be of great assistance, improving immunity and relieving pain of the nerve root.

Treatment

1 Vitamin C for its anti-viral effect and to increase immunity. This vitamin gives spectacular results when used intravenously for shingles. [1]
2 Vitamin B-complex for its effect on toning nerves.
3 Lymphatic herbs for dealing with congestion of lymph glands.
4 Magnesium phosphate for its effect in reducing nerve pain.
5 Selected homoeopathic remedies for reducing pain.

Case History

Arthur, a retired carpenter, developed shingles during 1986, and visited the clinic for treatment after eight weeks of suffering a stabbing pain on the right side of the chest along the path of the nerve trunk. He is also undergoing medical investigation for blood-stained sputum and is currently taking drugs for heart fibrillation (heart beat irregularities).

After one month of treatment his pain from the aftermath of shingles had completely disappeared. Treatment included vitamin B-complex, magnesium and potassium phosphate in a ratio of 2:1, liver and lymphatic herbs for cleansing, and a combination of homoeopathic ingredients which are specific for the herpes virus.

He is continuing treatment for the chest problem, but pain from the shingles has not returned.

Sinusitis

Sinus congestion is one of those very common ailments which although not life-threatening in any way, can make life a misery. It is a problem which can plague a person throughout their life with nasal blockage, facial pain, headaches and post-nasal drip. In some people it is continuous and in others it tends to occur after a cold.

Causes

The natural therapist usually finds a faulty metabolism and/or elimination as the prime cause for the problem. Inherited tendency through a tubercular or other inherited miasm features in our understanding of causes. The liver is often found to be sluggish and this in turn allows mucus to form. Environmental and nutritional causes are the eating of too much dairy produce and many toxins taken into the body, for example, the range of pesticides in our food chains.

Other biochemical causes are deficiencies of mineral salts like calcium phosphate, sodium sulphate, and iron phosphate, and deficiencies of vitamins A and C. [1]

Treatment

Nutritional changes may be very important for eradicating sinus problems; they involve removing dairy produce, and increasing raw foods in the diet. Specific remedies may include the following:

1 Vitamin C to increase immunity against infection and to reduce mucus.
2 Vitamin A to increase health of epithelial tissue lining the sinuses.
3 Iron phosphate and potassium chloride to reduce inflammation and exudate.
4 Potassium sulphate or calcium sulphate if mucus is green or yellow indicating bacterial infection following the cold virus.
5 Selected homoeopathic acute, constitutional, and miasmatic remedies.

Case Histories

John, aged thirty-one, visited with his girlfriend who was already undergoing treatment and he decided to have a general check-up. His main complaint was a history of sinus congestion which spanned many years. He had suffered from glandular fever two years prior to this date. His diet was good except for eight to ten coffees per day, and he took regular exercise in the form of running, cycling and swimming. Not many toxins were seen in the body via iris diagnosis, although some imbalance in the autonomic nervous system was found.

His first month of treatment included kyolic garlic, potassium sulphate, iron phosphate and potassium chloride. The three mineral salts covered the problem from the angle of inflammation and mucus, and vitamin C added to this action. Vitamin A was added to improve the general health of the epithelial tissues lining the nose. Homoeopathic Thuja 30 was given twice daily to remove inherited tendencies for sinus problems.

There was only intermittent improvement with the nose after the first month, and at the second visit lymphatic cleansing herbs were added to a repeat of the first prescription, and the potency of the Thuja was raised. After this second month of treatment, there was marginal improvement in all respects. By the fourth month, the nose had improved considerably and this improvement continued over the next three months until treatment was tapered off.

Judy, a teacher aged forty-eight, visited us with sinusitis and headache which she had suffered for years. Joint pains were also beginning. She felt the cold weather badly. In this case there were several problems which nevertheless are inter-related from the naturopathic viewpoint. If the sinus had been suppressed by cortisone sprays, there is no doubt the toxins in her system would have penetrated more deeply and the joints would have worsened as a result.

Her first month's treatment included vitamin C, catarrhal herbs, liver herbs, rheumatic herbs, magnesium and potassium phosphate for the headaches and nerve tone, and homoeopathic sinus drops in low potency. She reported less headaches and less pain in the joints. Supplements were repeated and during the second month she manifested influenza-like symptoms which often happens after one month's treatment. The influenza in this situation may be classed as a healing crisis.

Treatment was continued along the same line and during the fourth month she did use antibiotics as well as natural treatment for a severe bout of bronchitis. The nose and headaches were good the following month with a further relapse of catarrh the next month. Improvement continued the next month and when last seen, the nose was clear, there was no relapse with headaches, and no joint pains.

A phone call before writing this case history found that she had some relapse with the sinus since suspending treatment. This indicates that the treatment was not continued long enough for complete biochemical rebalancing of the body.

Stomach Ulcers

As this condition has been popularised through literature, most people are aware to some extent of the various types of burning and nagging pains which can accompany the problem. There can also be nausea, acidity in terms of acid rising into the throat, and poor appetite. Pains often occur when the stomach is empty.

Causes

These include poor diet, drugs such as the anti-inflammatory group, inherited tendencies, and stress. It is likely that both naturopaths and medical doctors will agree with this list. Naturopaths would be more inclined to emphasise mineral deficiencies as a significant cause.

Treatment

This will include specific attention to the diet. For the first few days of treatment the client may need to take vegetables juices only. A mixture of carrot, celery and cabbage is valuable. Cabbage has a factor known as vitamin U which appears to heal ulcers.[1] Generally speaking, the patient is encouraged to have a reasonable quantity of raw food so that the diet contains maximum enzyme activity. This is why juices are so valuable as they are raw without having the roughage which may cause bleeding in the acute stages of the ulcer.

Particular remedies may include the following:

1 Cabbage juice to heal stomach lining.
2 Zinc compounds to heal the ulcer.[2]
3 Sodium phosphate for its buffering effect in body tissues and fluids.[3]
4 Vitamin A for increasing resistance of epithelial tissue lining the stomach.[4]
5 Vitamin B-complex as a general nerve tonic and vitamin C in a buffered form for general immunity.
6 Herbs for liver and stomach may include melissa, angelica, marshmallow, dandelion, centaury, fringe tree and especially liquorice.[5]
7 Selected homoeopathic remedies for the particular individual.

Case Histories

John was one of my first patients in the early 1970s, and still visits occasionally for a tune-up. He was in his early thirties when diagnosed as having intercostal rheumatism and given a common anti-inflammatory drug. This diagnosis and treatment was disastrous because in fact he had a stomach ulcer, and the drugs made him 100 per cent worse in terms of the ulcer pain.

After one month of naturopathic treatment John was almost pain-free and feeling well. This first month's treatment included sodium phosphate, digestive herbs like angelica, marshmallow, melissa, dandelion and centaury, with a dash of trifolium for blood cleansing, magnesium phosphate for the ulcer pain, slippery elm powder to soothe the stomach lining, and vitamin B-complex as a general nerve tonic. (At the time of John's treatment I did not know about the value of liquorice.)

About six months' treatment at monthly intervals was given, and this was then tapered off. During the intervening years, John has also received a few months' treatment for an arthritic tendency in the cervical vertebrae, for patches of exhaustion when his newspaper job becomes too hectic, and for sinus. This pattern is typical of many of our clients who may visit us a couple of times each year after success with a particular ailment, returning at these times for both maintenance treatment and prevention.

As for the original stomach problem which John suffered, it has not returned except for a trace of heartburn from time to time as as result of stress. It is of note that in this case no constitutional or homoeopathic treatments were needed for the main ailment, although Bach flowers have been given to John at times for emotional stress. Stomach ulceration is a good example of the large range of moderately severe medical conditions which can be resolved with simple, and basic mineral, vitamin and herbal remedies.

Chris, an executive aged twenty-nine, presented with a dyspeptic condition. He had a sensation of a stone sitting under the heart, and flatulence. Iris diagnosis indicated his constitution was good, although toxins showed in the gastrointestinal area. His diet was good.

Given his basic constitution and good diet, progress was very fast and after three weeks he experienced 85 per cent improvement. Treatment over the next four months included sodium phosphate for the acidity, magnesium phosphate for spasm, flatulence and pain, B-complex as a general nerve tonic, and most importantly a herbal tonic of marshmallow, trifolium, angelica, melissa, wahoo and centaury. Except for the blood cleanser, trifolium, these are all herbs which tone the digestion.

It would have been advantageous for Chris to have continued for six months to consolidate his treatment but he went to work in New Zealand. The following year, I received a phone call from Chris requesting another course of treatment.

It may be imagined by some people with biochemical knowledge that the sodium phosphate has the same effect as sodium bicarbonate, and that relief from stomach conditions in these two cases is simply attributed to this salt as an antacid. Natural therapists do not find this so in clinical practice. This tissue salt is prepared in a homoeopathic manner in terms of the mixing process, and following cessation of its use, clients do not usually relapse. This is in contrast to the allopathic use of sodium salts.

In naturopathic philosophy, many bodily ailments commence in the stomach. It is appropriate to include a third case as gastrointestinal problems feature so markedly in our clinical practice.

Another John, aged thirty-one, visited me in 1982 with an X-ray diagnosis of an ulcer which he had suffered for eight months. John had a high pressure job in real estate. An earlier history of dyspepsia featured. The first month's treatment consisted of sodium phosphate compound, magnesium orotate for nerve stability and as an anti-spasmodic, a herbal tablet containing slippery elm, iron phosphate for inflammation of the stomach lining, papaya enzyme tablets, and Bach flowers for emotional stress.

On the second visit, John was feeling much better and the treatment was repeated with the addition of homoeopathic Calcium fluoride and Lycopodium as a further stomach tonic. In all he had eight months' treatment with no recurrence of stomach symptoms. Treatment was changed slightly from month to month. A zinc compound was included for a few months, and a herbal liver tonic replaced the previous slippery elm tablets. Some supplements in the way of gland tonics and regulators were included for thinning hair. The basic stomach supplements were continued for the full eight months.

Syphilis

As this is a venereal disease, naturopaths should only give treatment if the client is already undertaking medical treatment. Syphilis is included here because of the extraordinary effect the problem can have over many generations. Natural therapists who practise homoeopathy are familiar with the effects of even 'successfully' treated syphilis on future generations. Clients suffering from destructive tissue changes to any part of the body are understood to often need deep-acting homoeopathic remedies to remove this inherited taint or miasm.

A tendency to ulceration, and any destructive or deforming bone changes are two examples of this inherited problem. There is no suggestion that syphilis will actively recur in these clients, but rather that health can never be excellent while this inherited problem is present. Vitamins, minerals and herbs are fairly useless to remove the syphilitic taint. Only homoeopathic remedies have the capacity to penetrate the etheric energy pattern which is established at conception.[1] These deep acting remedies have the power to change the etheric pattern, but they must be individually selected.

Tachycardia

This is a cirulatory disturbance which manifests as very fast pulse and when occurring in bouts is often termed paroxysmal tachycardia. Palpitations is another term used for a racing pulse and this word is commonly employed when the heart 'races' in conjunction with emotional excitement.

Cause and Treatment

This can be summed up very briefly from the naturopathic point of view. Irregular or fast pulse is always associated with a magnesium deficiency. This element can be administered in a variety of ways including large doses of magnesium orotate, smaller doses involving magnesium phosphate, or homoeopathic doses of one of the magnesium salts. It is sometimes useful to also include anti-spasmodic herbs and Bach flower remedies. The latter therapy covers any emotional disturbances.

The subjective or more esoteric review of this problem considers the relation of the heart *chakra* or energy centre to heart function. There is a connection between the vagus nerve and the development of the heart centre and temporary problems can develop involving the interaction between the autonomic nervous system via the vagus nerve, and heart beat. Problems, however, are only likely to arise in clients who have a disturbance in magnesium assimilation.[1]

Case Histories

Bernard, a plumber aged forty-three, attended the clinic in 1980 for attacks of tachycardia during which he was unable to get his breath. At these times he lost concentration and his legs gave way when walking. He had suffered a coronary occlusion three years earlier and therefore his type of tachycardia involved some pathology as a contributing factor.

After one month on magnesium orotate, potassium phosphate, iron phosphate, liver herbs, kelp and vitamin B-complex, there were no further attacks. Due to his cardiac history, and the recurrence of slight chest pain at times, Bernard continued treatment for seven months. Slight changes were made during this time such as the addition of antispasmodic herbs and the reducing of the amount of magnesium to a smaller compound of magnesium phosphate. Treatment was tapered off after seven months.

John, aged twenty-eight, worked in the police force and was under a lot of stress from shift work. His particular work involved computerisation of information and records. He had suffered palpitations for seven years and this condition was worse at night. He awoke in the night shaking and in a hot sweat. Nausea accompanied the problem and at times he blacked out. Constipation was another problem. His iris revealed deficiencies in magnesium and calcium and inherited weakness in the bronchial area which often accompanies a lack of calcium.

Treatment for the first month included a calcium and magnesium compound, vitamin B-complex, and antispasmodic herbs. Liver herbs were given for the sluggish bowel, and Bach flowers for the solar plexus *chakra* which was obviously involved with the fear and panic experienced. A homoeopathic remedy called Ipecachuana was included for nausea in the drops, plus homoeopathic Chionanthus and Chelidonium for further liver toning.

On his return visit after one month, John reported the cessation of panic attacks in the night, improvement with the bowel, and intermittent improvement with the palpitations. There was still some nausea. The treatment was repeated plus vitamin C and a mineral compound for a respiratory virus. After the second month of treatment, he reported fewer palpitations, but complained of very light sleep at night and continuing nausea plus some vertigo. A new complaint involved upper chest pain.

I decided that the chest pains were of gastric origin and a herbal tablet consisting of slippery elm and other stomach herbs was given. The calcium and magnesium compound was replaced by larger daily doses of the magnesium in the orotate form. The other tablets and drops were continued. This seemed to be the turning point and John stabilised after these first three months. Sleep was very light at times but this problem was compounded by the wakefulness of his two small children. There were some palpitations depending on stress at work but no more unpleasant panic attacks during the night. Treatment was continued for another eight months and then tapered off.

Tapeworm

see Worms

Threadworms

see Worms

Thrush

This is the common name for Monilia or Candida Albicans. The condition affects thousands of women with a whitish plaque-like discharge which causes itching and soreness in the vagina. It can also manifest in newborn babies and in these cases can affect the oral cavity as a result from infection as the baby passes through the birth canal. The infecting organism is of a yeast type.

Causes

Natural therapists have their own understanding of this problem, although they accept the highly contagious nature of the yeast organism in certain mediums. The reader is referred to the section on vaginal discharges for a more comprehensive account of the inherited factors in pelvic problems from the naturopathic point of view.

The immediate cause of thrush is the provision of a suitable medium in which the yeast organism can flourish and it has been found that eating of refined sugar in many foods is a major contributing factor. Other factors which involve changes to the pH (acid/alkaline) balance in the gut and vagina result from the use of antibiotics, the contraceptive pill and pregnancy.[1]

Treatment

There must be strict attention to the diet involving the removal of all refined foods and an emphasis on vegetables, salad, and whole grain cereals. Even the use of honey and dried fruits is disallowed as they still provide the sugary medium in which the yeast organism flourishes. All foods containing yeast are eliminated. Specific supplements may include:

1 Acidophillus capsules to restore the normal flora of bowel and vagina.
2 Vitamin A to increase resistance of epithelial tissue lining these tracts.[2]
3 Vitamin C to improve immunity.
4 Herbs to cleanse the lymphatic system and tone the liver.
5 Specific homoeopathic remedies to antidote the Candida infection.
6 Zinc compounds have been found useful to increase immunity.
7 Garlic capsules inhibit the infecting organism.

Case Histories

It is difficult to find a clear-cut case of thrush as it tends to be a recurring problem in women if it has once been established. Robyn, aged twenty-nine, attended our clinic intermittently over several years for different health problems. Her thrush redeveloped while she was undergoing natural treatment towards the end of a gastrointestinal virus. This virus was followed by one in the respiratory tract which affected her throat, sinus and ears.

She was given lymphatic cleansing herbs including phytolacca, pennyroyal, burdock, echinacea, violet leaves, and dandelion. Potassium phosphate and iron phosphate were given for both the inflammation of respiratory organs and the vagina. It was of interest that the thrush was accompanied by a reappearance of warts as both these problems are a manifestation of the inherited miasm discussed under vaginal discharges. Homoeopathic Thuja was administered in the 200th potency for both warts and thrush.

All conditions cleared, and Robyn was next seen six months later suffering from 'morning sickness' in the second month of pregnancy. She was very tired. Thrush is often reactivated by the changing balance of hormones which takes place during pregnancy and which affects the vaginal pH (acid/alkaline ratio).

The treatment had to cover this aspect as well as being designed to cover the nausea. Initially, homoeopathic doses of liver herbs, a herbal liver tablet, and vitamin B6 were given for the nausea and vomiting, plus a high potency B-complex tablet and magnesium and potassium phosphate for the tiredness.

On her return after one month, Robyn reported the cessation of vomiting and less nausea. Another liver remedy was given for further improvement with the nausea and later, the usual supplements for pregnancy were added (see Pregnancy). In addition, lymphatic herbs were used to prevent recurrence of thrush. The pregnancy continued without disturbance and Robyn remained in good health.

Rita, aged thirty-one, suffered from recurrent thrush. She had recently been on the pill which by changing the hormonal levels, predisposes women to thrush. Other problems included abdominal bloating, recurrent ear infections, and right-sided lumbar-spine pain. She was also troubled by sluggish bowels and nasal catarrh. Several of these problems involve the lymphatic system and these include the thrush, sinus and ear ailments. Obesity was another problem.

The first prescription included iron phosphate, potassium chloride, sodium sulphate, liver herbs, B-complex, and magnesium and potassium phosphate for the nervous system. Homoeopathic doses of Hepar sulphuris and Kali muriaticum were given for both sinus and thrush. On her return visit, Rita reported disappearance of the thrush and a little more energy. Her second prescription included more emphasis on the digestion to resolve the bloating. Homoeopathic drops were included to balance the glands and hopefully to help weight loss as obesity was a continual problem. A kidney herbal tablet was included to help with the excess fluid Rita experienced in the abdominal area.

On her next visit, Rita reported occasional thrush, improvement in the stomach and she had lost one kilogram. She was suffering from another ear infection so treatment was adjusted for this aspect. During the subsequent year, she attended the clinic for various problems, but no recurrence of the thrush was reported.

Thyrotoxicosis

see Goitre

Tonsillitis

Natural therapists regard this common condition in young children as of particular importance because the tonsils are the gateway of the lymphatic system. We find that enlarged and infected tonsils respond quickly to natural therapies and consider surgery should only be undertaken after natural medication has been given a fair trial. I cannot remember a case during my practice which did not respond to natural remedies. Almost without exception, the lymphatic glands in the neck are enlarged in cases of recurrent tonsillitis.

Causes

The cause is directly related to a congested lymphatic system and this is often aggravated through dairy produce in the diet. Natural therapists do find inherited factors may also predispose a child in this direction. Slight mineral imbalances, and in particular deficiencies in vitamin C are contributing causes.

Treatment

1 Iron phosphate and potassium chloride for the inflammation and exudate.
2 Vitamin C for immunity and for its anti-bacterial action. [1]
3 Calcium phosphate or sulphate as indicated. [2]
4 Homoeopathic remedies, especially the mercury salts are fairly specific. [3]
5 Belladonna in homoeopathic potency is specific for high fevers assocated with tonsillitis.

It has been found that homoeopathic treatment for tonsillitis is as quick in effect as antibiotics, provided the remedies are taken when the tonsils first become inflamed.

Case History

Dean, aged six, had suffered tonsillitis since a baby. He had developed an associated problem with the ears and was becoming deaf. Antibiotics had been used extensively for his condition. His first prescription included calcium sulphate, iron phosphate and potassium chloride, vitamin C, lymphatic and liver herbs and homoeopathic drops which included the salt Mercurius biniodatum, plus Hepar sulphuris and Pulsatilla, also in homoeopathic potency.

This treatment was continued for over six months with minor adjustments as needed. There was no further tonsillitis, and hearing improved. He had a couple of months off treatment and the ears worsened following swimming in a chlorinated pool. Homoeopathic Thuja was then added to deal with the deep-seated tendency for mucus development, and this was followed by a further homoeopathic nosode to deal with an inherited tubercular tendency. During the following months there were no further colds.

Tuberculosis

This is one of the diseases that natural therapists are not permitted to treat. Like syphilis, however, it is important to mention because of its projection in the form of problems through many generations. It has already been stated in connection with respiratory problems that we often need to treat a tubercular taint. As with all inherited miasms, only a deep-acting homoeopathic nosode can eradicate a tubercular problem. We do not expect the person to ever manifest active tuberculosis. What natural therapists find is a tendency or weakness of the chest which makes the client prone to such conditions as asthma, recurrent bronchitis, and in some cases pneumonia.

It is of general interest that the chest weakness usually shows in the iris as a defect in the radial fibres in the position corresponding to the lungs or bronchials. This marking does not mean that the person will definitely manifest a clinical chest problem. Much will depend on their nutrition and life-style. It has been noted by natural therapists that persons with a tubercular taint are often unable to adequately assimilate calcium salts. There is no case history for this section as active TB has not been treated in the clinic.

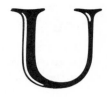

Ulcerative Colitis

This is now generally considered to be one of several disorders included under the term Bowel Inflammatory Disease (BID). The other main disease in this category is Crohn's disease and this is treated separately under that heading. Ulcerative colitis is usually confined to the large bowel and commonly extends from the rectum upwards. The inflammation is usually uniform in the part affected and there is ulceration and bleeding in the majority of cases. Malignancy may develop in chronic cases. The main symptoms are bloody diarrhoea and abdominal pain. In severe cases weight loss occurs.

Causes

From the medical viewpoint, the aetiology, as with Crohn's disease, is unknown. Some immunological and inherited factors have been considered as contributing factors, but this has not been found to be significant in all cases.

From our naturopathic viewpoint, many of the same factors would be relevant as for Crohn's disease. There are likely to be biochemical imbalances involving magnesium (tension of nerve and muscle fibres), zinc (ulceration), and the sodium status involving the pH factor (acid/alkaline levels). Digestive enzymes may be imbalanced and vitamin B-complex and C levels may be deficient. Poor nutrition may be a prominent factor and there will most likely be psychosomatic factors.

The psychosomatic connection functions through the solar plexus *chakra* as discussed in connection with other digestive problems. Our emotional life is directly expressed via this energy centre and any emotional stress, suppression or conflict will quickly affect organs associated with the digestive process. The general life-style is another area of great concern in this problem as lack of rhythm in the work, sleep, or eating patterns can profoundly affect the digestion via the autonomic nervous system — the link between the solar plexus *chakra* and the digestive organs.

Treatment

Attention to diet is the first cornerstone. The client will be advised to have at least four days on vegetable juices alone so that the inflammation of the bowel can subside. Suitable juices are carrot, celery, cabbage, and beetroot in small amounts, alternating with red grape juice. These juices should all be fresh and raw. This regime will be followed by a diet of fresh steamed vegetables, tofu (bean curd), millet meal, well-cooked brown rice, vegetable soups, and when tolerated without diarrhoea, fresh salads with cottage or ricotta cheese. White meats only will be allowed in moderate amounts.

Specific supplements will be similar to that for Crohn's disease, and will be applied to reduce spasm, heal inflammation and ulceration and generally tone the digestive system. They may include:

1 Vitamin B-complex as a general nerve tonic.
2 Magnesium salts in different strengths for spasm.
3 Iron phosphate for bleeding of mucosa.
4 Zinc chelate and vitamin A to heal ulceration. [1]
5 Selected homoeopathics for toning liver, pancreas, and mucosa of bowel. [2]
6 Bach flower remedies to cover emotional problems.
7 Constitutional homoeopathic remedies.

Case History

The following case is fairly typical of naturopathic findings with ulcerative colitis. John, an optometrist aged twenty-three, had been diagnosed as having the colitis five years earlier. He was taking a drug to affect the immune system, and antibiotics. Other problems involved tiredness and cystic acne which had manifested since puberty. At the time of his first visit he was having two bowel actions daily with a small amount of blood and mucus. He was concerned to have help with his general health and energy levels, and hoped to get off medical drugs.

The iris diagnosis revealed a heavily congested lymphatic system which would be a major cause for both the colitis and skin problems. The body was endeavouring to use both the skin and mucus membrane of the bowel as eliminative organs for the toxins, albeit rather unsuccessfully. In the case of John, his psychological attitudes were positive and hence, the toxic factor of the disease outweighed the psychological and nerve factor, although this still needed some attention. The Vega diagnosis was interesting as it showed involvement of both liver and bowel, and the biological index of the bowel corresponded approximately to a person of nearly fifty.

The first month of treatment included iron phosphate for inflammation and bleeding, homoeopathic drops for the lymphatic system and liver, and a small herbal mixture of digestive and blood cleansing herbs. As there were only two bowel actions per day, the herbal mixture was not expected to give any problem. Vitamin A for the epithelial lining of the bowel, and B-complex were included.

John was already booked for a colonoscopy during that first month to assess the extent of his problem. The diseased part of the bowel was found to be confined to the descending part of the colon. Unfortunately the investigation caused extensive haemorrhaging. As a result he was placed back on cortisone.

At his second visit following the investigation, the same remedies were repeated with the addition of a zinc compound to accelerate healing and to deal with any scarring in the bowel, plus magnesium phosphate for spasm. By the third visit, he was off the cortisone again and feeling considerably improved in terms of general health and energy. The Vega diagnosis revealed a considerable improvement in the health and function of the bowel.

The same prescription was repeated with the addition of vitamin B5 to boost the adrenal glands following withdrawal of the cortisone. John explained that when he goes off cortisone he temporarily suffers great stiffness and discomfort of joints. The pineapple enzyme bromelaine was added to prevent this occurrence. On his fourth visit, John reported no problems with the joints after the withdrawal of cortisone and he was feeling well in all respects. During the next month, John suffered two acute infections involving firstly the bowel and then the respiratory organs. This is probably a good sign and would be classed as an elimination crisis whereby accumulated toxins in the form of mucus are more speedily eradicated. Although the cortisone had to be resumed for a short time, once again, it was discontinued without any problems. Minor adjustments were made to the herbal and homoeopathic part of the treatment. John is convinced he is on the right road back to health as he feels generally so much better in himself. The immune suppressing drugs have now been discontinued by his medical doctor.

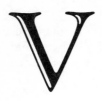

Vaginal Discharge

This term may include a variety of problems including thrush (monilia or candida albicans), trichomonas, and any infection which involves a discharge in that area of the body. These discharges may vary from being a bland, non-infected type of discharge, to acrid and painful discharges which can have a bad odour. The treatment will vary according to whether there is an infection or not and in keeping with the whole case.

The naturopathic approach to vaginal discharge is quite different. Firstly, it is a standard approach for natural therapists to be concerned not to suppress the discharge with antibiotics unless it is found to be of active venereal origin. The term active expresses the natural therapist's understanding that most vaginal discharges are related to the carrying of a venereal taint in the constitution. This inherited miasm may go back many generations and results from suppressive treatment of venereal diseases, in particular that of gonorrhoea. Subsequent generations are then born with a tendency to have pelvic inflammations and to develop pelvic adhesions easily.[1]

Natural therapists realise the need for speedy treatment of venereal problems with antibiotics. We stress, however, that the problem does not stop there, and that an inactive form of the disease penetrates deep into the organism to be expressed as perhaps ovarian cysts, blocked fallopian tubes, menstrual problems, or discharges in later generations. Problems of the lymphatic system involving the respiratory area also have their basic cause in this miasm, and may include bronchitis, asthma, and hay fever, and will involve both sexes.

From the naturopathic point of view, the only way to eradicate this inborn tendency is through the skilled use of homoeopathy. Subsequent generations will then be free of the tendency for pelvic and lymphatic problems. The following case is a perfect illustration of the whole sequence of events and the resolution of the problem.

Case History

Michelle, aged twenty-five, came to visit me with a painful and congested right breast, tenderness over the gall-bladder and a history of hay fever each year. Her iris indicated a great deal of lymphatic congestion and she had the typical 'lymphatic constitution' in terms of her body structure. The first month's treatment included lymphatic and liver herbs, vitamin C, mineral combination of iron phosphate and potassium chloride to work with the herbs to cleanse the lymphatic system, homoeopathic drops for the gall-bladder, and magnesium and potassium phosphate for general nerve toning.

One month later, Michelle was feeling better in herself and the lymphatic engorgment of the breast had reduced. The same prescription was repeated and improvement continued. The glands in the neck became enlarged as part of the normal retracing process. Similar treatment was continued and as the hay fever season was now in full swing, homoeopathic remedies of Kali bichromicum and Kali sulphuricum were given together with a homoeopathic mixture of several allergens. Of special importance was the miasmatic remedy for the lymph system which was given at this time in a high potency to work deeply into the system. This was Thuja in the 200th potency.[2]

Michelle continued with the treatment for the next few months and was well in all respects. Then after a few days in Sydney, she developed a vaginal discharge without any new sexual contacts, and with no apparent cause. From the naturopathic point of view, her system was retracing back to the original problem inherited from her forebears. She was very concerned because of wishing to commence a family this year. Apart from the discharge she had cramping in the pelvis and pains in the back, indicating that most of the reproductive area was involved.

At this next stage of her treatment, she was given a mixture to take four times daily; this contained burdock, violet leaves, clivers, trifolium, and echinacea. Kyolic garlic was also included and the homoeopathic Thuja was repeated. The potency of this was increased two weeks later as the problem had not completely resolved. At the next visit, all pelvic problems had cleared and it is expected that from now on the hay fever will not be such a problem.

Provided that Michelle has a good life-style, there is no reason why she should have any continuing lymphatic or pelvic problems, but it is possible that, with such a deep-seated tendency, one further healing crisis may be expected within the next few months. She is now in a much healthier state to start a family and hopefully her offspring will be free of these inherited lymphatic problems.

Varicose Veins, Varicose Eczema and Varicose Ulcers

Varicose veins is a common condition which natural therapists are asked to treat and is one area where surgery can often be avoided. The main problem with veins apart from aesthetic considerations is the aching legs which the person suffers, and more seriously, the possibility of thrombosis in bad cases. In older people, varicose eczema can become quite a problem, and varicose ulcers are the most serious problem usually involving the lower part of the leg. These ulcers can become seriously infected and even gangrenous due to the poor circulation which is often an associated condition.

Causes

As with haemorrhoids, causes are at least in part related to a familial incidence of mineral deficiency involving calcium fluoride.[1] Life-style will perhaps play a more prominent part than with haemorrhoids. Long hours spent standing still as is required in certain occupations will obviously aggravate this condition in which the elastic tissue of the veins is deficient. Due to the inherited incidence of the condition, dietary factors are inclined to be secondary. It is acknowledged, however, that constipation with consequent pelvic congestion, will aggravate a tendency to varicose veins. In cases of varicose ulcers, life-style factors are more involved and feature further mineral deficiencies such as zinc, and the need for improved circulation through exercise. There is also a toxic factor involved with ulcers and the lymphatic system is often found to be congested, together with arterial degeneration in many cases.

Treatment

In the case of varicose veins treatment will be similar to that for haemorrhoids, except for some difference in the homoeopathic remedies. Specific remedies will include therefore:

1 Calcium fluoride as the tissue salt for elastic tissue.
2 Vitamin E to improve circulation.
3 Liver herbs for detoxification of body.
4 Selected homoeopathic remedies.
5 Additions for varicose ulcers will include: Zinc salts and vitamin A for healing.[2]
6 Lymphatic cleansing herbs with emphasis on herbs like echinacea for its antibacterial action.

Case History

Quite often natural therapists will be treating several manifestations of circulatory imbalance together. In the case of Don, a forty-seven-year-old lecturer at a technical institute, there were problems of varicose veins, varicose eczema, the possibility of a varicose ulcer, and high blood pressure. Don is a tense person and has trouble 'switching off' with the result that he keeps very late hours. It was of interest that the iris revealed dark patches in the leg and kidney area and this has been noticed in a number of persons who have varicose eczema or ulcers on the lower leg.

Don had already placed himself on vitamins E, P, C, blood pressure herbs and garlic. Our main contribution to his treatment was in the form of blood cleansing herbs for the eczema, liver and kidney herbs for toning those organs to improve elimination, and magnesium orotate to relax the nervous system and thus reduce blood pressure. He was encouraged to continue his own supplements. After two months on this regime the eczema had improved to some extent.

Three months later, however, the varicose eczema began spreading and at this stage Lachesis, a homoeopathic remedy developed from snake poison, was introduced. This remedy is pertinent in conditions of the skin where a purple colour is manifesting, provided other constitutional signs are present. The eczema improved to some extent again after this month, but a small ulcer developed over the next few weeks. The basic treatment was continued, and a small homoeopathic mixture of Arnica, Lachesis and Sulphur proved healing for the ulcer and eczema.

Don continued to attend over a number of years and the skin on his lower leg gradually changed from purple to brown and then to a paler more normal hue. The skin became less fragile to knocks, and eczema abated. The underlying weakness of the veins was treated with various homoeopathic drops and calcium fluoride mineral tablets were taken over a long period of time. Liver, kidney and blood cleansing herbs were continued, and various magnesium compounds, vitamin B-complexes and nerve herbs were used for nervous tension.

Varicose problems, being a deep-seated inherited tendency, need treatment over a long time and Don attended the clinic for about five years; however, once he was stabilised I needed to see him only every two months. It was significant that at one stage during his treatment he needed attention to strained ligaments in his wrist thus indicating another facet of the problem with elastic tissue in his body. All his ailments were slow to respond, and this was not helped by the constant stress which he placed himself under in relation to work. When last seen, he had been working on developing a more relaxed life-style and the leg condition was almost negligible.

Venereal Herpes

see Herpes

Venereal Warts

This has become a modern epidemic. These warts are classed as a notifiable disease by the Health Department. As distinct from warts on the limbs, venereal warts can involve some discomfort and irritation and this is most likely because of their situation on mucus membrane. They are commonly found both on the external genitalia and also in the vagina.

Causes

We know that there is a virus associated with all warts, but only certain people seem to be vulnerable. Natural therapists understand that inherited factors make one more likely to develop warts and this is borne out by the finding that some clients with no sexual contacts have developed warts on their genitalia. Natural therapists do, however, accept the contagious aspect of venereal warts.

The more subtle factors involving imbalance of energies at the sacral level may be applied in the same way as in the discussion in the section on herpes.

Treatment

This will include very specific homoeopathic remedies to remove the inherited tendency and will be backed up by general treatment to cleanse the lymphatic system and tone the nervous system. Clients with this problem are usually very emotionally disturbed by the current medical approach and treatment. Female clients have had painful burnings to their warts on the genitals and vagina with liquid nitrogen. They also feel that they will be ostracised from all future sexual contact after reading dramatic and sensational accounts by the media and their medical advisers.

Case History

Shirley attended me for treatment following unsuccessful diathermy treatment for a veneral wart. She had suffered a great deal of pain immediately following the treatment and was horrified when the wart promptly grew again within weeks.

Her treatment included vitamin A, a mineral combination of sodium sulphate and potassium chloride, liver and lymphatic herbs for cleansing, and a high homoeopathic potency of nitric acid.[1] This latter remedy was the most specific part of the treatment; the other remedies would be negligible without its use. After one month's treatment, the wart was almost gone and the same selection of remedies was repeated. By the next visit the wart had completely disappeared and there was no recurrence. Treatment was continued for another two months to improve immunity and lessen the likelihood of any recurrence.

Considering the psychological anguish which can swamp lives afflicted by this problem, it is a great shame that natural medicine does not have more official support. Since it is a notifiable disease, natural therapists are not even in a position to treat the problem without the person first seeking medical advice. Medicine has admitted it can do nothing for specific venereal warts.[2]

Vertigo

see Meniere's Syndrome

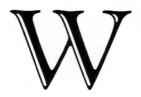

Warts

The strange thing about warts is that the worse the case, the quicker they often clear up. This follows the basic naturopathic concept that a vital person throws their health problems to the surface of the body. In the case of warts, while we acknowledge the presence of a virus, the natural therapist takes into account an inherited tendency which makes a person more vulnerable to the problem.

Case Histories

John was a teacher of retarded childen, and had suffered dozens of warts on the neck for two years. They returned after standard medical treatment. His life-style was only fair with a diet including some junk food, and he smoked fifteen cigarettes per day.

To his complete amazement, the warts disappeared after three weeks on liver and lymphatic herbs, potassium chloride, potassium phosphate, magnesium phosphate, and vitamin C. The main specific remedy for the warts was Thuja and this was given in the 30th potency each day. There are, however, many homoeopathic remedies which may be needed for warts and Thuja is not necessarily specific.

Margot, aged thirty-eight, had suffered multiple warts on the hands over a period of twelve months. She also had a history of eczema on the hands. The first month's treatment consisted of Thuja[1] in the 30th potency, a mineral combination of sodium sulphate and potassium chloride, vitamin C, and lymphatic and liver herbs. There was no change in the warts after this month.

During the second month, the basic treatment was continued

303

except for the changing of the homoeopathic Thuja to a higher potency. There was still not much change after this month. I concluded therefore that Thuja was not the correct homoeopathic remedy and this was replaced with a high potency of calcium carbonate during the third month. After another month with no change in the warts, the homoeopathic remedy was again changed to a high potency of Causticum which was continued for several months.

At her sixth visit, Margot reported that most of the warts had gone. There was a bit of a relapse with dry peeling palms; however this was an expected retracing back to a more acute form of skin manifestation. This recurrence of an old problem had disappeared by the next visit.

We often explain to clients that warts can take six months to clear up and this time period was accurate for Margot. In the previous case, a more severe crop of warts cleared up in a few weeks. This highlights comments at the beginning of this section; it indicates that the time taken to improve with natural medication is in direct proportion to the inherent vitality. In the case of John, his constitution was vital enough to manifest an inherent problem very strongly on the skin. Minimal treatment cleared the problem very quickly. Margot had a more complex situation requiring more complex treatment and a longer time-span; the cause was more deeply-seated and so there was less manifestation on the skin.

Margot came back for a general check-up one year later; there had been no re-occurrence of warts. She had just gone back into the workforce and we gave her general nerve toning for a few headaches which developed with the strain of readjusting to office work.

Whooping Cough

In spite of vaccination, I have treated many vaccinated children for whooping cough over the last fifteen years. Epidemics appear to go in cycles of seven years. The medical explanation for this is that due to the virus changing its protein coat every seven years or so, the previous batches of prepared sera are then no longer suitable. Natural therapists do not like mass vaccination and not all medical scientists agree with the procedure. Several very eminent scientists have condemned immunisation programmes outright.[1]

Causes

The immediate infective organism is the pertussis virus. Certain constitutions are more vulnerable including especially those children with a tubercular taint in the family tree. The anthroposophical group of doctors have a unique explanation for the problem of whooping cough. They explain that in these children the astral body is in a poor relationship to the etheric/physical part of the constitution. The normal rhythm of the psychic life is disturbed and the child is unable to adequately exhale the astral nature which in turn affects the breathing rhythm.[2] Herbal remedies are given which normalise these processes. This coincides with naturopathic findings in clinical practice that the children most affected are very short of the mineral most needed for stabilisation of the nervous system — magnesium phosphate.

Treatment

1 Magnesium phosphate in very regular doses.
2 Vitamin C to improve immunity and eliminate mucus.[3]
3 Iron phosphate and potassium chloride to reduce lymphatic glandular swelling.
4 Herbal lung tonic and cough mixture including especially tincture of drosera which is specific for whooping cough.[4]
5 Homoeopathic herbs for the liver.

Case History

Sophie, aged three, and her brother, aged five, had been 'whooping' for weeks with no relief from standard medical treatment. So many children had whooping cough at their school that parents were not even bothering to keep the children home after the intitial infectious period was over. They were attending school still 'whooping' and I was told that a mop and bucket had become standard classroom equipment.

These children only needed a couple of weeks' treatment to give them complete relief. Treatment included in particular magnesium phosphate for its anti-spasmodic effect, liver herbs, and a cough mixture containing the drosera. They were also given the magnesium phosphate in homoeopathic potency.

Worms

This is a very common problem and includes threadworms, round worms and tape worms. Other types of parasites occurring less frequently will not be discussed. Threadworms occurring in children are the most common worm infestation which confronts the natural therapist. In many cases the standard pharmaceutical products have been administered, and the worms have returned within a few weeks. The most common symptoms of thread-worms in children are general irritability and itching around the anus, especially at night. As the worms tend to come outside the anus in the warmth of the bed, confirmation is found by inspection after the child is asleep. Threadworms look like small pieces of cotton as the name implies.

Causes

The natural therapist can offer a very logical explanation as to why worms are more prevalent in some children and adults than others. The basis of all naturopathic philosophy centres on a balance of flora in the gastrointestinal tract. Due to incorrect nutritional habits, many people upset the acid/alkaline balance. The balance is also disturbed by antibiotics and other drugs. Accumulation of waste due to faulty metabolism and poor elimination is another major cause for the proliferation of thread-worms. Correct the imbalances and the worms disappear. It is true that infection is easy through children ingesting the eggs from contact with infected children, but the worms do not breed except in a suitable medium.

Treatment

Attention to the diet is essential with a reduction in all products containing white flour and sugar so that the bowel contents become more alkaline. An increase of vegetables and salad is encouraged for the same reason. Specific supplements include:

1 Sodium phosphate to increase alkalinity.
2 Calcium phosphate is usually found to be necessary.
3 Homoeopathic liver drops to tone the digestive organs.
4 Homoeopathic Cina[1] is specific for threadworms and homoeopathic Male fern for tapeworm.

Case History

In 1973, I treated two small boys who had been living in India with their mother. Both boys, who were aged three and six, had returned to Australia with bad bronchial conditions and worms. There was considerable enlargement of lymph nodes in the necks of both children. It is of interest that the tubercular constitution may manifest all these problems, including worms.

The boys were given calcium phosphate, a tubercular homoeopathic nosode, lymphatic cleansing and liver herbs in homoeopathic doses, a herbal cough mixture, vitamin C, and the useful mineral combination of iron phosphate and potassium chloride to eradicate mucus. Cina drops were also included. The worms were gone within one month and the bronchial condition within two months.

Notes

1 What does Natural mean?

[1] Burr, H. S., *Blueprint for Immortality*. Neville Spearman (London, 1972); Coleby, S., 'New Controversial Theory on Growth Could Revolutionise Cancer Diagnosis', *University of Sydney News*, 5 August 1986.

[2] Bradley, F. J., 'Vaccination: Its Effect on the Immunological System, Cancer and Cot Deaths', *J. of Alternative Medicine*, May 1986, 4 (5) 18.

[3] Stone, I., *The Healing Factor — Vitamin C Against Disease*. Grosset & Dunlap (New York, 1972); Dettman, G., 'Aboriginal Infant Health and Mortality Rates' (Letter to Ed.), *Med. J. of Aust.*, 7 April 1973, 711; and Turkel, H., 'Vitamin C & Immunisation' (Letter to Ed.), *Medical Tribune*, February 1983.

[4] Kiester, E., 'Lizards & Shakespeare Explain Fever', *The Age*, 8 April 1985.

[5] Jacka, J., *A Philosophy of Healing*. Inkata Press (Melbourne, 1979).

[6] Kenyon, J. (ed.), *Short Manual of Vegatest-Method*. Vega (Greishaber, W. Germany, 1981).

2 The Subtle Causes of Disease

[1] Capra, F., *The Turning Point*. Bantam (New York, 1983).

[2] Briggs, J. P. and Peat, D., *Looking Glass Universe*. Fontana (London, 1985).

[3] Bailey, A. A., *Esoteric Healing*. Lucis Press (London, 1953).

[4] Bailey, A. A., *A Treatise on Cosmic Fire*. Lucis Press (London, 1953).

[5] Moss, T., *The Body Electric*. J. P. Tarcher (New York, 1979); Reich, W., *The Cancer Biopathy*. Farrar, Straus & Giroux (New York, 1973); Husemann/Wolff, *The Anthroposophical Approach To Medicine*. Anthroposophic Press (New York, 1982); Burr, H. S., *Blueprint For Immortality*. Spearman (London, 1972); Jacka, J., *Vivaxis — A Science of Life Energies*. Southern School of Natural Therapies (Melbourne, 1984).

[6] Kenyon, J., *Modern Techniques of Acupuncture*, vol. I. Thorsons (London, 1985).

[7] Miller, C., 'Ancient Idea is Revolutionary', *The Age*, 8 September 1986.

[8] 'New Controversial Theory on Growth Could Revolutionise Cancer Diagnosis', *University of Sydney News*, 5 August 1986.

[9] Bailey, A. A., *Esoteric Healing*.

[10] Maslow, A., *Religions, Values and Peak Experiences*. Viking (New York, 1970).

[11] Bailey, A. A., *Esoteric Psychology*, volumes 1 and 2. Lucis Press (London, 1942).

[12] Pfieffer, C., *Zinc and Other Micro-Nutrients*. Keats (New Canaan, 1978) 6–7.

[13] Petersdorf, R. G. *et al. Harrison's Principles of Internal Medicine*, 10th edn. McGraw-Hill (Sydney, 1983) 739.

[14] Karagulla, S., *Breakthrough to Creativity*. De Vorss (California, 1967); Tansley, D., *Subtle Body*. Thames & Hudson (London, 1977).

3 The Cornerstones of Treatment

[1] Mount, J. L., *The Food and Health Of Western Man*. Precision Press (Buckshire, U. K., 1979) 1–21.

[2] Ibid., 72–90.

[3] Regtop, H., 'Is Magnesium the Grossly Neglected Mineral?', *Int. Clin. Nutr. Rev.* (1983) 3 (3) 10–20.

[4] Fisher, P. *et al.*, 'Effect of Zinc Supplementation on Copper Status in Adult Men', *Am. J. Clin. Nutr.* (1984) 40, 743–6.

[5] Callinan, P. J., *The Mechanism of Iron Absorption*. Dee Why Printing (Sydney, 1975).

[6] Boericke, W. and Dewey, W., *The Twelve Tissue Salts*. Set Dey & Co. (Calcutta, 1959).

[7] Buist, R., 'Vitamin Toxicities, Side Effects and Contraindications', *Int. Clin. Nutr. Rev.* (1984) 4 (4) 159–71.

[8] Stone, I., *The Healing Factor — Vitamin C Against Disease*. Grosset & Dunlap (New York, 1972).

[9] Draper, H. H. and Bird, R. P., 'Antioxidants and Cancer', *J. Agricultural and Food Chem.* (1984) 32 (3) 433–5.

[10] Abstract, 'Alpha-tocopherel Influences Tissue Levels of Vitamin A and Its Esters', *Nutrition Reviews* (1985) 43, 55–6.

[11] Lesser, M., *Nutrition and Vitamin Therapy*. Grove Press (New York, 1980).

[12] Ibid.

[13] Wren, R. C., *Potter's New Cyclopaedia of Botanical Drugs and Preparations*. Health Science Press (Rustingdon, Sussex, 1968).

[14] Grossinger, R., *Planet Medicine*. Anchor Books (New York, 1980).

[15] Weeks, N., *The Medical Discoveries of Edward Bach, Physician*. C. W. Daniel (Ashingdon, 1940).

[16] Nixon, F., *Search for Vivaxis*, parts 1 & 2. Magnetic Publishers (Chemainus, 1982) (o.p.).

[17] Callinan, P. J., *The Mechanism of Iron Absorption*.

[18] Morris-Owen, R. M., 'Placebo Effect and Homoeopathic Effect', *Br. J. Homoeopathy* (1980) 69 (4) 216–20.

Acne

[1] Darling, C., Moore, J., Besser, G. *et al.*, 'Androgen Status in Women with Late Onset or Persistent Acne Vulgaris,' *Clin. Exp. Dermatol.* (1984) 9, 28–35.

[2] Jensen, B., *Iridology — The Science and Practice in the Healing Arts*. Bernard Jensen Publishing (California, 1982); Jaquin, N., *Practical Palmistry*. D. B. Taraporevala Sons & Co. (Bombay, 1964); Campbell, D. C., 'Hair Analysis: A Diagnostic Tool for Measuring Mineral Status in Humans', *J. Orthomolecular Psychiatry* (1985) 14 (4) 276.

[3] Hahnemann, S., *The Chronic Diseases*. Ringer & Co. (Calcutta, N.D.).

[4] Kloss, J., *Back to Eden*. Woodbridge Press (California, 1974).

5 Fisher, L., *Mineral Compounds and Human Disease*. Blackmores Books (Sydney, 1978).
6 Pfieffer, C., *Zinc and Other Micro-Nutrients*. Keats (Connecticut, 1978).
7 Stone, I., *The Healing Factor — Vitamin C Against Disease*. Grosset & Dunlap (New York, 1972).
8 Kugen, A., Mills, O., Leyden, J. *et al.*, 'Oral Vitamin A in Acne Vulgaris', *Arch. Dermatol.* (1982) 118, 891–4.
9 Kent, J. T., *Lectures on Homoeopathic Materia Medica*. Boericke and Tafel (Philadelphia, 1956) 981.

Abdominal Migraine

1 Boericke, W. and Dewey, W., *The Twelve Tissue Remedies of Schussler*, 6th edn. B. Jain (New Delhi, 1981) 88–95.

Addison's Disease

1 Petersdorf, R. G. *et al.*, *Harrison's Principles of Internal Medicine*, 10th edn. McGraw-Hill (Sydney, 1983) 651.
2 Bott, V., *Anthroposophical Medicine*. Rudolf Steiner Press (London, 1978) 132–42.

Alcoholism

1 Guenther, R. N., 'The Role of Nutritional Therapy in Alcoholism Treatment', *Int. J. Biosocial Res.* (1983) 4, 5–18.
2 Williams, R., *Nutrition Against Disease*. Bantam Books (New York, 1971); Das, I., Burch, R. E. and Hahn, H. K. J., 'Effects of Zinc Deficiency on Ethonal Metabolism and Alcohol and Aldehyde Dehydrogenase Activities', *J. Lab. Clin. Med.* (1984) 104, 610–17.
3 Kalokerinos, A., *Every Second Child*. Thomas Nelson (Melbourne, 1974) 127–8.
4 Yunice, A. A., Hsu, J. M., Fahmy, A., and Henry, S., 'Ethanol-ascorbate inter-relationship in Acute and Chronic Alcoholism in the Guinea Pig', *Proc. Soc. Exp. Biol. Med.* (1984) 177, 262–71.
5 Dutta, S. K., Miller, P. A., Greenberg, L. B. *et al.*, 'Selenium and Acute Alcoholism', *Am. J. Clin. Nutr.* (1983) 38, 713–8.

Allergies

1 Philpott, W. and Philpott, K., 'Principles of Bio-Ecological Medicine', *J. Orthomolecular Psych.* (1982) 11(3) 208–15.
2 Laird, D., 'Using Biofeedback to Uncover Food Sensitive Persons', *J. Orthomolecular Medicine* (1986) 1(2) 78–83.
3 Bott, V., *Anthroposophical Medicine*. Rudolf Steiner Press (London, 1978) 117–21.
4 Reynolds, R. D. and Natta, C. L., 'Depressed Plasma Pyridoxal Phosphate Concentrations in Adult Asthmatics', *Am. J. Clin. Nutr.* (1985) 41, 684–8.

Amenorrhoea

1 Albert-Puleo, M., 'Fennel and Anise as Estrogenic Agents', *J. Ethnopharmacology* (1980) 2, 337–44.

Anaemia

1 Bott, V., *Anthroposophical Medicine*. Rudolf Steiner Press (London, 1972) 107–8.
2 Callinan, P. J., *The Mechanism of Iron Absorption*. Dee Why Printing (Dee Why, N.S.W., 1975).
3 Ibid.

Angio-neurotic Oedema

[1] Bott, V., *Anthroposophical Medicine*. Rudolf Steiner Press (London, 1978) 117–21.

[2] Wheeler, C. E., *An Introduction to the Principles and Practice of Homoeopathy*. Health Science Press (London, 1948) 69–75.

Ankylosing Spondylitis

[1] Petersdorf, R. G. *et al.*, *Harrison's Principles of Internal Medicine*, 10th edn. McGraw-Hill (Sydney, 1983) 1987.

Anorexia Nervosa

[1] Abstract, 'Evidence for Zinc Deficiency in Anorexia Nervosa', *Int. Clin. Nutr. Rev.* (1985) 5 (3) 143.

Anxiety

[1] Drury, Neville (ed.), *The Bodywork Book*. Harper & Row (Sydney, 1984).

[2] Fisher, L., *Mineral Compounds and Human Disease*. Blackmores Books (Sydney, 1978).

[3] Lesser, M., *Nutrition and Vitamin Therapy*. Grove Press (New York, 1980).

Arthritis

[1] Airola, P., *There is a Cure for Arthritis*. Parker Pub. (New York, 1968).

[2] Kloss, J., *Back to Eden*. Lifeline Books (California, 1974) 536.

[3] Schwartz, E. R., 'The Modulation of Osteoarthritic Development by Vitamins C & E', *Int. J. Vitamin & Nutrition Res.* (1984) suppl. 26, 141–6.

[4] Harper, *Review of Physiological Chemistry*, 16th edn (Langs, 1977) 618.

[5] Fisher, L., *Mineral Compounds and Human Disease*. Blackmore Books (Sydney, 1978).

[6] Petersdorf, R. G. *et al.*, *Harrison's Principles of Internal Medicine*, 10th edn. McGraw-Hill (Sydney, 1983) 1974.

[7] Abstract, *Int. Clin. Nutr. Rev.* (1983) 3 (1) 50.

[8] Stone, I., *The Healing Factor*. Grosset & Dunlap (New York, 1972) 108–12.

[9] Macneill, A. D., 'Rheumatoid Arthritis. Report on an Ongoing Trial', *Br. Homoeopathic J.* (January 1977) LXVI (1) 13–19.

Asthma

[1] Allen, D. A., 'Environmental Factors in the Provocation of Asthma and Hayfever', *Australian Family Physician* (1985) 14 (3) 172–6.

[2] Wilson, G., *The Hazards of Immunisation*. Athlone Press (University of London, 1967).

[3] Freedman, B. J., 'A Diet free from Additives in the Management of Allergic Disease', *Clin. Allergy* (1977) 7, 417–27.

[4] Bock, S. A., 'Food Related Asthma and Basic Nutrition', *J. Asthma* (1981) 20, 377–81.

[5] Bott, V., *Anthroposophical Medicine*. Rudolf Steiner Press (London, 1978) chapter 10.

[6] 'Dairy, Migraine and Asthma', *Int. Clin. Nutr. Rev.* 4 (4) 203. Extract from *Israeli J. Med. Sc.* (1983) 19, 806–9.

[7] Dawson, W. *et al.*, 'Actions of Sodium Ascorbate on Smooth Muscle', *Br. J. Pharmacology & Chemotherapeutics* (1967) 31, 269–75.

[8] Collip, P. J. *et al.*, 'Pyridoxine Treatment of Childhood Asthma', *Ann. Allergy* (1975) 35, 93–7; Simon, S. W., 'Vitamin B12 Therapy in Allergy and Chronic Dermatosis', *J. Allergy* (1951) 2, 183–5.

[9] Foreman, J. C., 'Mast Cells — The Action of Flavanoids', *J. Allergy Clin. Immunol.* (1984) 73, 769–74.

[10] Brunner, E. H. *et al.*, 'Effect of Parental Mg. in Pulmonary Function, Plasma, cAMP and Histamine in Bronchial Asthma', *J. Asthma* (1985) 22, 3–11.

[11] Foubister, D. M., 'Constitutional Types', *Br. Homoeopathic J.* (October 1987) 70 (4) 197–202.

[12] Ibid.

Atherosclerosis

[1] Higuchi, M., Hashimoto, I., Yamakawa, K. *et al.*, 'Effect of Exercise Training on Plasma High-density Lipoprotein Cholesterol Levels at a Constant Weight', *Clin. Physiol.* (1984) 4, 125–33.

[2] Tanner, T., 'Effects of Dietary Fish and Fish Oil Supplements on Health', *Int. Clin. Nutr. Rev.* (1986) 6 (1) 14.

[3] Renaud, S., Blache, D., Dumont, E. *et al.*, 'Platelet Function after Cigarette Smoking in Relation to Nicotine and Carbon Monoxide', *Clin. Pharmacol. Ther.* (1984) 36, 389–95.

[4] Potter, J. D., Topping, D. L. and Oakebnful, D., 'Soya Saponins and Plasma Cholesterol', *Lancet* (1979) 1, 223–4; Yudin, J., 'Dietary Factors in Atherosclerosis: Sucrose', *Lipids* (1978) 13, 370–2.

[5] Arnesen, E., Forde, O. H. and Thele, D. S., 'Coffee and Serum Cholesterol', *Br. Med. J.* (1984) 288, 1960.

[6] Malinow, M. R., 'Alfalfa', *Atherosclerosis* (1973) 30, 27–43.

[7] Regtop, H., 'Is Magnesium the Grossly Neglected Mineral?', *Int. Clin. Nutr. Rev.* (1983) 3 (3) 10–20.

[8] Khan, A. R., Seedarnee, F. A., 'Effect of Ascorbic Acid on Plasma Lipids and Lipoproteins in Healthy Young Women', *Atherosclerosis* (1981) 39, 89–95.

[9] Arora, R. C. and Arora, S., 'Comparative Effect of Clofibrate, Garlic and Onion on Alimentary Hyperlipemia', *Atherosclerosis* (1981) 39, 4, 447–52.

[10] Steiner, M. and Anastasi, J., 'Vitamin E — An Inhibitor of Platelet Release Action', *J. Clin. Invest.* (1976) 57, 732–7; Okuma, N., Takayama, H. and Uchino, H., 'Generation of Prostacyclin-Like Substance and Lipid Peroxidation in Vitamin E Deficient Rats', *Prostaglandins* (1980) 19, 527–36.

[11] Krumdieck, C. and Butterworth, C. E., 'Ascorbate-cholesterol-lecithin Interactions: Factors of Potential Importance in the Pathogenesis of Atherosclerosis', *Atherosclerosis* (1976) 24, 1–18.

[12] Taussig, S. J. and Nieper, H. A., 'Bromelain: Its Use in Prevention of Cardio-Vascular Disease — Present Status', *J. Int. Act. Prev. Med.* (1979) VI, 139–50.

Atherosclerosis — Angina

[1] Bailey, A. A., *Esoteric Healing.* Lucis Press (London, 1953).

[2] Green, E. and Green, A., *Beyond Biofeedback.* Delacorte Press (U.S.A., 1977).

Atherosclerosis — Coronary Artery Disease

[1] Editorial, 'Blood Cholesterol and Coronary Artery Disease', *Lancet* (1984) 1, 317–18.

[2] Seelig, M. S. and Heggtveit, H. A., 'Magnesium Interrelationship in Ischemic Heart Disease: A Review', *Am. J. Clin. Nutr.* (1974) 27, 59–79;

Turlapaty, P.D.M.V. and Altura, B. M., 'Magnesium Deficiency Produces Spasms of the Coronary Arteries: Relationship to Etiology of Sudden Death Ischemic heart Disease', *Sci.* (1980) 208, 199–200.

[3] Hanline, M., 'Hypomagnesaemia Causes Coronary Artery Spasm', *J. of AMA* (1985) 253, 342.

[4] Jenkins, M., 'An Approach to Ischemic Heart Disease', *Br. Homoeopathic J.* (1977) LXVI (2) 71–8.

Auto-immune Disorders

[1] Petersdorf, R. G. *et al.*, *Harrison's Principles of Internal Medicine*, 10th edn. McGraw-Hill (Sydney, 1983) 350.

[2] Gawler, I., *You Can Conquer Cancer*. Hill of Content (Melbourne, 1984); Hildebrand, G., 'Immunity Can be Improved by Meditation', *J. Alternative Med.* (1986) 4 (2) 16–17.

[3] Cooper, M. R. *et al.*, 'Stimulation of Leukocyte Hexose Monophosphate Shunt Activity by Ascorbic Acid', *Infection and Immunity* (1971) 3, 851–3.

Bell's Palsy

[1] Gaby, A., *The Doctor's Guide to B6*. Rodale Press (Emaus, Pa., 1984).

[2] Fisher, L., *Mineral Compounds and Human Disease*. Blackmore Books (Sydney, 1978).

Blood Pressure — Hypertension

[1] Lang, T. *et al.*, 'Relationship between Coffee Drinking and Blood Pressure: Analysis of 6,321 Subjects in the Paris Region', *Am. J. Card.* (1983) 52, 1238–42; Schroeder, K. L. and Chen, M. S., 'Smokeless Tobacco and Blood Pressure', *N.E.J.Med.* (1985) 312, 919.

[2] De Boni, V. *et al.*, 'Neurofibrillary Degeneration induced by Systemic Aluminium', *Acta Neuropath* (1976) 35, 285–94; Pierkle, J. L. *et al.*, 'The Relationship between Blood Lead Levels and Blood Pressure and its Cardiovascular Risk Implications', *Am. J. Epid.* (1985) 121, 246–58.

[3] Freis, E., 'Salt, Volume and the Prevention of Hypertension', *Circ.* (1976) 53, 589–95.

[4] Malinow, M. R., 'Alfalfa', *Atherosclerosis* (1973) 30, 27–43.

[5] Rao, R. *et al.*, 'Effect of Polyunsaturated Oils on Blood Pressure and Essential Hypertension', *Cli. Exp. Hypertension* (1981) 3, 27–38; Steiner, M. and Anastasi, J., 'Vitamin E — An Inhibitor of Platelet Release Reaction', *J. Clin. Invest.* (1976) 57, 732–7.

[6] Graham, J. D. P., 'Cratageus Oxyacantha in Hypertension', *Br. Med. J.* (1939) 11, 951–3.

[7] Dyckner, T. and Wester O., 'Effect of Magnesium on Blood Pressure', *Br. Med. J.* (1983) 286, 1847–9.

Bronchiectasis

[1] Boericke, W. and Dewey, W., *The Twelve Tissue Remedies of Schussler*, 6th edn. B. Jain (New Delhi, 1981).

[2] Counsell, J. N. and Hornig, D. H., *Vitamin C (Ascorbic Acid)* Applied Science (London, 1981) 249–70.

[3] Dreizen, S., 'Nutrition and the Immune Response — A Review', *Int. J. Nutr. Res.* (1979) 49, 220–8.

Bronchitis

[1] Jensen, B., *Iridology — The Science and Practice*. Bernard Jensen (California, 1982).

[2] Ogle, K. A. and Bullocks, J. D., 'Children with Allergic Rhinitis and/or Bronchial Asthma Treated with Elimination Diet: A Five year Follow Up', *Ann. Allergy* (1980) 44, 137–8.

[3] Cheraskin, E., Ringsdorf, M. and Sisley, G., *The Vitamin C Connection*. Harper & Row (New York, 1983) 37–40.

[4] Somner, A., Katz, J. *et al.*, 'Increased Risk of Respiratory Disease and Diarrhoea in Children with Pre-existing Mild Vitamin A Deficiency', *Am. J. Clin. Nutr.* (1984) 40, 1090–5.

Cancer

[1] Mount, S. J. L., 'Diet, Cancer and Life', *Br. Homoeopathic J.* (1978) LXVII (3) 185–207.

[2] Husemann, F. and Wolff, O., *The Anthroposophical Approach to Medicine*, vol. 1. The Anthroposophic Press (New York, 1982) 187–92.

[3] Ibid.

[4] Burr, H. S., *Blueprint For Immortality*. Neville Spearman (London, 1972).

[5] Jacka, J., *Cancer: A Physical and Psychic Profile*. Privately printed (Melbourne, 1977).

[6] Leroi, R., 'Viscum Album Therapy of Cancer', *Br. Homoeopathic J.* (July 1978) 37 (3) 167–84.

[7] Sobers, P., *Deliciously Natural*. Greenhouse (Melbourne, 1986); Draper, H. H. and Bird, R. P., 'Antioxidants and Cancer', *J. Agriculture and Food Chem.* (1984) 32 (3) 432–5.

[8] Gawler, I., *You Can Conquer Cancer*. Hill of Content (Melbourne, 1984).

[9] Simonton, C. O. and Simonton, S., *Getting Well Again*. Bantam Books (New York, 1978).

[10] Gerson, M., *A Cancer Therapy*. Totality Books (California, 1975).

[11] Leroi, R., 'Vicum Album . . .?'

[12] Gerson, M., *A Cancer Therapy*.

[13] Romney, S. L. *et al.*, 'Plasma Vitamin C Levels and Cervical Dysplasia', *Am. J. Obstet. & Gyn.* (1985) 151 (7) 976–80.

[14] Wilie-Rosett, J. A., Romney, S. L., Slagle, N. S. *et al.*, 'Influence of Vitamin A on Cervical Dysplasia and Carcinoma in Situ', *Nutrition & Cancer* (1984) 6 (1) 49–57.

[15] Husemann/Wolff, *The Anthroposophical Approach . . .*, 379–92.

Carpal Tunnel Syndrome

[1] Ellis, J., Folkers, K., Shizukuishi, S. *et al.*, 'Response of Vitamin B6 deficiency and the Carpal Tunnel Syndrome to Pyridoxine', *Proc. Nat. Acad. Sci.* (1982) 79, 7494–8.

Cataracts

[1] Fisher, L. H., *Mineral Compounds in Human Disease*. Blackmore Books (Sydney, 1978); Skalka, H. and Prchal, J., 'Cataracts and Riboflavin Deficiency', *Am. J. Clin. Nutr.* (1981) 34, 861–3; Consul, R. N. and Nagpal, P. N., 'Quantitative Study in the Variations of the Levels of Glutathione and Ascorbic Acid in Human Lenses with Senile Cataract', *Eye Ear Nose and Throat Monthly*, (1968) 47, 336–9.

Chicken-pox

[1] Pearson, D. and Shaw, S., *Life Extension — A Practical Scientific Approach*. Warner Books (New York, 1984) 408–11.

Chilblains

[1] Fisher, L., *Mineral Compounds and Human Disease*. Blackmore Books (Sydney, 1978).

Coeliac Disease

[1] Petersdorf, R. G. *et al.*, *Harrison's Principles of Internal Medicine*, 10th edn. McGraw-Hill (Sydney, 1983) 1733.

[2] Abstract from *Lancet* 1, 320–2, appearing in *Int. Clin. Nutr. Rev.* (1983) 3 (4) 30–1.

[3] Ibid., 31. See also Abstract, *CMA Journal* (1985) 127, 963–5.

Common Cold

[1] Stone, I., *The Healing Factor — Vitamin C Against Disease*. Grosset & Dunlap (New York, 1972) 64–76.

[2] Somer, A., Katz, J. *et al.*, 'Increased Risk of Respiratory Disease and Diarrhoea in Children with Pre-existing Mild Vitamin A Deficiency', *Am. J. Clin. Nutr.* (1984) 40, 1090–5.

Constipation

[1] Abstract, 'Dietary Fibre and Protection From Chronic Diseases in Western Society', *Int. Clin. Nutr. Rev.* (1983) 3 (2) 32–3.

[2] Lindlahr, H., *The Practice of Nature Cure*. Godbolay (Poona, India, 1954) 222–30.

[3] Savitz, D. A., *Case-Control Study of Childhood Cancer and Residential Exposure to Electro-Magnetic Fields*. Department of Epidemiology, Uni. of N. Carolina (1986).

Corneal Ulceration

[1] Boyd, T. A. *et al.*, 'Influence of Ascorbic Acid in the Healing of Corneal Ulcers in Man', *Br. Med. J.* (1950) 2, 1145–8.

Cramps

[1] Regtop, H., 'Is Magnesium the Grossly Neglected Mineral?', *Int. Clin. Nutr. Rev.* (1983) 3 (3) 18.

[2] Stuart, M. (ed.), *Encyclopedia of Herbs and Herbalism*. Orbis (London, 1979).

Crohn's Disease

[1] Abstract, 'Nutritional Supplementation to Restore Growth in Crohn's Disease', *Int. Clin. Nutr. Rev.* (July 1983) 3 (3) 21.

[2] Boyd, H., 'Gastrointestinal Disease', *Br. Homoeopathic J.* (January 1978) LXVII (T) 13–19.

Cystitis

[1] Stone, I., *The Healing Factor — Vitamin C Against Disease*. Grosset & Dunlap (New York, 1972) 138–45.

[2] Blackie, M., 'Urinary Remedies', *Br. Homoeopathic J.* (January 1978) LXVII (1) 46–58.

Depression

[1] Maurizi, C., 'Disorder of the Pineal Gland Associated with Depression, Peptic Ulcer and Sexual Dysfunction', *Southern Med. J.* (1984) 77, 1516–18; Rosenthal, N., Sack, D., Carpenter, C. *et al.*, 'Antidepressant Effects of Light in Seasonal Depressive Disorders', *Am. J. Psychiat.* (1985) 142, 163–70.

[2] Lesser, M., *Nutrition and Vitamin Therapy*. Grove Press (New York, 1980) chapter 3.

[3] Clover, A., 'Homoeopathy and the Operative Concepts in Depression', *Br. Homoeopathic J.* (1978) LXVII (4) 230–8; Blackie, M., 'Depression', *Br. Homoeopathic J.* (1978) LXVII (4) 238–47.

Dermatitis

[1] Sampson, K., 'Role of Immediate Food Hypersensitivity in the Pathogenesis of Atopic Dermatitis', *J. Allergy Clin. Immunol.* (1983) 71, 473–80.

[2] Abstract of Swedish paper, 'Selenium for Treatment of Skin Disorders', *Int. Clin. Nutr. Rev.* (1984) 3 (4) 18–19.

[3] Boyd, H. W., 'Skin Problems', *Br. Homoeopathic J.* (1977) LXVI (1) 33–7.

Diabetes

[1] Petersdorf, R. G. *et al.*, *Harrison's Principles of Internal Medicine*, 10th edn. McGraw-Hill (Sydney, 1983).

[2] Burkitt, D. and Trowell, H., *Western Diseases, Their Emergence and Prevention*. Harvard University Press (Cambridge, Mass., 1981).

[3] Ibid.

[4] Pederson, O., Beck-Neilson, H. and Heding, L., 'Increased Insulin Receptors after Exercise in Patients with Insulin Dependent Diabetes Mellitus', *New Eng. J. Med.* (1980) 302, 866–92.

[5] Stone, I., *The Healing Factor — Vitamin C Against Disease*. Grosset & Dunlap (New York, 1972) 146–52.

[6] Oliver-Beever, R. and Zahnd, G. R., 'Plants with Oral Hypoglycaemic Action', *Quart. J. Crude Drug. Res.* (1979) 17, 139–96.

[7] Abstract, *Int. Clin. Nutr. Rev.* (1982) 3 (4) 47; Editorial, 'Beneficial Effects of Chromium Supplementation', *J. of AMA* (1982) 247, 3046–7; Tadros, S. *et al.*, 'Protective Effect of Trace Elements (Zn, Co, Mn, Cr) on Allaxan Induced Diabetes', *Ind. J. Exp. Biol.* (1982) 20, 93–4.

[8] Simpson, H. C. R., 'A High Carbohydrate Leguminous Diet Improves all Aspects of Diabetic Control', *Lancet* (1981) 1, 1–5.

Diarrhoea

[1] Fisher, L., *Mineral Compounds and Human Disease*. Blackmore Books (Sydney, 1978).

[2] Boyd, H., 'Gastrointestinal Disease', *Br. Homoeopathic J.* (January 1978) LXVII (1) 13–19.

Diverticulitis

[1] Boericke, W., *The Twelve Tissue Remedies of Schussler*. Stet Dey & Co. (Calcutta, 1959) 34–40.

Down's Syndrome

[1] Abstract, 'Zinc — Some Recent Developments', *Int. Clin. Nutr. Rev.* (1983) 3 (2) 41.

Ear Infections

[1] Saarinen, U. M., 'Prolonged Breast Feeding a Prophalaxis for Otitis Media', *Acta Pediatr. Scand.* (1982) 71, 567–71.

Eczema

[1] Petersdorf, R. G. *et al.*, *Harrison's Principles of Internal Medicine*, 10th edn. McGraw-Hill (Sydney, 1983) 258.

[2] Sampson, H., 'Role of Immediate Food Hypersensitivity in the Pathogenesis of

Atopic Dermatitis', *J. Allergy Clin. Immunol.* (1983) 71, 473–80.

Jacka, J., *A Philosophy of Healing.* Inkata Press (Melbourne, 1978) chapter 6.

Endometriosis

[1] Thomson, A. D. and Cotton, R. E., *Lecture Notes on Pathology.* Blackwell Scientific Publications (London, 1968) 610.

Epilepsy

[1] Petersdorf, R. G. *et al.*, *Harrison's Principles of Internal Medicine*, 10th edn. McGraw-Hill (Sydney, 1983) 2018.

[2] Abstract, 'Role of Magnesium Deficiencies in Convulsive Syndromes in Children', *Int. Clin. Nutr. Rev.* (1985) 5 (1) 50.

[3] Allen, R. B., 'Nutritional Aspects of Epilepsy', *Int. Clin. Nutr. Rev.* (1983) 3 (3) 3–8.

Fibroids

[1] Foubister, D. M., 'Constitutional Types', *Br. Homoeopathic J.* (1981) 70 (4) 197–202.

Fluid Retention

[1] Chapman, J. B., *Dr Schussler's Biochemistry.* New Era Laboratories (London, 1973) 31.

Fractures

[1] Regtop, H., 'Is Magnesium the Grossly Neglected Mineral?', *Int. Clin. Nutr. Rev.* (1983) 3 (3) 10–20.

[2] Robertson, W. Van B., 'The Biochemical Role of Ascorbic Acid in Connective Tissue', *Annals N. Y. Academy of Sciences* (1961) 92, 148–58.

Gallstones

[1] Twentyman, L. R., 'The Liver and Depression', *Br. Homoeopathic J.* (1980) 69 (1) 12–14.

[2] Ross, G., 'Chelidonium Majus', *Br. Homoeopathic J.* (1981) 70 (4) 206–7.

[3] Boericke, W., *Pocket Manual Homoeopathic Materia Medica*, 9th edn. B. Jain (New Delhi, 1979).

Gastritis

[1] Williams, R., *Biochemical Individuality.* University of Texas Press (London, 1975).

[2] Tyler, M. L., *Homoeopathic Drug Pictures.* Health Science Press (Bradford, Devon, 1942) 575–9.

German Measles

[1] Vargos, M., 'Vitamin C in the Treatment of Influenza', *El Dia Medica* (1963) 35, 1714–15; Dalton, W. L., 'Massive Doses of Vitamin C in the Treatment of Viral Disease', *J. Indiana State Med. Assoc.* (1962) 55, 1151–4.

[2] Allen, B., 'Rubella Immunisation', *Aust. J. Med. Tech.* Special issue (November 1973).

Glandular Fever

[1] Dalton, W. L., 'Massive Doses of Vitamin C in the Treatment of Viral Disease', *J. Indiana State Med. Assoc.* (1962) 55, 1151–4.

Glaucoma

[1] Petersdorf, R. G. *et al.*, *Harrison's Principles of Internal Medicine*, 10th edn. McGraw-Hill (Sydney, 1983) 105.

[2]   Fishbein, S. and Goodstein, S., 'The Pressure Lowering Effect of Ascorbic Acid', *Annal Opthalmol.* (1972) 4, 487–91.

Glomerulonephritis

[1]   Petersdorf, R. G. *et al.*, *Harrison's Principles of Internal Medicine*, 10th edn. McGraw-Hill (Sydney, 1983) 1628.

[2]   Fisher, L., *Mineral Compounds and Human Disease*. Blackmore Books (Sydney, 1978) 31.

Goitre, Grave's Disease, Simple Goitre

[1]   Petersdorf, R. G. *et al.*, *Harrison's Principles of Internal Medicine*, 10th edn. McGraw-Hill (Sydney, 1983) 626.

[2]   Tyler, M. L., *Homoeopathic Drug Pictures*. Health Science Press (Bradford, Devon, 1952) 432–6.

Gonorrhoea

[1]   Jacka, J., *A Philosophy of Healing*. Inkata Press (Melbourne, 1979) chapter 6.

[2]   Allen, H. A., *The Chronic Miasms*. Roy and Co. (Bombay, 1960).

Gout

[1]   Boericke, W. and Dewey, W., *The Twelve Tissue Remedies of Schussler*, 6th edn. B. Jain (New Delhi, 1981).

Growing Pains

[1]   Roberts, H. A., *The Principles and Art of Cure by Homoeopathy*. Health Science Press (London, 1942) 208–28.

[2]   Kent, J. T., *Lectures on Homoeopathic Materia Medica*. Boericke & Tafel, (Philadelphia, 1956) 196–209.

Haemophilia

[1]   Walker, H. K., Hall, W. D. and Hurst, J. W., *Clinical Methods*. Butterworth (Sydney, 1980) 387–8.

Haemorrhoids

[1]   Boericke, W. and Dewey, W., *The Twelve Tissue Remedies*. Set Dey & Co. (Calcutta, 1959) 34–40.

Hallucinations

[1]   Hoffer, A., 'Foreword. A Journey into the World of Schizophrenia', *J. Orthomolecular Psychiatry* (1984) 13 (4) 262–8.

Hay Fever

[1]   Dawson, W. and West, G. B., 'The Influence of Ascorbic Acid on Histamine Metabolism in Guinea Pigs', *Br. J. Pharmacology* (1965) 24, 725–34.

[2]   Rodale, J., *The Complete Book of Vitamins*. Rodale Books (Pennsylvania, 1971) 111–42.

Headache

[1]   Boericke, W. and Dewer, W., *The Twelve Tissue Remedies of Schussler*, 6th edn. B. Jain (New Delhi, 1981) 74 and 88.

Heart Disease

[1]   Boericke, W. and Dewey, W., *The Twelve Tissue Salts*. Set Dey & Co. (Calcutta, 1959) 35–40.

[2]   Manthey, J., 'Magnesium and Trace Metals: Risk Factors for CHD', *Circulation* (1981) 64, 722–9.

Hepatitis

[1] Twentyman, L. R., 'The Liver and Depression', *Br. Homoeopathic J.* (1980) 69 (1) 12–14.

[2] Boericke, W., *Pocket Manual of Homoeopathic Materia Medica*, 9th edn. B. Jain (New Delhi, 1979) 446.

[3] Stuart, M. (ed.), *The Encyclopedia of Herbs and Herbalism.* Orbis (London, 1979) 58–60.

[4] Lesser, M., *Nutrition and Vitamin Therapy.* Grove Press (New York, 1980) 33.

Hernia

[1] Petersdorf, R. G. *et al.*, *Harrison's Principles of Internal Medicine*, 10th edn. McGraw-Hill (Sydney, 1983) 1696.

[2] Boericke, W. and Dewey, W., *The Twelve Tissue Remedies.* Set Dey (Calcutta, 1959) 34–40.

Herpes

[1] Petersdorf, R. G. *et al.*, *Harrison's Principles of Internal Medicine*, 10th edn. McGraw-Hill (Sydney, 1983) 1633.

[2] Ibid.

[3] Terezhealmy, G. *et al.*, 'The Use of Water Soluble Bioflavanoid-ascorbic Acid Complex in the Treatment of recurrent Herpes-labialis', *Oral Surg.* (1978) 45, 56–62.

[4] Fitzherbert, J., 'Genital Herpes and Zinc', *Med. J. Aust.* (1979) 1, 399.

[5] Griffith R., Delong, D. and Nelson, J., 'Relation of Arginine-Lysine Antagonism to Herpes Simplex Growth in Tissue Culture', *Chemotherapy* (1981) 27, 209–13.

Hiccoughs

[1] Boericke, W. and Dewey, W., *The Twelve Tissue Remedies of Schussler*, 6th edn. B. Jain (New Delhi, 1981).

Hypoglycaemia

[1] Airola, P., *Hypoglycaemia: A Better Approach.* Health Plus (Arizona, 1977).

[2] Wright, D. W. *et al.*, 'Sucrose-Induced Insulin Resistance in the Rat: Modulation by Exercise and Diet', *Am. J. Clin. Nutr.* (1983) 38, 879–83.

[3] Regtop, H., 'Is Magnesium the Grossly Neglected Mineral?', *Int. Clin. Nutr. Rev.* (July 1983) 3 (3) 10–20.

[4] Editorial, 'Beneficial Effects of Chromium Supplementation', *J. of AMA* 247, 3046–7.

[5] Black, D. A. K. *et al.*, *Lancet* (1952) 1, 224.

Impetigo

[1] Boericke, W. and Dewey, W., *The Twelve Tissue Remedies of Schussler.* B. Jain (New Delhi, 1981).

Insomnia

[1] Kaplan, H. and Sadock, B., *Modern Synopsis of Comprehensive Textbook of Psychiatry*, vol. IV. Williams and Wilkens (Baltimore, Mass., 1985) 558–74.

[2] Boericke, W. and Dewey, W., *The Twelve Tissue Remedies of Schussler*, 6th edn. B. Jain (New Delhi, 1981).

[3] Leatherwood, D. et al., 'Aqueous Extract of Valerian Root (Valeriana officinalis L.) Improves Sleep Quality in Man', Pharm. Biochem. Behav. (1982) 17, 65–71.

Kidney Stones
[1] Petersdorf, R. G. et al., Harrison's Principles of Internal Medicine, 10th edn. McGraw-Hill (Sydney, 1983) 1675.
[2] Rose, G. and Westbury, E., 'The Influence of Calcium Content of Water, Intake of Vegetables and Fruit and of other Food Factors on the Incidence of Renal Calculi', Urol. Res. (1975) 3, 61–6; Rao, N., Gordon, C., Davis, D. and Blacklock, N., 'Are Stone Formers Maladaptive to Refined Carbohydrates?', Br. J. Urol. (1982) 54, 575–7.
[3] Lemann, J., Piering, W. and Lennon, E., 'Possible Role of Carbohydrate Induced Hypercalciuria in Calcium Oxalate Kidney Stone Formation', New Eng. J. Med. (1969) 280, 232–7; Shaw, P., Williams, G. and Green, N., 'Idiopathic Hypercalciuria: Its Control with Unprocessed Bran', Br. J. Urol. (1980) 52, 426–9.
[4] Wunderlich, W., 'Aspects of the Influence of Magnesium Ions on the Formation of Calcium Oxalate', Urol. Res. (1981) 9, 157–60; Will, E. and Bijvoet, L., 'Primary Oxalosis: Clinical and Biochemical Response to High Dose Pyridoxine Therapy', Metab. (1979) 28, 542–8.
[5] Bott, V., Anthroposophical Medicine. Rudolf Steiner Press (London, 1976) chapter 12.
[6] Boericke, W., Pocket Manual of Homoeopathic Materia Medica, 9th edn. B. Jain (New Delhi, 1979).
[7] Blackie, M. G., 'Urinary Remedies', Br. Homoeopathic J. (January 1978) 38 (1) 46–57.

Laryngitis
[1] Kaul, T. N., Middleton, E. and Ogra, P. L., 'Anti Viral Effects of Bioflavanoids on Human Viruses', J. Med. Virol. (1985) 15, 71–9.

Leukaemia
[1] Lasagna, L., 'One-A-Day Plus C', J. N. Y. Academy Sci. (1981) 21 (9) 35.

Measles
[1] Paez de la Torre, J. M., 'Ascorbic Acid in Measles', Archives Argentinos de Pedeatria (1945) 24, 225–7.
[2] Wilson, G., The Hazards of Immunisation. Athlone Press (University of London, 1967); Coulter, H. and Fisher, B., A Shot in the Dark. Harcourt, Brace & Javanovich (New York, 1985).

Melanoma
[1] Abstract, 'Selenium Indicator of Cancer', Int. Clin. Nutr. Rev. (1985) 5 (2) 102.

Meniere's Disease
[1] Petersdorf, R. G. et al., Harrison's Principles of Internal Medicine, 10th edn. McGraw-Hill (Sydney, 1983) 2154.
[2] Jacka, J., Vivaxis — A Science of Life Energies. Privately printed (Melbourne, 1984).

Menopause
[1] Husemann, F. and Wolff, O., The Anthroposophical Approach to Medicine, vol. 1. Anthroposophic Press (New York, 1982) 186.

[2] Bailey, A. A., *Esoteric Healings*. Lucis Press (London, 1953) 58–60.

Menstrual Cramps

[1] Petersdorf, R. G. *et al.*, *Harrison's Principles of Internal Medicine*, 10th edn. McGraw-Hill (Sydney, 1983) 486.

[2] Boericke, W. and Dewey, W., *The Twelve Tissue Remedies*. Set Dey & Co. (Calcutta, 1959) 177.

Migraine

[1] Petersdorf, R. G. *et al*, *Harrison's Principles of Internal Medicine*, 10th edn. McGraw-Hill (Sydney, 1983) 18–20.

[2] Ibid.

[3] Buist, R., 'Migraine and Food Intolerance', *Int. Clin. Nutr. Rev.* (1983) 4 (2) 52–3.

Motion Sickness

[1] Petersdorf, R. G. *et al.*, *Harrison's Principles of Internal Medicine*, 10th edn. McGraw-Hill (Sydney, 1983) 2154.

[2] Von Keller, G., 'Cocculus', *Br. Homoeopathic J.* (1980) 69 (2) 95–103.

Mouth Ulcers

[1] Henkin, R. J., 'Zinc in Wound Healing', *New England J. Med.* (1974) 291, 665–74.

[2] Dreizen, S., 'Nutrition and the Immune Response — A Review', *Int. J. Nutr. Res.* (1979) 49, 220–8.

Multiple Sclerosis

[1] Petersdorf, R. G. *et al.*, *Harrison's Principles of Internal Medicine*, 10th edn. McGraw-Hill (Sydney, 1983) 2098.

[2] Boericke, W. and Dewey, W., *The Twelve Tissue Remedies*. Set Dey & Co. (Calcutta, 1959) 88–95 and 72–82.

Mumps

[1] Dalton, W. L., 'Massive Doses of Vitamin C in the Treatment of Viral Diseases', *J. Indiana State Med. Assoc.* (1962) 55, 1151–4.

Neuralgia

[1] Boericke, W. and Dewey, W., *The Twelve Tissue Remedies*. Set Dey and Co. (Calcutta, 1959) 245.

[2] Hui Bon Hoa, J., 'Facial Neuralgia: An Analysis of 33 Cases Responding to Homoeopathic Treatment, *Br. Homoeopathic J.* (1977) LXVI (3) 144–56.

Neuritis

[1] Ellis, J., Folkers, K., Wataber, T. *et al.*, 'Clinical Results of A Crossover Treatment with Pyridoxine and Placebo of the Carpal Tunnel Syndrome', *Am. J. Clin. Nutr.* (1979) 32, 2040–6.

Neuroses

[1] Abstract, 'Pharmacological Doses of Vitamins B1, B3, and B6 for Agrophobia', *Int. Clin. Nutr. Rev.* (1983) 3 (3) 33.

[2] Ward, J. L., 'To Be or Not to be Subclinical Pellagra', *J. Orthomolecular Psych.* (1977) 6 (2) 183–5; Barr, W., 'Pyridoxine Supplements in the Premenstrual Syndrome', *Practitioner* (1984) 228, 425–7.

[3] Gilka, L., 'The Biochemistry of the Schizophrenias', *J. Orthomolecular Psych.* (1978) 7 (1) 6–16.

[4] Chancellor, P. M., *Handbook of the Bach Flower Remedies*. C. W. Daniel & Co. (London, 1971).

[5] Dhawale, M. L., *Principles and Practice of Homoeopathy*, vol. 1. Karnatak (Bombay, 1967) 289–303.

Obesity

[1] Mount, J. L., *The Food and Health of Western Man*. Precision Press (London, 1979) chapter 11.

Osteoporosis

[1] Petersdorf, R. G. *et al.*, *Harrison's Principles of Internal Medicine*, 10th edn. McGraw-Hill (Sydney, 1983) 1949.

[2] Husemann, F. and Wolff, O., *The Anthroposophical Approach to Medicine*. Anthroposophic Press (New York, 1982) 177.

Ovarian Cysts

[1] Boericke, W. and Dewey, W., *The Twelve Tissue Remedies*. Set Dey & Co. (Calcutta, 1959) 213.

[2] Ibid., 40–50.

Paget's Disease

[1] Petersdorf, R. G. *et al.*, *Harrison's Principles of Internal Medicine*, 10th edn. McGraw-Hill (Sydney, 1983) 1960–3.

Pancreatitis

[1] Petersdorf, R. G. *et al.*, *Harrison's Principles of Internal Medicine*, 10th edn. McGraw-Hill (Sydney, 1983) 1836–44.

Parkinson's Disease

[1] Boericke, W. and Dewey, W., *The Twelve Tissue Remedies*. Set Dey & Co. (Calcutta, 1959) 72–94.

Pleurisy

[1] Cooper, M. R. *et al.*, 'Stimulation of Leukocyte Hexose Monophosphate Shunt Activity by Ascorbic Acid', *Infection and Immunity* (1971) 3, 851–3.

[2] Kloss, J., *Back to Eden*. Lifeline Books (California, 1974) 360.

Pneumonia

[1] Cheraskin, E., Ringsdorf, W. M. and Sisley, E., *The Vitamin C Connection*. Harper & Row (New York, 1983) 35–40.

[2] Jacobsen, M., *J. Organic Chem.* (1967) 32 (5) 1646–7.

[3] Dreizen, S., 'Nutrition and the Immune Response — A Review', *Int. J. Nutr. Res.* (1979) 49, 220–8.

Premenstrual Tension

[1] Piesse, J., 'Nutrition Factors in the Premenstrual Syndrome', *Int. Clin. Nutr. Rev.* (1984) 4 (2) 54–80.

[2] Abstract, 'Nutrition and Premenstrual Tension', *Int. Clin. Nutr. Rev.* (January 1963) 3 (1) 30.

[3] Abraham, G. E., 'Nutritional Factors in the Etiology of the Premenstrual Tension Syndrome', *J. Reproductive Med.* (1983) 28, 446–64.

[4] Barr, W., 'Pyridoxine Supplements in the Premenstrual Syndrome', *Practitioner* (1984) 228, 1390, 425–7.

Prolapse

[1] Boericke, W. and Dewey, W., *The Twelve Tissue Salts*. Set Dey & Co.

(Calcutta, 1959) 34–40.
[2] Tyler, M., *Homoeopathic Drug Pictures*. Health Science Press (Bradford, Devon, 1952) 738–49.

Prostatitis

[1] Heston, W., 'Prostate Inflammation Linked to Zinc Shortage', *Prevention* (June 1977) 113; Fahim, M., Fahim, Z., Der, R. and Harman, J., 'Zinc Treatment for the reduction of Hyperplasia of the Prostate', *Fed. Proc.* (1976) 35, 361.
[2] Mount, L. J., *The Food and Health of Western Man*. Precision Press (London, 1975) 114.
[3] Horton, R., 'Benign Prostatic Hyperplasia: A disorder of Androgen Metabolism in the Male', *J. Am. Geri. Soc.* (1984) 32, 380–5.

Psoriasis

[1] *Circulating Medical File*. Special Research Project, Psoriasis, Supplement. The Edgar Cayce Foundation, (Virginia Beach, 1976) 5016–1.
[2] Vorhees, J. G., Chakranarti, S. G., Batero, F. *et al.*, 'Zinc Therapy and Distribution in Psoriasis', *Arch. Derm.* (1969) 100, 669–73.
[3] Tyler, M., *Homoeopathic Drug Pictures*. Health Science Press (Bradford, Devon, 1952) 546–56.

Raynaud's Syndrome

[1] Green, A. and Green, E., *Beyond Biofeedback*. Delacorte Press (New York, 1977) 40–1.

Rheumatic Fever

[1] Taylor, S., 'Scurvy and Carditis', *Lancet* (1937) 1, 973–9.

Rickets

[1] Arneil, G. C., *Dietary Study of 4365 Scottish Infants*, Scottish Health Service Studies, no. 6. Scottish Home and Health Dept. (Edinburgh, 1967).

Scabies

[1] Hahnemann, S., *The Chronic Diseases*. Ringer & Co. (Calcutta, n.d.) 36–49.

Scarlet Fever

[1] Hornig, D. H. and Counsell, J. N., *Vitamin C*. Applied Science Publishers (London, 1982) 249–72.

Schizophrenia

[1] Kahan, F. H., 'Out of the Quicksands', *J. Orthomolecular Psych.* (1977) 6 (2) 87–164.
[2] Gilka, L., 'Biochemistry of the Schizophrenias', *J. Orthomolecular Psych.* (1978) 7 (1) 6–16.
[3] Hawkins, D., 'Diagnosing the Schizophrenias', *J. Orthomolecular Psych.* (1977) 6 (1) 18–26.
[4] Smith, T., 'A Homoeopathic Approach to Schizophrenia', *Br. Homoeopathic J.* (1979) LXVIII (1) 20–8.

Scleroderma

[1] Petersdorf, R. G. *et al.*, *Harrison's Principles of Internal Medicine*, 10th edn. McGraw-Hill (Sydney, 1983) 2004.
[2] Husemann, F. and Wolff, O., *The Anthroposophical Approach to Medicine*. Anthroposophic Press (New York, 1982) 181.

Scurvy

[1] Stone, I., 'Eight Decades of Scurvy. The Case History of a Misleading Dietary Hypothesis', *J. Orthomolecular Psych.* (1979) 8 (2) 58–62.

Senile Dementia

[1] Terry, B. D. and Katzman, R., *The Neurology of Ageing*. F. A. Davis & Co. (Philadelphia, 1983) 51–85.

[2] Perl, D. P., 'Alzheimer's Disease: X-ray Spectrometric Evidence of Aluminium Accumulation in Neurofibrillary Tangle-bearing Neurones', *Science* (1980) 208, 297–9.

[3] Hoffer, A. and Walker, M., *Nutrients to Age Without Senility*. Keats (New Canaan, 1980).

[4] Bailey, A. A., *Death the Great Adventure*. Lucis Press (London, 1984).

Shingles

[1] Zureick, 'Treatment of Herpes and Shingles with Vitamin C Intravenously', *J. des Practiciens* (1950) 64, 586.

Sinusitis

[1] Ruskin, S., 'The Epinephrine Potencity Effect of Sodium Ascorbate in Allergy', *Ear Nose and Throat Monthly* (1948) 27, 63–9; Dreizen, S., 'Nutrition and the Immune Response — A Review', *Int. Vit. Nutr. Res.* (1979) 49, 220–8.

Stomach Ulcers

[1] Cheney, G., 'Rapid Healing of Peptic Ulcers in Patients Receiving Fresh Cabbage Juice', *Cal. Med.* (1949) 70, 10–14.

[2] Formmer, D. J., 'The Healing of Gastric Ulcers by Zinc Sulphate', *Med. J. Aust.* (1975) 2, 793.

[3] Boericke, W., *Pocket Manual of Homoeopathic Materia Medica*, 9th edn. B. Jain (New Delhi, 1979) 403.

[4] Abstract, 'Vitamin A and Gastric Ulcers', *Int. J. Tissue Reactions* (1983) V 301–7.

[5] Marle, J., Aarson, P. *et al.*, 'Deglycyrrhizinised Liquorice (DGL) and the Renewal of Rat Stomach Epithelium', *Eur. J. Pharm.* (1981) 72, 219.

Syphilis

[1] Roberts, H. R., *The Principles and Art of Cure by Homoeopathy*. Health Science Press (London, 1942) chapter 28.

Tachycardia

[1] Regtop, H., 'Is Magnesium The Grossly Neglected Mineral?', *Int. Clin. Nutr. Rev.* (1983) 3 (3) 10–20.

Thrush

[1] Galland, L., 'Nutrition and Candidiasis', *J. Orthomolecular Psych.* (1985) 14 (1) 50–60.

[2] Beisel, W. R. *et al.*, *J. of AMA* (1981) 245–53.

Tonsillitis

[1] Caels, F., 'Contribution to the Study of the Effect of High Doses of Vitamin C in Oto-Rhino-Laryngological Infections', *Acta Oto-Rhino Laryngologica Belgica*, vol. 7 (Brussels, 1953) 395–410.

[2] Boericke, W. and Dewey, W., *The Twelve Tissue Salts*. Set Dey & Co. (Calcutta, 1959) 288.

3 Boger, C. M., *A Synoptic Key of the Materia Medica*. Jain, (New Delhi, n.d.) 252–7.

Ulcerative Colitis

1 Henkin, R. J., 'Zinc in Wound Healing', *N. E. J. Med.* (1974) 291; 665–74.

2 Boyd, H., 'Gastro-intestinal Disease', *Br. Homoeopathic J.* (1978) LXVII (1) 13–19.

Index

Note: Symptoms are denoted by all lower case, upper case denotes the disease state.

abdomen, *see also* stomach
abdominal distension, 113–16
Abdominal Migraine, 49–51
abdominal pain, 49–51, 116–17, 139–42, 246–9, 293–5
acid foods, regurgitation, 195–7
acid urine, 128–30
acidity, stomach, 282–5
Acne, 45–9
acupressure, xv, 4
acupuncture, xv, 16
Addison's Disease, 51–2
Adrenal Glands,
    degeneration, 51–2
    related energy centre (*chakra*), 27–8
air pollution, 45–6, 74–9
Air Sickness, 230
Ajna *chakra*, 25, 28
albumen, in urine, 170–4
Alcoholism, 52–3
Alexander Technique, xv, 4
Allergies, 53–6, 113–16, 132–5, 146–8, 186–8
    air pollution, 45–6, 74–9
alternative medicine, methods, 29–38
Alzheimer's Disease, 276–8
Amenorrhoea, 57–8
Anaemia, 58–9
Androgen, imbalance, 46
Angina, 81–6
Angio-neurotic Oedema, 60–1
ankles, swollen, 157–8

Ankylosing Spondylitis, 61–2
Anorexia Nervosa, 62–4
anthroposophical medicine, 14
anus,
    bleeding, 183–5
    itching, 183–5, 306–7
Anxiety, 64–6
arms, pain, 264–6
aromatherapy, xv, 36
Arterial diseases, 79–86
Arthritis, 67–74, 108–9
    juvenile, 70–4
    peripheral, 61–2
Ascorbic acid deficiency, 276
Asthma, 74–9, 149–50
astral body, xv, 17–18
Atherosclerosis, 79–86, 124–6
atma, xv, 17–19
Auto-immune Disorders, 70–4, 86–8, 170–4

Bach flowers, xv, 35–6
back, pain in lower, 61–2, 245–6, 258–60
base *chakra*, 27–8
Bell's Palsy, 89–90
bile duct, stones, 160–3
bio-functional diagnosis, xvi, 10, 14
'bioplasma', 13, 15–16
birth, care before, 253–4
bladder,
    inflammation, 128–30
    pain, 256–8

blood in urine, 128–30, 170–4, 183, 211–13, 258–60
Blood pressure, 90–6
high, 79–86
blood sugar, high, 136–9
Body Fluids, retention of, 157–8, 254–6
bones,
deformity, 245–6, 267–8
degeneration, 241–2
fractured, 158–9
bowel,
bleeding, 293–5
constipation of, 119–22
inflammation, 126–8, 293–5
looseness, 139–42
pain, 256–8
spasm, 116–17
ulceration, 293–5
Bowel Inflammatory Disease (BID), 126–8, 293–5
breasts, soreness, 157–8
breathing difficulties, 74–9, 98–100, 149–50, 250–1
breathlessness, 58–9, 286–8
Bronchial diseases,
asthma, 74–9
bronchiectasis, 96–8
bronchitis, 98–100, 149–50
bruising, 276
buddhi, xvi, 17–19

calcium deficiency, 241–2
calculi,
common bile duct, 160–3
gall-bladder, 160–3
kidney, 211–13
Cancer, 101–8
cervical, 105–8
effect of meditation, 12–13
Candida, 288–90
Car Sickness, 230
Carcinoma, 101–8
Cardiovascular Diseases, 79–86, 191–2, 286–8
Carpal Tunnel Syndrome, 108–9
Cataracts, 109–10
cereals, allergies, 113–16
Cerebrovascular Disease, 110–11
Cervical Dysplasia, 105–8

chakras, xvi, 16, 21, 22–8, 23
Ajna, 25, 28
base, 27–8
crown, 27, 28
heart, 26–7
sacral, 22–4
solar plexus, 25–6
throat, 22, 24
Chest diseases, see Respiratory diseases
chest pain, 81–6
'chi', xvi, 13, 15–16
Chicken-pox, 111–12
Chilblains, 112–13
Children,
abdominal pain, 49–51
arthritis, 70–4
immune systems, 7–9
leg pain, 181–2
Cholelithiasis (gall stones), 160–3
Cholestasis (jaundice), 210
cholesterol in blood, 79–86
chronic disease, development, 7–9
'chronic miasms', 6–7
circulation, disorders, 112–13, 263, 298–300
see also Vascular diseases
Climacteric, 223–4
Coeliac Disease, 113–16
Cold, Common, 117–19
cold sensitivity, 112–13, 263, 273–6
Colic, 116–17, 160–3
Colitis, 126–8
ulcerative, 293–5
colon,
diverticulitis, 142–3
enlargement, 142–3
see also bowel
common bile duct, stones, 160–3
congestion, nasal, 186–8, 280–2
consciousness, loss of, 110–11
consciousness, seven levels of, 16–21, 22–8
Constipation, 119–22
as symptom, 49–51, 142–3
convulsions, 152–4
Corneal Ulcer, 122–4
Coronary Diseases, 79–86, 191–2
Coronary Occlusion 84–6
Cough, Whooping, 304–6

coughing, 96–8, 98–100
Cramps, 124–6
    menstrual, 225–6
Crohn's Disease, 126–8
Croup, 214–16
crown *chakra*, 27, 28
Cystic Acne, 45–9
Cystitis, 128–30
Cysts, ovarian, 242–4

deafness, 145–6
de-armouring, xvi
dehydration, 139–42
Dementia, senile, 276–8
Demyelinating Disease, 231–4
Depression, 131–2
    as symptom, 202–4, 254–6
Dermatitis, 132–5, *see also* Eczema
Diabetes, 136–9
diagnosis, methods, 9–10, 14–15
diaphragm,
    hernia, 195–7
    nerve irritation, 200–1
Diarrhoea, 139–42
    as symptom, 49–51, 126–8, 166,
        293–5
diet,
    allergens in, 53–6, 74–9
    and constipation, 119–22
    fats in, 160–3
Digestion, related disorders, 119–22
disease, development, 7–9, 11–15
Diseases, *see* under name of the
    disease
Diverticulitis, 142–3
dizzy spells, 219–22
Down's Syndrome, 144
Drug addiction, alcohol, 52–3
dust, allergic reactions, 186–8
Dysmenorrhoea, 225–6
Dysplasia, cervical, 105–8

Ear Infections, 145–6
Eczema, 132–5, 146–8
    relation to asthma, 75
    varicose, 298–300
elimination of wastes,
    excessive, 139–42
    lack of, 119–22
emotional depression, 131–2

Emphysema, 149–50
endocrine glands,
    related energy centre (*chakra*), 16,
        22–8
Endometriosis, 150–2
energy centres, 13, 15–16, 22–8, 23
    Ajna, 25, 28
    base, 27–8
    crown, 27, 28
    heart, 26–7
    sacral, 22–4
    solar plexus, 25–6
    throat, 22, 24
energy fields, 13–15
energy, lack of, 94–6
    see also tiredness
Enteritis, regional, 126–8
environment, allergens in, 53–6, 74–9
Epilepsy, 152–4
Eruptions, skin, 45–9
etheric body, xvi, 13, 15–16
exhaustion, 94–6, 136–9, 168–9
extremities, sensitivity to cold,
    112–3, 263, 273–6
eyes,
    itching, 186–8
    pain, 169–70
    sight deterioration, 109–10
    ulceration, 122–4
    weeping, 186–8

face,
    Herpes, 197–200
    pain, 235–6, 280–2
    paralysis, 89–90
    skin lesions, 197–200
    swelling, 60–1
fatigue, 51–2, 58–9, 192–5, 202–4
feet, swollen, 157–8
fever, 111–12, 218–19, 222–3, 234,
    266–7, 270–1
Fibroids, 155–7
fibrosis, skin, 273–6
fingers,
    sensitivity to cold, 112–3, 263,
        273–6
    swollen, 157–8
    tingling pain, 108–9
Fluid retention, 157–8
    as symptom, 254–6

food additives, 53–6, 74–9
food allergies, 53–6, 113–16
Fractures, 158–9
Frostbite, 112–13

Gallstones, 160–3
Gastro-intestinal Infections, 139–42, 163–6
  Gastritis, 163–6
  Gasto-enteritis, 166
genes, immune response, *see* Auto-immune diseases
Genetic Disorders, 70–4, 144, 183
genetic influences, 6–7
Genital Herpes, 197–200
genitals, skin lesions, 197–200
German electro-acupuncture, xvi, 14
German Measles, 167–8
gland, prostate, diseases, 258–60
glands,
  related energy centre (*chakra*), 16, 22–8
  swollen, 168–9, 234
Glandular Fever, 168–9
Glaucoma, 169–70
Glomerulonephritis, 170–4
Glucose Tolerance Test, 203
Glycosuria, 136–9
Goitre, 174–8
gonads, related energy centre (*chakra*), 22–4
Gonorrhoea, 178–9
Gout, 179–81
'grand-mal' (Epilepsy), 152–4
Granuloma, Hodgkin, 201–2
Grave's Disease, 175, 177–8
groin area, pain, 242–4
Growing Pains, 181–2
gums,
  bleeding, 276
  ulcers, 231

Habits, compulsive, 52–3, 62–4
Haematuria, 183
Haemophilia, 183
Haemorrhoids, 183–5
Hallucinations, 185–6
  as symptom, 271–3
hands, pain, 264–6
Hay Fever, 186–8

Head Colds, 117–19
Headache, 188–91
  as symptom, 110–11, 222–3, 226–9, 280–2
health, seven levels of consciousness, 16–21, 22–8
hearing loss, 145–6
heart *chakra*, 26–7
Heart Disease, 79–86, 191–2, 286–8
Heartburn, 163–6
Hepatitis, 192–5
herbalism, xvi, 30, 32–3, 43
Hernia, 195–7
Herpes, 197–200
  zoster, 278–80
Hiatus hernia, 195–7
Hiccoughs, 200–1
high blood pressure, 79–86, 91–4
Hodgkin's Disease, 201–2
holistic medicine, 11–15, 29–38
homoeopathy, xvi, 30, 33–5
homoeostasis, xvii, 3–4, 5
hormonal imbalance, 57–8, 223–4
hot flushes, 223–4
Hypersensitivity, 53–6
Hypertension, 79–86, 91–4
Hyperthyroidism, 175, 177–8
Hypoglycaemia, 202–4
Hypotension, 94–6
Hypothyroidism, 175, 176–8
Hysteria, 64–6

Immune system, breakdown, 70–4, 86–8, 170–4
  Deficiency Disorders, 205–6
immunity, 7–9, 276
Impetigo, 206–7
Indigestion, 163–6, 195–7
infants, immune system, 7–8
Infectious diseases,
  Chicken pox, 111–12
  Glandular fever, 168–9
  Hepatitis, 192–5
  Herpes, 197–200
  Impetigo, 206–7
  Measles, 218–19
  Meningitis, 222–3
  Mumps, 234
  Rheumatic fever, 266–7
  Rubella, 167–8

Scabies, 269–70
Scarlet fever, 270–1
Shingles, 278–80
Thrush, 288–90
Whooping cough, 304–6
Infectious Mononucleosis, 168–9
infertility, female, 150–2, 155–7
inflammation, see body site of
    inflammation
Influenza, 117–19
    as symptom, 186–8, 192–5
insecurity, 64–6
Insomnia, 207–9
    as symptom, 64–6, 223–4, 254–6
Insulin-dependent Diabetes, 136–9
interviews, patient, 38–9
Intestinal Diseases, see abdomen,
    bowel, colon, diarrhoea,
    gastro-intestinal infections
iron deficiency, 58–9
iron phosphate, 43
irritability, 254–6, 306–7
Ischaemic Heart Disease, 79–86
itching,
    anal area, 183–5, 306–7
    eyes, 186–8
    fingers or toes, 112–13
    skin, 111–12, 132–5, 146–8, 269–70

Jaundice, 192–5, 210
joints,
    fusion, 61–2
    inflamed, 179–81
    pain in, 67–74, 179–81, 266–7
    stiffness, 266–7
    swollen, 67–74

Kidney Stones, 211–13
kidneys, pain, 211–13
kinesiology, xvii, 10
Kirlian photography, xvii, 14
Kundalini fire, 28

Laryngitis, 214–16
legs, aching, 298–300
legs, pain in children's, 181–2
Leukaemia, 216–7
life fields, 13–15
limbs, fractured, 158–9
liver, 43,
    inflamed, 192–5

loss of weight, 62–4
low blood pressure, 94–6
lungs, inflammation, 250–1
Lymphatic system, 43
    glands, enlarged, 167–8, 291–2
    glands, malignant diseases, 101–7,
        201–2
    nodes, swelling, 278–80
lymphocyte deficiency, 86–8
Lymphomas, 101–8

Measles, 218–19
    German (Rubella), 167–8
medicine,
    alternative, 29–38
    anthrosophical, 14
    holistic, 11–15
meditation, as therapy, 19–21
Melanoma, 219
Meniere's Disease, 219–22
Meningitis, 222–3
Menopause, 223–4
Menstrual Cycle,
    absence, 57–8
    and body fluids, 157–8
    before period, 254–6
    cessation, 223–4
    cramps, 225–6
    headaches, 226–9
    interrupted, 242–4
    pain, 150–2, 225–6
Mental disorders, see Psychological
    disorders
metabolism, over-active, 175, 177–8
metabolism, under-active, 175, 176–7
Middle ear infection, 145–6
Migraine, 226–9
mineral deficiencies, 58–9, 124–6,
    241–2
minerals, 30–1
Mongolism, see Down's Syndrome
Monilia, 288–90
Mora therapy, xvii, 14
Morbilli (Measles), 218–19
morning sickness, 253–4
Motion Sickness, 230
Mouth Ulcers, 231
mucus, in lungs, 149–50
Multiple Sclerosis (MS), 231–4
Mumps, 234

muscle, over-use disorders, 108–9, 264–6
muscle wastage, 236–7
muscular cramp, 124–6
myelin sheath, destruction, 231–4

nasal passages, blocked, 186–8, 280–2
natural therapy, methods, 29–38
natural therapy, philosophy, 11–28
nausea, 139–42, 166, 192–5, 226–9, 230, 282–5
neck stiffness, 222–3
Neoplasms, 101–8
Nephritis, 170–4
nerve pain, 278–80
nerves, inflammation, 236–7
Nervous disorders, 62–6
Nervous System Diseases, 231–4, 236–7, 276–8
Neuralgia, 235–6
Neuritis, 236–7
Neuroses, 64–6, 237–8, see also Anxiety
numbness, 108–9, 236–7
    fingers or toes, 263, 273–6
nutrition, clinical, 29

Obesity, 239–41
Occupational diseases, 264–6
Oedema, angio-neurotic, 60–1
orgonomy, xvii, 14
Osteitis deformans, 245–6
Osteoarthritis, 67–70
Osteoporosis, 241–2
Otitis Media, 145–6
Ovarian Cysts, 242–4
over-weight, 239–41
oxalate stones, 211–13

Paget's Disease, 245–6
pain,
    abdominal, 49–51, 116–17, 139–42, 246–9, 293–5
    above groin, 242–4
    arms, 264–6
    bowel and bladder, 256–8
    breathing, 250–1
    chest, 81–6
    cramping, 124–6, 225–6

ear, 145–6
eye, 169–70
face, 235–6
facial, 280–2
gall-bladder, 160–3
hands, 264–6
head, 188–91, 226–9
joints, 67–74, 179–81, 266–7
kidneys, 211–13
legs, 181–2
lower back, 61–2, 245–6, 258–60
menstrual, 150–2
nerve, 278–80
shoulder, 160–3
stomach, 163–6, 282–5
tingling, 236–7
wrist and hands, 108–9
palpitations, 175, 177–8, 286–8
Palsy, Bell's, 89–90
pancreas, inflammation, 246–9
pancreas, related energy centre (chakra), 25–6
Papillomas, 249
papules, 111–12
paralysis, 89–90, 110–11, 231–4
Paralysis Agitans, 249–50
Parkinson's Disease, 249–50
Paroxysmal Tachycardia, 286–8
patient/therapist relationship, 38–9
Peptic Ulcer, 282–5
Personality disorders, 271–3
Pertussis, 304–6
pineal gland, related energy centre (chakra), 28
pituitary gland, related energy centre (chakra), 25
placebo effect, 39
Pleurisy, 250–1
PMT (Premenstrual Tension), 254–6
Pneumonia, 96–8, 252–3
pollen, allergic reactions, 186–8
posture, degeneration, 245–6, 249–50
potassium chloride, 43
'prana', xvii, 13, 15–16
Pregnancy, 253–4
Premenstrual Tension, 254–6
prescribing remedies, 36–8
Prolapse, 256–8
Prostate diseases, 258–60

Psoriasis, 260–2
Psychological Disorders, 64–6,
    131–2, 185–6, 237–8, 271–3,
    276–8
    see also habits
pulmonary disorders, *see* Respiratory
    Diseases
pulse, rapid, 175, 177–8, 286–8
pulse, slow, 175, 176–7
pustules, 111–12

rashes, 111–12, 167–8, 218–19,
    270–1, 278–80
Raynaud's Syndrome, 263, 273–6
regurgitation, *see* indigestion or
    vomiting
remedies, 29–38
Renal Calculi, 211–13
Renal Diseases, 170–4, 211, 273–6
renal pain, 211–13
Repetitive Strain Injury, 264–6
    see also Carpal Tunnel Syndrome
reproductive glands, related energy
    centre (*chakra*), 22–4
Respiratory Diseases, 74–9, 96–100,
    250–1, 252–3, 291–2, 304–6
    see also Upper Respiratory Tract
    Infections
Rheumatic Fever, 266–7
Rheumatoid Arthritis, 70–4
Rhinitis, allergic seasonal, 186–8
Rickets, 267–8
Round Worms, 306–7
RSI (Repetitive Strain Injury),
    264–6
Rubella, 167–8

sacral energy centre (*chakra*), 22–4
Sarcoma, 101–8
Scabies, 269–70
Scarlet Fever, 270–1
Schizophrenia, 271–3
Scleroderma, 273–6
Sclerosis, multiple, 231–4
Sclerosis, progressive systemic, 273–6
Scurvy, 276
Sea sickness, 230
Senile Dementia, 276–8
Shingles, 278–80
shoulder pain, 160–3

Sinusitis, 280–2
skeleton deformity, 245–6
skeleton rigidity, 249–50
Skin,
    blemishes, 45–9
    cancer, 219
    diseases, 146–8, 260–2
    eruptions, children, 206–7
    fibrosis, 273–6
    inflammation, 132–5
    itching, 111–12, 132–5, 146–8,
        269–70
    leathery, 273–6
    lesions, 197–200, 260–2
    scaling patches, 260–2
    yellow, 192–5, 210
sleep, inability to, 207–9
solar plexus, related energy centre
    (*chakra*), 25–6
spasm, bowel, 116–17
Spondylitis, ankylosing, 61–2
spots, white, 288–90
sputum, accumulation, 96–8
sterility, *see* infertility
Stomach,
    distension, 113–16, 163–6
    pain, 163–6, 282–5
    Ulcers, 282–5
stones, gall, 160–3
stones, kidney, 211–13
Streptococcal Infections, 266–7,
    270–1
Stress related disorders, 64–6, 79–86,
    91–4
Stroke, 110–11
struvite stones, 211–13
sugar, craving for, 202–4
Sugar diabetes, 136–9
swelling, *see* body site of swelling
Syphilis, 285

Tachycardia, 286–8
Tapeworm, 306–7
Tenosynovitis, 264–6
therapist/patient relationship, 38–9
therapy,
    prescribing, 36–8
    relation to seven levels of
        consciousness, 16–21, 22–28
    types, 29–38

Theratest, xvii, 14
thirst, abnormal, 136–9
Threadworms, 306–7
throat, sore, 168–9, 214–16, 266, 270–1, 291–2
thrombosis, 298–300
Thrush, 288–90
thymus gland, 86–8
related energy centre (chakra), 26–7
thyroid gland, 174–8
overactive, 175, 177–8
related energy centre, 24
swollen, 174–8
under-active, 175, 176–7
Thyrotoxicosis, 175, 177–8
tinnitus, 219–22
tiredness, 51–2, 58–9, 192–5, 202–4
toes, inflammation around, 179–81
toes, sensitivity to cold, 112–3, 263, 273–6
tongue, swollen, 60–1
Tonsillitis, 291–2
touch-for-health, xviii, 4
Travel Sickness, 230
Tuberculosis, 292
Tumours, 101–8
benign, 155–7

Ulcerative Colitis, 293–5
ulcers,
bowel, 293–5
corneal, 122–4
mouth, 231
peptic, 282–5
stomach, 282–5
varicose, 298–300
unconsciousness, 152–4
Upper Respiratory Tract Infections, 117–19, 145–6, 186–8, 214–16
ureter, stones, 211
uric acid, excess, 179–81
uric acid stones, 211–13
urination,
difficult, 258–60
excessive, 136–9
painful, 128–30
urine,
acid, 128–30
albumen in, 170–4

blood in, 128–30, 183, 170–4, 211–13, 258–60
dark, 210
pus in, 128–30
uterus,
bleeding from, 154
disorders related to, 150–2, 155–7
prolapse, 256–8

Vagina, itchy, 288–90
Vaginal Discharge, 288–90, 296–8
Varicella, 111–12
Varicose Eczema, 298–300
Varicose Ulcers, 298–300
Varicose Veins, 298–300
anal area, 183–5
Vascular Disorders, 79–86, 110–11, 112–13, 263
Vega diagnosis, xviii, 14, 242–3
Veins, varicose, 298–300
Venereal Diseases, 178–9, 197–200, 285, 301–2
Venereal Herpes, 197–200
Venereal Warts, 301–2
Vertigo, 219–22
vesicles, 111–12, 197–200, 206–7
Viral hepatitis, 192–5
vision, impaired, 122–4, 169–70, 231–4
vision, loss of, 109–10
Vitamins, 31–2
C, 43
C deficiency, 276
D deficiency, 267–8
Vivaxis techniques, xviii, 14, 36
voice, loss of, 214–16
vomiting, 139–42, 192–5, 226–9, 230

wakefulness, 207–9
Warts, 301–2, 303–4, see also Papillomas
weight gain, 157–8, 175, 176–7, 239–41
weight loss, 113–16, 126–8, 136–9, 175, 177–8
wheezing, 74–9, 98–100
Whooping Cough, 304–6
Worms, 306–7
wrist pain, 108–9

yellow skin, 192–5, 210